The Reorganized National Health Service

Sixth edition

Ruth Levitt
Office for Public Management
London, UK

Andrew Wall
Visiting Senior Fellow
Health Services Management Centre
University of Birmingham, UK

John Appleby
Director, Health Systems Programme
King's Fund, London, UK

Stanley Thornes (Publishers) Ltd

First edition published in 1976 by Croom Helm, revised July 1976.
Second edition published in 1977 by Croom Helm, revised 1979.
Third edition published in 1984 by Croom Helm.
Fourth edition published in 1992 by Chapman & Hall.
Fifth edition published in 1995 by Chapman & Hall.

Sixth edition published in 1999 by:
Stanley Thornes (Publishers) Ltd
Ellenborough House
Wellington Street
Cheltenham
Glos.
GL50 1YW
United Kingdom

00 01 02 03 / 10 9 8 7 6 5 4 3 2

A catalogue record for this book is available from the British Library

ISBN 0 7487 3894 0

Typeset by Acorn Bookwork, Salisbury, Wiltshire
Printed and bound in Great Britain by Martins the Printers Ltd, Berwick upon Tweed

ealth Service

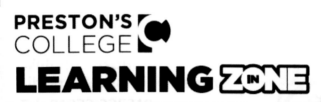

CONTENTS

PREFACE

The National Health Service reached its 50th anniversary in July 1998. This is a remarkable achievement that has been made possible by a unique combination of political, professional, social and cultural values in the UK. In this book we explain clearly and critically what the NHS is, how it works, why it looks and works the way it does, how it has come to its present state and what its future options are.

Reorganization has become a constant feature for the NHS, as politicians, professionals and the public seek to influence or improve the structure and operations of the NHS and to shape the outcomes it can produce. Strategic thinking is always a challenge for the NHS, and we indicate where there are some persistent problems which still need to be resolved. Providing health services publicly and privately raises important questions about the key goals of effectiveness, efficiency and quality. These questions are increasingly in focus, as the social and ethical priorities for proper distribution of appropriate services have to be argued.

We acknowledge with thanks the use of copyright material quoted from HMSO, The Stationery Office and other sources.

Ruth Levitt
Andrew Wall
John Appleby
March 1999

SELECTED ABBREVIATIONS

ACAS	Advisory, Conciliation and Arbitration Service
ACC	Association of County Councils
ACHCEW	Association of Community Health Councils for England and Wales
ADC	Association of District Councils
AIDS	Acquired immune deficiency syndrome
ALA	Association of Local Authorities
AMA	Association of Metropolitan Authorities
ASC	Action for Sick Children (formerly NAWCH)
ASH	Action on Smoking and Health
BDA	British Dental Association
BMA	British Medical Association
BSI	British Standards Institution
BTS	Blood Transfusion Service
BUPA	British United Provident Association
CDSC	Communicable Diseases Surveillance Centre
CE	Chief Executive
CEPOD	Confidential Enquiry into Perioperative Deaths
CHC	Community health council
CHD	Coronary heart disease
CHI	Commission for Health Improvement
CMDS	Core minimum data set/Community contract minimum data set
COHSE	Confederation of Health Service Employees (see UNISON)
CPN	Community psychiatric nurse
CSO	Central Statistical Office
CSSD	Central sterile services department
CT	Computed tomography
D&C	Dilatation and curettage
DGH	District general hospital
DGM	District general manager
DH	Department of Health
DHA	District health authority
DHSS	Department of Health and Social Security
DMC	District medical committee
DMO	District medical officer
DMU	Directly managed unit
DN	District nurse
DoH	Department of Health
DPH	Director of Public Health

DRG	Diagnosis-related group
DSS	Department of Social Security
EBS	Emergency Bed Service (London)
ECR	Extracontractual referral
EFL	External financing limit
EL	Executive letter
ENB	English National Board for Nursing, Midwifery and Health Visiting
ENT	Ear, nose and throat
FCE	Finished consultant episode
FHS	Family health services
FHSA	Family health services authority (formerly FPC)
FPA	Family Planning Association
FPC	Family practitioner committee
GDC	General Dental Council
GDP	General dental practitioner
GDP	Gross domestic product
GDS	General dental services
GHS	General household survey
GIFT	Gamete intra-fallopian transfer
GM	General manager
GMC	General Medical Council
GMP	General medical practitioner
GMS	General medical services
GMSC	General Medical Services Committee
GPFH	General practice fundholder
HA	Health authority
HAA	Hospital Activity Analysis
HAS	Health Advisory Service
HAZ	Health action zone
HC	Health circular
HCHS	Hospital and community health services
HES	Hospital episode system
HFEA	Human Fertilisation and Embryology Authority
HIP	Health improvement programme
HIPE	Hospital Inpatient Enquiry
HIV	Human immunodeficiency virus
HMO	Health maintenance organization (USA)
HR	Human resources
HRG	Healthcare related groups/Healthcare resource group
HSC	Health and Safety Commission
HSI	Health service indicator
HVA	Health Visitors Association
IBD	Interest-bearing debt
ICD	International Classification of Diseases
ICU	Intensive care unit
IPR	Individual performance review

IVF	In vitro fertilization
JCC	Joint consultative committee
LHG	Local health group
LoS	Length of stay
MCA	Medicines Control Agency
MDS	Minimum data set
MDU	Medical Defence Union
MIT	Minimally invasive therapy
MMR	Measles, mumps and rubella (vaccine)
MRC	Medical Research Council
MRI	Magnetic resonance imaging
MSF	Manufacturing, Science and Finance (technical staff trade union)
NALGO	National and Local Government Officers' Union (see UNISON)
NAO	National Audit Office
NCEPOD	National Confidential Enquiry into Peri-operative Deaths (formerly CEPOD)
NCT	National Childbirth Trust
NHS	National Health Service
NHSAR	National Health Service Administrative Register
NHSE	National Health Service Executive
NHSME	National Health Service Management Executive (now National Health Service Executive)
NICE	National Institute for Clinical Excellence
NMR	Nuclear magnetic resonance
NPF	National performance framework
NPUS	National patient and user survey
NSF	National service framework
NUPE	National Union of Public Employees (see UNISON)
NVQ	National Vocational Qualification
OECD	Organization of Economic Cooperation and Development
OPCS	Office of Population Censuses and Surveys
P&T	Professional and technical
PAC	Public Accounts Committee
PACT	Prescription analysis and cost tabulation
PAS	Patient administration system
PCG	Primary care group
PCT	Primary care trust
PDC	Public dividend capital
PDP	Personal development plan
PES	Public Expenditure Survey
PHLS	Public Health Laboratory Service
PPP	Private Patients Plan
PREP	Post registration and practice

PRP	Performance-related pay
PSS	Personal social services
QA	Quality assurance
QALY	Quality-adjusted life year
R&D	Research and development
RAWP	Resource Allocation Working Party
RCCS	Revenue consequences of capital schemes
RCN	Royal College of Nursing
RGM	Regional general manager
RHA	Regional health authority
SFF	Service and financial frameworks
SHA	Special health authority
SHARE	Scottish Health Authorities Revenue Equalization
SHHD	Scottish Home and Health Department
SIFTR	Service increment for teaching and research
SMR	Standardized mortality ratio
TQM	Total quality management
UGM	Unit general manager
UKCC	United Kingdom Central Council for Nursing, Midwifery and Health Visiting
UNISON	Public sector union, amalgamation of COHSE/NALGO/NUPE
WHO	World Health Organization
WTE	Whole time equivalent

MINISTERS OF HEALTH AND SECRETARIES OF STATE

MINISTERS OF HEALTH

1919–21	Dr Christopher Addison
1921–22	Sir Alfred Mond
1922–23	Sir Arthur Griffith-Boscawen
1923	Neville Chamberlain
1923–24	Sir William Joynson-Hicks
1924	John Wheatley
1924–29	Neville Chamberlain
1929–31	Arthur Greenwood
1931	Neville Chamberlain
1931–35	Sir E. Hilton-Young
1935–38	Sir Kingsley Wood
1938–40	Walter Elliot
1940–41	Malcolm MacDonald
1941–43	Ernest Brown
1943–45	Henry Willink
1945–51	Aneurin Bevan
1951	Hilary Marquand
1951–52	Harry Crookshank
1952–55	Ian Macleod
1955–57	Robin Turton
1957	Dennis Vosper
1957–60	Derek Walker-Smith
1960–63	Enoch Powell
1963–64	Anthony Barber
1964–68	Kenneth Robinson

SECRETARIES OF STATE FOR SOCIAL SERVICES

1968–70	Richard Crossman
1970–74	Sir Keith Joseph
1974–76	Barbara Castle
1976–79	David Ennals
1979–81	Patrick Jenkin

1981–87	Norman Fowler
1987–88	John Moore

Secretaries of State for Health

1988–90	Kenneth Clarke
1990–92	William Waldegrave
1992–95	Virginia Bottomley
1995–97	Stephen Dorrell
1997–	Frank Dobson

INTRODUCTION

Many people regard the National Health Service as the great success of the United Kingdom's welfare state experiment since 1945. They see the NHS as a benevolent and social institution caring for the public when they become sick and doing so without direct charge. Few other countries in the world have attempted this degree of state altruism. But such an idealistic perspective risks creating myths, which need more rigorous analysis. The first edition of this book explored the policies that had formed and sustained the NHS over its first 25 years. Its continuing political history and ever-changing organizational arrangements have been considered in subsequent editions, to explain the nature and disposition of its resources and its future. This new edition examines the NHS as it is now and discusses the major intractable problems as well as the reasons why it still represents a remarkable political and social achievement.

Governments have three choices in funding health care: direct, indirect or not at all. Most developed countries mix these approaches. The UK puts the greatest emphasis on direct funding. In most other countries indirect funding is more popular, whereby people pay insurance premiums, directly or through their employers, for cover in the event of sickness. This method allows a degree of choice in the level of contributions and the level of services. It fails to provide cover for those who are unable to pay the premiums; state funding is therefore necessary for them. At the other end of the scale, the wealthy can afford their own private arrangements, paying for services whenever they need them without the cushioning effect of publicly subsidized insurance. They may pay directly or through a private insurance scheme. Such people are always a small minority. Between them and those that pay nothing at all there is a significant group of people who pay for a single treatment, usually a surgical procedure, in order to avoid the inconvenience of waiting to have it on the NHS. This group has been getting larger.

By carrying the financial risks attached to illness, the NHS is in fact a state insurance scheme. The people pay for the NHS largely through general taxes so there is no direct link between what they pay and what they receive. The condition for receiving care is need, not the ability to pay. The two great advantages of this system are that it not only removes the profit motive from the transaction but also allows patients to be referred to whatever specific service best meets their need.

There is no doubt that the NHS, despite its shortcomings, represents comparatively good value for money. There are at least two main reasons for this. First, the service costs are not inflated by the need to provide investors or owners with dividends or profits. Second, the staff, particularly medical staff, receive relatively low salaries compared to those in other developed countries.

Important though value for money is, the NHS must be judged ultimately on whether or not it contributes to improvement in the health of the people. One way to check this is to consider a snapshot of life in 1948, on the eve of the new NHS, and see how that compares with nearly 50 years later (see Table 1.1).

Table 1.1

Then and now (England and Wales)

	1948	1996	Difference
Life expectancy at birth			
Men	66.4	74.4	+8.0
Women	71.2	79.6	+8.4
Perinatal mortality*	38.5	8.6	−29.9
Maternal mortality+	102	6	−96.0
Deaths from infectious diseases			
TB	23 175	416	−22 759
Diphtheria	156	0	−156
Whooping cough	748	0	−748
Measles	327	0	−327
Polio	241	1	−240
AIDS	0	476	+476

Stillbirths and deaths within 7 days per 1000 still and live births (the definition changed in 1993 from born dead after 28 weeks' to born dead after 24 weeks' gestation)
+*per 100 000 deliveries*
Sources: compiled using statistics from Department of Health Statistics Division; Office of National Statistics; Office of Health Economics (1997). *Compendium of Health Statistics*. OHE, London

Although people now live longer, the NHS can scarcely claim sole credit for this increase. Improvements in living conditions generally have been a significant factor. The reduction in infant mortality and the decrease in deaths from most infectious diseases are also important.

In 1948 people's usual contact with the NHS was through their family doctor. He or she would generally be working in a single-handed practice with little support from others. But he or she would be prepared to do home visits, and was regarded as a family friend. The range of available treatments was limited (the pharamaceutical explosion was yet to come): traditional potions and lotions were what people expected. The situation is very different 50 years later. The majority of GPs work in group practices with an impressive range of supporting staff and facilities. The post-war vision of a comprehensive network of health centres replacing the haphazard distribution of surgeries and local authority clinics did not materialize. In their stead, well-equipped surgeries became the rule rather than the exception. Appointment systems also came to be expected. Patients are more confident and questioning than before. They have come to expect medications to relieve many of their symptoms.

Up to 1948, access to hospital treatment was very different from how it is today. For someone who was acutely ill, the voluntary hospital was available if they had contributed in some way to an insurance scheme. Those who had not went to the local authority hospital. Voluntary hospitals were reckoned to have better medical staff.

The length of stay in hospital was on average over four times as long as it is today (more than 20 days in the 1950s, 5 in 1998). Patients were accommodated in large 'Nightingale' style wards whose 26 or more patients were all in the same room, the very sick with the less sick. There was often a pecking order which allowed those getting well to progress physically up the ward further away from Sister's office. Pity the patient who progressed down to the corner bed next to Sister's office: their condition was likely to be grave indeed.

Patients requiring surgery needed to be assessed carefully for their suitability for anaesthesia. Elderly patients, and others with poor lung capacity, were often considered too great a risk. Today age is no bar to anaesthesia. This is a major change given the growing number of very elderly people who can benefit from orthopaedic surgery. One of the most notable advances has been the ability of surgeons to replace hips and other joints in elderly people suffering from osteoarthritis.

Hip replacements came in the 1950s following the pioneering work of Charnley at Wrightington Hospital, Lancashire, but even in the 1960s, access to these operations was often rationed by the hospital management's budget for prostheses

The advance of medical science and technologies has been dramatic, although developments have been erratic and not always successful. The availability of antibiotics and other powerful pharmaceutical medicines has fundamentally transformed the repertoire of treatments. Transplant surgery, unthinkable in 1948, is very much part of the scene 50 years later, even though its overall success rate is variable. Kidney transplants are now routine and have a high success rate but heart and lung transplants are still problematic.

The experience of mothers and children in 1948 was very different from today. Maternity arrangements were particularly chaotic at the end of the war. Mothers could have their babies at home, in a nursing home or in a hospital. Fewer than 50% chose an institutional setting and the risk was correspondingly greater. Wherever mothers were delivered, they were expected to lie-in for several days after the birth. Today mothers are encouraged to get up sooner to decrease the risk of a blood clot forming.

Children were more likely to be admitted to hospital because of infectious diseases and other childhood ailments. Once there, they were isolated from their family, whose visiting rights were restricted in the belief that too much visiting would upset the child. Children requiring surgery were often admitted to adult wards. Today such a practice is expressly forbidden. The admission of a child to hospital is to be avoided if at all possible but where it is inevitable there is great emphasis on creating a child-friendly environment and parents are encouraged to stay with their children.

At the other end of life, the elderly person in 1948 might find that they had to spend their last years in a long-stay hospital. These hospitals were usually former workhouses, typically built in the 1840s following the Poor Law Amendment Act 1834. Imposing but intimidating institutions, they provided a poor environment for care. Patients were often confined to bed as day rooms were in short supply. The wartime Hospital Survey[1] depicted a service that had failed to keep up with the times. Matters are quite different 50 years later. The long-stay hospitals for elderly patients no longer exist. Most of the workhouse buildings have been closed or modernized and converted for much more active regimes. Unwell elderly people are still admitted to hospitals but for an average stay of under 20 days, undergoing assessment by a multi-disciplinary team headed by a geriatrician. Those requiring long-term nursing care are then either supported at home or admitted to an independently run nursing home whose amenities are likely, on the whole, to be much higher than those previously provided by the NHS in hospital.

There is one major change in caring for elderly people that has punctured the NHS's claim to be free at the point of use: many elderly patients now have to pay directly for their nursing care. Under the arrangements negotiated between health authorities and social services departments of local authorities, elderly patients in nursing homes are assessed for their ability to contribute to the costs of their care. In 1998 anyone with capital over £16 000 was expected to pay for their nursing care. This is not the case if they are able to stay at home and receive care from district nurses. This is a major policy shift (see Chapter 9). It marks a significant and, some would say unforgivable, compromise of the founding principles of the NHS.

The mental hospitals in 1948 were even worse environments than long-stay hospitals for the physically frail. Possibly as a result of the war, the numbers of people in hospital with mental illnesses reached a peak in the early 1950s: 150 000 patients were housed in Victorian lunatic asylums, some of which had over 2000 beds, with over 60 patients living and sleeping in each ward. Many of the wards were locked, men and women were segregated, and nursing staff were allocated to one or the other and managed separately. Yet such institutions were not wholly bad. Because of their geographical isolation the hospitals were often largely self-sufficient and had their own programmes of sport and entertainment. Workshops were also provided so that at least some patients could develop or maintain manual skills. Horticulture and farming and work in the laundry provided others with worthwhile activity. Today's attempts to employ outside hospital people who have recurring mental illnesses have not been very successful.

Similarly the institutions for people with learning disabilities (then called mental deficiency) were isolated and self-sufficient. For the most disabled, conditions were often appalling and the care was no more than basic feeding and minimal personal hygiene. But there were also significant numbers of inmates whose intellectual ability was only marginally impaired, and they were able to make use of the recreational facilities: it was not uncommon for there to be a weekly dance, filmshow and outings for the more competent. The better hospitals of this kind also had good sports facilities, including a swimming pool.

Today the situation has changed fundamentally. Care in the

community, a major policy shift initiated in the 1980s, has meant that institutional care only persists for those people with mental illnesses who need acute intervention or whose level of illness makes community care impossible. The number of hospital places for mentally ill people is now less than a third of that of the 1950s and the average length of stay is a matter of days, not months or years.

For people with learning disabilities there is practically no specific hospital provision, only that required to treat other illnesses arising in the ordinary course of events. It is now largely accepted that people with learning disabilities can live in small groups in the community and benefit from the general amenities of those communities. Learning disabilities are not now seen as illnesses and the services are run by social services departments working with health, housing and education agencies as appropriate. There is little doubt that most people with learning disabilities now have an immeasurably improved quality of life.

For people with mental illnesses progress is less easy to assess. The rise in drug abuse, the continuing problem of alcoholism and the persistent level of some psychotic illnesses means that many people still need active care from health professionals of various kinds. The emphasis on care in the community has sometimes abandoned these patients to the streets and to hopelessness. In 1998 the Labour government announced a review of this situation and it seems likely that there will now be some modifications to what were, for a time, seen as the most appropriate policies for caring for people with mental illnesses. The growing number of very elderly people has also increased the problems of caring for elderly people with mental confusion, often referred to as dementia, or Alzheimer's disease.

For most people the last 50 years have seen major improvements. They are likely to live longer and have a higher overall quality of life. They are now likely to be treated with a much higher level of expertise, by more knowledgeable staff, who have considerable technological and pharmacological support at hand. They are also more likely to be involved in discussing their own condition and making choices about their own care. If they are admitted to hospital the level of amenity will be higher, with more emphasis on privacy and social comfort.

But there is another side to this. It can be argued that the creation of the NHS, far from being a manifestation of a socialist dream, as the myth persistently portrays it, was actually only one stage in the difficult and continuing process of organizing health care provision:

> *...it may be highly misleading to think of the Health Service as a social welfare measure at all. Its chief objective ... was to improve a remarkably inefficient and inadequate set of services, its chief means of doing so organizational rationalization and the use of central and regional planning.*
>
> Eckstein 1964[2]

There is no doubt that the various arrangements for providing health care in the 1940s were unsatisfactory and inefficient. Launching the NHS in 1948 resolved some of these difficulties and had the support of most people at the time. The conditions that existed then are not at all the same ones facing British society today. The NHS has begun to crumble, partly because the old values of universality of access and equity are no longer being upheld.

Some go further and say that the NHS is positively failing. Waiting lists, those manifestations of apparently irresistible demand, keep on rising and successive governments' attempts to control them continue to be unsuccessful. Although the proportion of the country's wealth, the gross national product, spent on the NHS appears low by international comparison, the finances are not in good shape and poor levels of staffing and badly maintained buildings show just how far financial compromises have been made. There has been constant political tinkering, demonstrating an obsessive concern for organizational change at the expense of attention to achieving lasting clinical and service improvements. This has fuelled widespread cynicism among professional and managerial staff who feel that morale has never been lower.

Faced with this level of criticism is it possible to maintain that the NHS is a good system and has an assured future? This book attempts to put the good features and the bad in perspective, describing how the NHS has reached its present state and what is likely to happen to it. One thing is certain: an institution so deeply embedded in the experience of the UK's people is unlikely to fade away. It is therefore important that both expert and layman understand the issues.

REFERENCES

1. Ministry of Health (1945 & 1946) *Hospital Survey*. HMSO, London.
2. Eckstein, H. (1964) *The English Health Service – Its Origins, Structure and Achievements*. Harvard University Press, Cambridge, MA, USA.

BACKGROUND TO TODAY'S NATIONAL HEALTH SERVICE

What is the National Health Service? Its three basic elements are the hospital service, the family practitioner services and community-based services. They each have separate origins, and the great achievement of the 1946 National Health Service Act[1] was to bring them together legislatively. The Labour government of the day was forced to make compromises during the final preparations before launching the NHS. The outcome was less than ideal, because this framework had failed to integrate the three elements sufficiently thoroughly. This explains the persistence of many of the NHS's subsequent difficulties and limitations.

The first attempt to unify the NHS organizationally took place in 1974[2]. This structure was simplified in 1982[3]. In 1984/85 the introduction of 'general management' helped to prepare the ground for a market-orientated approach which was a major characteristic of the 1990 legislative changes[4]. Following the general election of 1997 the new Labour government tried to capitalize on the perceived successes of the 1990 reorganization while repudiating the market ideology[5] that had informed it.

2.1 HEALTH SERVICES BEFORE 1948 – A BRIEF HISTORY

2.1.1 Hospitals

Hospitals have their origins in religious and charitable institutions in the Middle Ages. Indeed, St. Bartholomew's Hospital, London, was founded in 1123. But institutional care was at best haphazard until the mid-eighteenth century, when there were moves to open better hospitals supported by voluntary subscriptions. In London and elsewhere purpose-built small hospitals were established and many of them still survive today as names and even sometimes as buildings. By 1800 these hospitals were providing 4000 beds, half of them in London.

During the course of the next 150 years voluntary hospitals grew in number and size. During the nineteenth century a significant number of specialized hospitals were created too, notably eye infirmaries and children's hospitals. This was followed by the development of cottage hospitals.

Voluntary hospitals represented a philanthropic approach to helping those sick people who could not afford to have the personal attendance of their doctor at home. But they were open only to those who were covered by some sort of contributory or insurance scheme or who were sponsored. Many people therefore had to seek their hospital treatment elsewhere.

One of the earliest cottage hospitals opened in Cranleigh, Surrey, in 1859; there were 180 by 1880, serving small towns and rural communities. By 1948 there were 1 143 voluntary hospitals supplying around 90,000 beds, each with about 80 beds on average; only 75 had more than 200 beds. Many were in poor financial health, and buildings, some of which had been damaged in the war, were often in a bad state of repair. There was a sense of crisis

Box 2.1

Legislation, government papers and significant reports mentioned in this chapter

1601	Poor Law Act
1834	Poor Law (Amendment) Act
1902	Midwives Act
1911	National Insurance Act
1913	Mental Deficiency Act
1920	Dawson report [*national health service organization*]
1929	Local Government Act
1942	Beveridge report [*the need for a welfare state*]
1944	A National Health Service [*white paper*]
1945/46	Hospital Survey [*the state of hospitals*]
1946	National Health Service Act
1954	Bradbeer report [*management of hospitals*]
1956	Guillebaud report [*financing of the NHS*]
1959	Cranbrook report [*maternity services*]
1959	Mental Health Act
1962	A Hospital Plan for England and Wales
1962	Porritt report [*management of health services*]
1963	Gillie report [*GPs' role*]
1966	Salmon report [*nursing management*]
1967	'Cogwheel' report [*medical management*]
1968	First green paper [*reorganization*]
1968	Seebohm report [*social work*]
1968	Redcliffe–Maud report [*local government*]
1969	Bonham-Carter report [*district general hospitals*]
May 1971	Second green paper [*reorganization*]
Aug1972	National Health Service Reorganisation [*white paper*]
Sept 1972	Management Arrangements [*the 'Grey Book'*]
1973	National Health Service Reorganisation Act
1974	Democracy in the NHS [*came into force July 1975*]
July 1979	Royal Commission on the NHS
Dec 1979	Patients First [*NHS reorganization*]
Oct 1983	Griffiths report [*management*]
April 1986	Primary Health Care
Nov 1987	Promoting Better Health Care
March 1988	Community Care [*second Griffiths report*]
Jan 1989	Working for Patients
Nov 1989	Caring for People
June 1990	National Health Service and Community Care Act
Oct 1991	Patient's Charter
June 1992	The Health of the Nation
Oct 1992	Managing the new NHS
April 1997	Primary Care Act
Dec 1997	The new NHS [*white paper*]
Feb 1998	Our Healthier Nation
June 1998	A First Class Service [*quality*]
March 1999	Royal Commission on Long Term Care
April 1999	Primary Care Groups operational

The need to support those sick people unable to work and support themselves had been recognized as early as 1601, when the first Poor Law Act was passed. For over two centuries the indigent sick could expect some degree of help but this system progressively failed, until the Poor Law Amendment Act was passed in 1834. This major piece of legislation attempted to provide a nationwide system for looking after the poor. Many new workhouses were built in the next two decades and each provided sick wards in addition to the other accommodation. In the 1860s there were 600 provincial workhouses looking after over 40,000 sick and indigent people. The amenities in workhouses were still very basic. By the end of the century some were beginning to develop the sick wards into comprehensive hospitals providing a service for those unable to obtain admission to voluntary hospitals.

> **Key reference:** Hodgkinson, R. (1967) *The Origins of the National Health Service: The Medical Services of the Poor Law 1834–1871.* Wellcome Institute, London.

The Local Government Act of 1929 repealed the Poor Law acts and gave local authorities the opportunity to develop hospitals comparable to those in the voluntary sector. Some authorities, such as Middlesex, did so but other county councils did little more than continue to provide long-term care in what were then called Public Assistance Institutions. Very low standards were endured by many long-term patients still being looked after in buildings that had seen little modernization since being built a century earlier.

Things might have been better had the voluntary hospitals and local authorities co-operated more, but this seldom happened. Furthermore, governments of the 1930s became increasingly concerned about a serious shortage of beds overall: in the event of war and a rise in the need for emergency treatment there could be a sudden crisis. Accordingly the Emergency Hospital Service (also known as the Emergency Medical Service – EMS) was set up to plan and provide substantial additional beds accommodated in hastily built huts, sometimes on new sites, sometimes attached to existing hospitals. Not all of these beds were in the right place and not all were ultimately needed, but they provided a stop-gap pending systematic redevelopment of all the hospitals after the Second World War. The Hospital Survey[6], which studied the whole of England and Wales as ten regions, was conducted during the war and published in 1945 and 1946. This depicted a sorry state of affairs. Only an integrated national health service could undertake the mammoth task of renewing facilities on a nationwide basis.

The institutional care and treatment of people with mental disorders dates back to 1403, with the first recorded admissions of insane people to Bethlem Hospital, London, a religious establishment founded in 1247; in the eighteenth century this hospital, popularly known as Bedlam, became a tourist attraction. By the end of the century a more humane approach to treating the insane was developing under such doctors as William Tuke, a Quaker, who opened The Retreat in York in

1796. Following legislation in 1807 and later in the nineteenth century, a national network of asylums was gradually developed. Then significant progress came with the Mental Deficiency Act, 1913, which finally separated people with what are now called learning disabilities from those with mental illnesses. Under that Act people with learning disabilities were subdivided into four categories: idiots, imbeciles, feeble-minded and moral defectives. This led to many inappropriate admissions to hospitals of people who were released only after the Mental Health Act 1959 had been passed, and by moves to resettle people in the community, which developed in the 1980s.

Of the specialized hospitals for infectious diseases, sanatoria for the care and treatment of patients with tuberculosis were the most important. In the 1940s there were over 30,000 beds for these patients, although even that was considered insufficient. By 1958 deaths from TB had dropped by 80% with effective mass radiography and the development of streptomycin. There were similar breakthroughs with such other infectious diseases as polio. Infectious diseases beds were released for other patients but were often in unsuitable institutions in remote locations.

2.1.2   Family practitioner services

At the heart of community-based health care was – and is – the general practitioner. Before the large-scale development of hospitals all doctors worked in the community but in due course some doctors chose to specialize in hospital work. Those who remained in the community were less well paid and, until training for general practice was made mandatory in the 1980s, they were often relatively poorly trained. Nevertheless, experience in treating common ailments and their knowledge of family circumstances meant they were held in high esteem by their patients.

These were the patients able to pay either directly or through friendly societies, trades unions or other similar schemes. Not until the National Insurance Act 1911 was there overall entitlement to free treatment from a GP and then only for working people on the doctor's panel. Others had to rely on hospital outpatient departments or health and welfare clinics set up by some local authorities. Before the NHS the distribution of GPs reflected supply and demand, so the more deprived areas were likely to be least well served. GPs guarded their independent status jealously and the prospect of losing it made many of them antagonistic to the proposal for a national health service. In the event the government compromised, and GPs have managed to retain their independent contractor status ever since.

2.1.3   Community-based services

The development of doctors' 'panels' under the 1911 Act did much to improve GP services, but there was still no comprehensive approach to health care. Although the 1920 Dawson report[7] was ignored at the time, its wide-ranging proposals were ultimately influential. It recommended

See Chapter 11 for further details

domiciliary services from doctors, pharmacists and local authority staff, primary health centres with beds under the control of GPs with diagnostic facilities, outpatient clinics, dental, ancillary and community services, secondary health centres for specialist diagnosis and treatment, supplementary services for infectious and mental illness, teaching hospitals with medical schools, the promotion of research, standardized medical records, and the establishment of a single authority to administer all medical and allied services with medical representation and local medical committees. In retrospect this report proved to set the agenda for the rest of the twentieth century!

Key reference: Ministry of Health, Consultative Council on Medical and Allied Services (1920) *Interim Report on the Future Provision of Medical and Allied Services (Dawson report)*. HMSO, London.

A more professional approach to nursing in the community developed from the mid-nineteenth century and was gradually formalized under the Queens Institute, founded in Liverpool, and by accredited training for health visitors. The Midwives Act of 1902 established a roll of approved midwives. Under the 1911 National Insurance scheme only registered pharmacists could dispense medicines (except in remote areas, where GPs did their own dispensing). Similarly there was a gradual acceptance of the professional status of opticians with their own register established in 1923.

Despite the scope of these services, community health care overall was fragmented, particularly as local authorities offered very variable standards of provision.

2.2 CREATION OF THE NATIONAL HEALTH SERVICE

It is customary to depict the UK's National Health Service as the supreme achievement of a post-war socialist government. A less idealistic view is that the country's economy could not be rebuilt after the war unless its population was relieved from reliance on fragmented, financially crippled and under-resourced health services often operating out of century-old buildings in a bad state of repair. The shortcomings had already been analysed in Sir William Beveridge's report[8], which was dedicated to slaying the 'five giants': want, ignorance, disease, squalor and idleness. The recommendations of the Beveridge report formed the foundation of the UK's welfare state.

For health Beveridge envisaged a comprehensive service, meaning that the full range of medical and nursing services should be available to every citizen as and when they needed them. The wartime coalition government accepted this broad aim and in 1944 Henry Willink, Minister of Health, published a white paper called *A National Health Service*[9].

Key references: Timmins, N. (1995) *The Five Giants – a Biography of the Welfare State*. HarperCollins, London; Webster, C. (1988 and 1996) *The Health Services since the War*, Vol.1 1948–57, Vol.2 1958–79. The Stationery Office, London.

Box 2.2

A National Health Service – 1944 white paper

- Central control by Ministry of Health.
- Advised by Central Health Services Council.
- Local health boards incorporating local authority hospitals and clinics.
- Contracting arrangement with voluntary hospitals.
- Contracting arrangements with GPs.
- Regulated distribution of GPs.

During discussion of the white paper, the idea of a two-tier regional and local administrative system was proposed. A sticking point was the remuneration of doctors. The 1944 Labour Party Conference had decided in favour of a full-time salaried service but in the final negotiations following Labour's landslide electoral victory in 1945 the new Minister of Health, Aneurin Bevan, eventually compromised, leaving GPs as independent contractors and allowing salaried hospital doctors to undertake private work outwith their NHS contract. The British Medical Association (BMA) only agreed to take part in the new NHS at the eleventh hour, with these concessions won.

The National Health Service Act[10] was passed in November 1946 and the new arrangements were launched on 5 July 1948, 'the appointed day', free to patients at the point of use. The Minister of Health was made personally responsible to Parliament for the provision of all hospitals and specialist services on a national basis, and for the Public Health Laboratory Service, the Blood Transfusion Service and research concerned with the prevention, diagnosis and treatment of illness. He also had indirect responsibility for family practitioner and local authority health services. The Central Health Services Council and its professional Standing Committees were established to keep the Minister well informed.

All hospitals were nationalized under 14 (subsequently 15) regional boards (England and Wales), each of which had at least one medical school in their region. Thirty-six teaching hospitals associated with medical schools were designated and were run by Boards of Governors who were directly responsible to the Ministry of Health. Within the regions, 377 hospital management committees (HMCs) were created. Their size and responsibilities varied.

Local health authorities (60 counties and 78 county boroughs) continued to be responsible for community services including maternal and child welfare, health visiting, district nurses, vaccination and immunisation, health centres (where they existed), and the care of those people with mental deficiency (learning disabilities) or mental illnesses who were not in hospital. The third part of the NHS, family practitioner

Four mental hospitals were allowed to remain private: Cheadle Royal, Manchester; The Retreat, York; St. Andrew's, Northampton; and St. Luke's, north London

See Chapter 7 for arrangements in Scotland, Wales and Northern Ireland

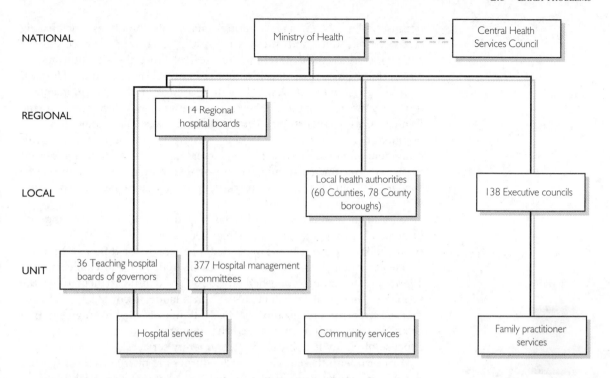

NATIONAL

Ministry of Health ---- Central Health Services Council

REGIONAL

14 Regional hospital boards

LOCAL

Local health authorities (60 Counties, 78 County boroughs)

138 Executive councils

UNIT

36 Teaching hospital boards of governors

377 Hospital management committees

Hospital services

Community services

Family practitioner services

Figure 2.1

The National Health Service 1948–74 (England and Wales)

services, was administered by 138 executive councils, which were financed directly by the Ministry of Health to administer the contracts of GPs, dentists, pharmacists and opticians.

Although it had been intended to forbid charitable donations to the NHS, this was changed and voluntary organizations were in some cases absorbed and in others continued to provide aid-supported services. The school medical service remained outside the NHS, being run by education authorities, and environmental health services remained directly run by local authorities. The Industrial Health Service was the responsibility of the Ministry of Labour. The armed services retained their own separate health service.

2.3 EARLY PROBLEMS

The cost of the new NHS very quickly became a financial problem to the Labour government faced with numerous spending demands. The key principle of a free service was first breached in 1951 with the introduction of charges to some people for spectacles and dentures. Charges for medicines were introduced by the incoming Conservative government a year later, abolished by the new Labour government in 1965 and reintroduced in 1968. But such income was a drop in the ocean, particularly as around 60% of patients were exempt from the charges.

Equally problematic was the poor state of health services

premises. The NHS had inherited many old buildings and hastily erected EMS huts and there was considerable war damage in the main cities. Piecemeal developments scarcely met the situation and in 1962 the Minister of Health, Enoch Powell, published *A Hospital Plan for England and Wales*[11], which approved the development of district general hospitals. Their role was further developed in the Bonham-Carter report of 1969[12]. These hospitals would serve a population of around 125,000 people, but subsequently this catchment population was greatly increased. The recommendations of these two documents dominated hospital development until the 1990 changes encouraged a free market approach allowing collaboration with private finance.

The main financial problems stemmed from the ever-increasing rise in demand. Patients' expectations had been stimulated by the availability of the NHS, and no real allowance had been made for this. The Minister of Health set up a review committee, chaired by C.W. Guillebaud, in 1953, but its report, published in 1956[13], did little to help solve the problem. One of its members, Sir John Maude, recorded his concern that the tripartite organization of the NHS not only led to fragmentation of services but unduly emphasized the importance of the hospitals at the expense of family health care and community services.

Concern with these divisions grew during the next ten years. In 1962 the Porritt report[14] suggested a unified service run by area health boards. The Gillie report[15] a year later suggested that GPs should commission services on behalf of their patients. This now proves to have been an interesting anticipation of ideas that have become current.

See Chapter 11 for further details

The three Cogwheel reports were nicknamed from the design on their front covers

Gradual changes in administration within the hospital service were encouraged by the Bradbeer report[16]. Hospital administrators took over the housekeeping services – domestic, catering, laundry and linen, and residences – from the matrons, who in turn were developing their own professional role. This culminated in the Salmon report in 1967[17], the foundation for a new (and subsequently much reviled) hospital nursing management structure under the control of a chief nursing officer. Hospital doctors were urged to involve themselves in management. The reports known as Cogwheel[18] proposed medical specialty groupings, as a way to introduce more self-management by clinical teams. Clinical methods were also advancing, enabling more sophisticated interventions and achieving better outcomes as well as reducing lengths of stay. The Cranbrook report 1959[19] changed maternity services profoundly by unequivocally favouring hospital confinements, at that time only 60% of all births, and by heavily criticizing the fragmented maternity services split across the three parts of the NHS. Even more radical was the Mental Health Act 1959[20], which reduced the number of compulsorily admitted patients and led to a wholesale review of hospitalized people with mental illness and mental subnormality (the then new term for mental deficiency). Over the next 30 years the hospital population of these groups of patients reduced by 65% and almost all the old asylums and mental hospitals closed.

2.4 PREPARING FOR THE FIRST REORGANIZATION

In the late 1960s, it had become clear that the tripartite divisions of the NHS were creating difficulties and that a new-look organization might resolve this. The independent Porritt report[21] had already suggested structural changes, largely ignored in 1962, but in July 1968 Kenneth Robinson, the Minister of Health, published what became known as the first green paper: *The Administrative Structure of Medical and Related Services in England and Wales*[22]. He proposed 40–50 area boards replacing existing regional hospital boards, boards of governors and hospital management committees in direct contact with the Ministry of Health and serving populations of between 750,000 and 3 million.

At the same time major reviews of social work and local government were in progress by the Committee on Local Authority and Allied Personal Services (chaired by Frederick Seebohm)[23] and a Royal Commission on Local Government (chairman Lord Redcliffe-Maud)[24], respectively. Meanwhile Richard Crossman had succeeded Robinson and had become the first Secretary of State for Social Services, leading the new Department of Health and Social Security (DHSS). A second green paper, *The Future Structure of the National Health Service*[25] published in February 1970, proposed a two-tier structure for England, with regions responsible for hospital and specialist planning and 90 area health authorities matching local authority boundaries. The general election in June 1970 did not return a Labour government and a year later Sir Keith Joseph, the new Secretary of State, issued a consultative document for England[26], which retained the proposals to incorporate the local authority health services into the duties of the new area authorities and to match health and local authorities' boundaries. The duties of regions were to be enhanced. A new proposal was the formation of Community Health Councils to represent the consumer.

The consultative document also announced that two 'expert studies' had been commissioned by the DHSS: Brunel University's Health Service Organizational Research Unit carried out work on the roles and relationships in the NHS and McKinsey conducted pilot schemes and examined the internal organization of the DHSS itself.

The fruits of Brunel University's HSORU's work are contained in two books: *Hospital Organization*, 1973 and *Health Services*, 1978, Heinemann, London

May 1971	Consultative document.
August 1972	White paper *National Health Service Reorganization*.
November 1972	NHS reorganization bill before Parliament.
September 1972	'Grey Book' published.
End of 1972	Commission established to manage staff changes.
5 July 1973	National Health Service Reorganization Act.
February 1974	New Labour government.
1 April 1974	New reorganized NHS starts.
July 1975	Revised Labour proposals for authority membership.

Box 2.3

Timetable of changes

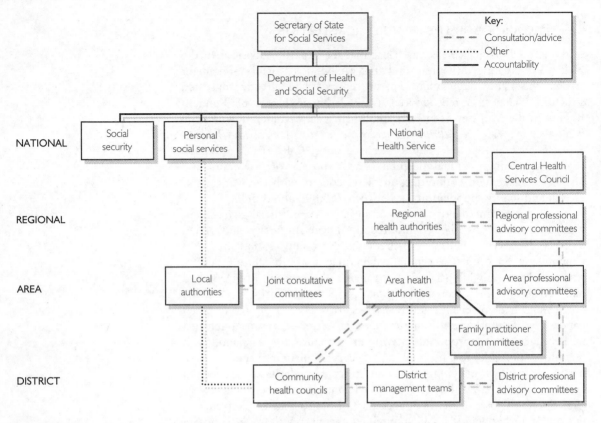

Source: adapted from *Management Arrangements for the Reorganised National Health Service* (1974). HMSO, London

Figure 2.2

The reorganized National Health Service 1974.

2.5   THE NEW ARRANGEMENTS

Under the new arrangements 90 area health authorities (AHAs) were responsible for planning services and appointed district management teams (DMTs) to carry them out. At area level there was an area team of officers (the ATO) comprising an administrator, a nurse, a public health doctor and a finance officer. The DMT comprised administrator, nurse, public health doctor, finance officer, GP and consultant. The last two were nominated by their local peers. The DMT was not accountable to the ATO but could be monitored by them. Most (66%) areas had more than one district. Relationships between the two types of teams were often poor and the rather remote health authorities, made up of non-executives, had difficulty in keeping abreast with activity on the ground.

Relationships between authorities were also problematic, and the attempt to separate planning from operational functions was equally troubled. Furthermore there was tension arising from the administrative demarcation of areas to match local government boundaries and the more natural and better-established catchment areas of particular district general hospitals (DGHs).

The new arrangements took over two years to implement. At the same time there was an unprecedented increase in industrial disputes by health service workers. Barbara Castle, the new Secretary of State, also tried to restrict private practice facilities within the NHS and this led to a particularly bitter dispute with doctors.

It was clear that the 1974 reorganization was not proving as successful as hoped and accordingly Barbara Castle asked Sir Alec Merrison to chair a Royal Commission on the NHS[27], the first wide-ranging review since the Guillebaud committee 20 years previously. It reported in 1979 that 'we need not be ashamed of our health service and that there are many aspects of which we can be justly proud'. But it did criticize the number of administrative tiers and the consequent increase in bureaucracy. This fuelled the incoming Conservative government's desire to simplify the structure of the NHS. In December 1979 it issued *Patients First*[28].

See Chapter 12 for more details

The changes were finalized in July 1980 in circular HC(80)8 *Health Services: Structure and Management*[29] and came into force on 1 April 1982

- District health authorities to replace AHAs.
- Professional consultative machinery to be simplified.
- Unit management to replace functional management.
- Simplified planning system.
- Future of CHCs to be reviewed.

Box 2.4

Patients first

2.6 INTRODUCTION OF 'GENERAL MANAGEMENT'

The team or consensus management approach had been a deliberate characteristic of the 1974 reorganization. In addition, in the 1980s, government enthusiasm for privatization insisted that health authorities contracted out support services, and implemented much more stringent efficiency controls and financial and manpower cuts. The management arrangements attracted heavy criticism for failing to hold one member of the DMT accountable for making and implementing decisions. Perhaps the alleged procrastination was more a consequence of the inherent complexity of the decisions to be made.

The Secretary of State, Norman Fowler, asked Roy Griffiths, managing director of the supermarket chain Sainsbury's, to set up a team to advise him privately on how the NHS could be better managed. Its report was well received and published in October 1983[30]. Griffiths identified a lack of drive in the NHS, and he and his team said this was because at each level of management no one person was accountable for action. In addition, professionals and functional managers had been given too much scope. When the appointment of general managers started, following the authorizing circular HC(84)13[31], the Minister of Health, Kenneth Clarke, attempted to bring new management blood into the NHS. In the event applicants from elsewhere were not particularly numerous and the few who were appointed were not always successful, finding the complex environment difficult to master.

Clarke succeeded Fowler as Secretary of State in 1988; he later steered the 1990 Act through Parliament and introduced the GPs' new contract

---

Key reference: DHSS (October 1983) *The NHS Management Inquiry* (Griffiths report). DHSS, London.

Griffiths also proposed changes at the DHSS. A Supervisory Board would be responsible for determining the objectives of the health service, approving overall budgets and monitoring performance. The Secretary of State was to chair the Board, which would include the Permanent Secretary of the DHSS, the Chief Medical Officer and the Chairman of a Management Board, and who were to act as an executive board accountable to the Supervisory Board. The Supervisory Board was duly appointed but its role and influence remained obscure. The Management Board was much more prominent, and it started the gradual erosion of the traditional division between civil servants, who serve Parliament and its ministers, and the public servants, in this case the officers of the regional health authorities, who through districts ran the services on the ground.

The initial antagonism to Griffiths from doctors and nurses, who feared an over-authoritarian management style, largely evaporated. But the government was still wanting to limit the insatiable financial demands made by the NHS and its ability to attract public support to embarrass the political leaders. The Prime Minster, Mrs Thatcher, set up another private review in 1988, which resulted in two white papers: *Working for Patients*[32] in January 1989 and *Caring for People*[33] in November 1989.

An example of this embarrassment was the government's discomfort at the media interest in a baby who had been denied a heart operation in Birmingham

2.7   *Working for Patients and Caring for People*

The white papers *Working for Patients* and *Caring for People* led to the National Heath Service and Community Care Act, 1990, which came into effect after 1 April 1991. These reforms were among the most radical since the inception of the NHS, and were part of the Thatcher government's reappraisal of the public sector and the welfare state.

Although the Conservatives had won a third general election in 1987 and had given assurances about the future of the NHS in their manifesto,

Box 2.5

Working for Patients

- Introduction of the 'internal market' by separating 'purchasing' and 'providing' functions.
- Creation of NHS trusts with greater freedom to set pay levels and borrow for capital projects.
- New corporate boards of management at regional, health authority and trust levels with joint executive and non-executive membership.
- Fundholding for larger GP practices allowing them to purchase certain patient services direct from providers.
- Consultants' contracts held by trusts (previously held by regions).
- Family health services authorities to replace family practitioner committees.
- Tax relief on private medical insurance for elderly people.
- Extension of medical audit.
- Extension of hospital clinical budgeting.
- 'Indicative prescribing' to contain GP drug costs.

they found themselves beset with the continuing financial problems and resulting cuts in service. These problems were not only a result of government policy; they also arose from growing public expectations, advances in medical technology and an ageing population. But the Conservatives believed that it was wise to attempt to limit the apparently insatiable demand by introducing much more rigorous means of controlling costs and by encouraging those who could afford it to pay more towards their care. This meant enabling private practice to develop and limiting the public provision of long-term care for elderly people. This forced them into independent and private-sector nursing homes, where they had to pay for their own care until their money ran out.

Caring for People was a long-awaited response to three reports on community care issued between 1986 and 1988[34-36]. Its major proposal was to separate 'health' from 'social' care. The former was free if provided by NHS staff, the latter was means tested. Social services departments were also expected to transfer their own direct provision of residential care to the private or charitable sector. This in turn needed a more extensive inspection system to regulate those providers. These changes took some time to implement and the demarcation between health and social care proved to be a continuing problem, often leading to disputes.

The subsequent Labour government set up a Royal Commission in 1998 to investigate the care of the elderly and its funding; see Chapter 9

The Conservatives also believed that a great deal of effort and many resources were being wasted, particularly through bureaucratic management. They were convinced that the NHS would benefit from less government intervention. Much influenced by economists from the USA, in particular Alain Enthoven, the government decided to subject the NHS to the disciplines of the market. Competition between providers of health care would not only improve patient choice but would also give health authorities and individual hospitals incentives to work efficiently and become more flexible and adaptable to a discerning market. It followed that provider units would need to be smaller and that the monolithic health districts in place since 1982 would need to be broken up.

> **Key reference:** Enthoven, A. (1985) *Reflections on the Management of the NHS,* Nuffield Provincial Hospitals Trust, Occasional Paper 5. NHPT, London. This essay was highly influential in introducing the concept of the 'internal market' to the NHS.

Stricter control of professionals was another goal of the new arrangements. Professionals were frequently criticized by the Thatcher government for pursuing their own interests in preference to those of their clients. Unsurprisingly, therefore, *Working for Patients* was opposed by doctors and nurses alike, who claimed it gave too much power to managers, rather than themselves, at the expense of patients' interests. The public were inclined to support the professionals' view. At the time, the Secretary of State, Kenneth Clarke, was also negotiating a new contract with GPs, which led to further bad relations. Notwithstanding the resulting unpopularity, the government proceeded to introduce the new arrangements, separating health authorities (the purchasers of health care) from the providers (the newly created trusts). Despite the complexities and the initial uncertainties, the changes had been fully implemented by 1996. Political opponents accused the Conservatives of preparing to dismantle the NHS. The government insisted that this was not so. Insofar as it had rejected other ways of funding the NHS, for instance by insurance, it could be believed.

At the top of the NHS organization the Policy Board superseded the Supervisory Board. More significant was the new NHS Management Executive, which was renamed the NHS Executive (NHSE) in 1993. Its members are led by the chief executive and include career civil servants and NHS managers, together with one or two outsiders brought in for their special expertise. Separating the executive wing (transferred to Leeds) from the policy wing (remaining in London) brought about fundamental changes in the way the DoH worked.

At the next level were regions, with similar boundaries as before for the time being (although in 1998 an all-London region was set up, disbanding the awkward Anglia and Oxford region in the process). Until 1996, regions and the new health authorities were led by corporate boards, with a non-executive chairman, five other non-executives and up to five executive directors. The appointment of the non-executives was ultimately in the hands of the Minister of Health, advised by districts and regions.

The new health authorities became the purchasers and commissioners of care. They were responsible for assessing need, planning services, contracting with providers, and monitoring those contracts which were on a yearly basis. This permitted much more stringent control of providers' performance as contracts could be withdrawn where performance was unsatisfactory.

A significant late addition to *Working for Patients,* somewhat inconsistent with its other proposals, was the scheme for GP fundholding. Under this option, GPs were given their own budgets to manage and this offered them considerable leverage over hospital providers. The inconsistency arose from the fact that they were also service providers. But fundholding did alter the power balance between general practice and hospital medical services. Even non-fundholder GPs enjoyed greater authority over providers now that heath authorities could determine the future contracts with those providers. Fundholding also encouraged patients to demand better care from their GPs, knowing that the GPs could no longer so easily blame others for unsatisfactory performance.

The DoH was able to issue only general guidance on the implementation of the 1990 Act: it was left to NHS managers to work out the details. This gave them even more power than they had assumed under Griffiths, but also exacerbated tensions between them and their clinical colleagues despite the increased opportunities for doctors themselves to become involved in managerial decision-making.

Despite the radical nature of the 1990 changes, they were essentially evolutionary too. For patients the changes were a mixed blessing. In

The appointment arrangements became more formalized from July 1996 in line with a new code of practice issued by the Commissioner for Public Appointments[37]

Purchasing and commissioning were initially synonymous terms; subsequently they took on separate meanings; see Chapter 4

some respects their interests were enhanced by fundholding and the increased responsiveness of the new health authorities and NHS trusts. But for those patients not in a fundholding GP practice, there was the real risk of becoming second-class citizens wherever hospitals attempted to please fundholders, who had the greater purchasing power, before they responded to non-fundholders. This criticism of a two-tier or two-class system was made much of by the Labour opposition.

2.8   THE HEALTH OF THE NATION

An accurate observation about the NHS since 1948 is that it is more of a 'national sickness service', giving too little attention and resources to improving the health of the population. The white paper *The Health of the Nation*[38] was published in July 1992, in an attempt to counter this criticism. It introduced a new national strategy, focusing on health rather than health care. It was designed to be the start of a continuous process of target-setting, monitoring and reviewing a health strategy that would address key areas of concern over time. The first five areas, identified because they represented major causes of premature death or avoidable morbidity, and involved effective interventions which could be monitored, were:

- coronary heart disease;
- cancers;
- mental illness;
- HIV/AIDS and sexual health;
- accidents (particularly among young men).

See Chapter 9 for more detailed discussion

Targets were set for each of these, to be achieved by 2000.

2.9   THE 1990 CHANGES IN PRACTICE

The 1990 changes to the running of the NHS were ambitious. How successful were they in practice? Did the new arrangements increase the ability of the NHS to respond to patients' needs more effectively? Did the separation of functions provide improved incentives and sharpen the focus of health authorities', trusts' and fundholders' endeavours? Were consumers of the health services more satisfied?

2.9.1   Separation of functions

The 1990 Act separated purchasers, the health authorities, from providers, the NHS trusts. The rationale behind this split was that purchasers in the past allegedly had spent too much time on operational matters and had therefore been unable to take a more strategic look at the needs of their populations: the urgent problem could drive the more important issue off the agenda. To a certain extent this was true, but perhaps more due to the way management was practised rather than to the structure. Nevertheless the purchaser–provider split was felt by the majority of those in the NHS to have been successful and was retained by the incoming Labour government in 1997.

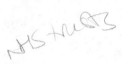

The creation of NHS trusts was less successful. There were few restraints, in order to get the process going, and any configuration of service providers who wanted to become an NHS trust could do so, except joint hospital and community trusts. These were discouraged on the grounds that, without the tension caused by forcing a competitive market approach between them, primary care would continue to be disadvantaged. The shortcoming of this liberal approach was that trust sizes and boundaries were not always suited to longer-term needs. Soon there were a significant number of trust mergers.

Concurrent with the separation of purchasers and providers, and greatly facilitated by it, was the new emphasis on primary care and associated attempts to limit the apparently insatiable demand for secondary care resources. This originated in the 1980s, when it became increasingly evident that three factors were causing primary or community care to be insufficiently in focus. First, the more ambitious managers tended to work in secondary care, while family health services authorities had not attracted the more able people. Second, it was an important manifestation of the unequal status between hospital consultants and GPs. Despite improved conditions of service following the new GPs' Charter in 1966, they were still regarded professionally as second rank. Third, the main impetus for refocusing the NHS on primary care was to tackle GPs' tendency to refer patients too readily and sometimes inappropriately for hospital care, causing unnecessary expense.

The enhanced status of primary care was also greatly helped by fundholding, which enabled GPs to make more detailed decisions about each patient and his or her needs. They were now aware of the price tag on passing each patient into the hospital system.

At first purchasers were largely left to their own devices while the trusts were given all the attention. In due course this changed but the opportunities for health authorities to alter established patient referrals were limited and where they tried this had destructive organizational consequences. Managing the internal market did not bring about the expected dividends.

The white paper *Choice and Opportunity* in 1996[39] was followed by The Primary Care Act, 1997[40], which was rushed onto the statute book days before the general election. This attempted to free primary care from some of the statutory impediments which were making innovation difficult. It allowed GPs to be employed directly rather than as contractors. Another provision that was endorsed by the new government was the unification of practice budgets.

2.9.2   Too many managers?

The 1974 reorganization had been criticized for requiring increasing numbers of administrators to try to make it work. Although the 1982 changes removed the area tier, they had perpetuated the separation between the hospital sector and the rest of the services, and so-called functional management within districts. This had tended to segment the whole organization into functional and professional hierarchies. Griffiths

In 1997 the East Norfolk and Suffolk HAs drove the Anglian Harbours Trust out of business by reallocating contracts to other trusts

See Chapters 4 and 8 for details of practice budgets

had tried to simplify the structure by having one unambiguous leader. But the split still continued within the units. The 1990 Act did nothing to resolve the perception that there were too many managers in the system. Indeed, its requirements forced a further increase in their number. The creation of service contracts, which had grown significantly for support services in the early 1980s, burgeoned under the 1990 Act into wholesale contracting between purchasers and providers for all patient care. A substantial increase in managerial staff, to implement these processes was inevitable. 'Management' always tends to be unpopular, and becomes especially so at election times when political scapegoats are sought for perceived shortcomings.

The increase in non-clinical managers was accompanied by the rising numbers of doctors who, willingly or not, have had to undertake managerial work. Fundholders sometimes relished the opportunity to control their destinies but many also complained of the managerial consequences. In a few instances GP practices opted out of fundholding for that reason. The other main reason for needing more managers was the work associated with ensuring the NHS becomes demonstrably more efficient and effective. Providing the necessary evidence involves considerable managerial input.

2.9.3 Consumerism

It is a tenet of a market economy that the consumer is empowered to make choices. In health services this is difficult because consumers' knowledge is usually deficient; they therefore have difficulty in deciding what is the 'best buy' for them. Formerly consumer interests had been preserved by community health councils, created in the 1974 reorganization. They were not always paid much attention by health authorities and trusts, but used well they could be a valuable resource, undertaking research into public opinion and improving the dialogue between the service and its public. They were never the sole means of establishing patients' and the general public's attitudes to their health services. In 1991 the government published the *Patient's Charter*[41], which set out standards by which the NHS could be judged by its users.

See Chapter 13 for more about community health councils

Three more factors have put further pressure on clinical and managerial staff to provide better services: the development of technology, media coverage of new treatments and drugs, and the ability of more and more patients to access the Internet to educate themselves about their health, ailments and treatment options. This expansion of people's expectations cannot be satisfied by the NHS alone, but recent surveys of public opinion suggest that popular regard for the NHS is declining from its former high point.

2.10 *The new NHS*

The first Labour government for 18 years was elected on 1 May 1997. In opposition, Labour had been highly critical of the market approach to health care and of fundholding, which in its view had led to a two-class service as non-fundholders' patients had to wait longer because their GPs had less leverage with trusts. The new Secretary of State, Frank Dobson, issued a white paper, *The new NHS*[42], in December 1997. The government was in some difficulty because it wished to retain significant elements of the 1990 Act reforms but also wanted to appear to be making its own important innovations. The internal market was therefore replaced by 'integrated care', a term that reinstated planning into the NHS. Planning seemed to have become incompatible with the prevailing market philosophy. The white paper acknowledged the need to retain GPs' involvement through fundholding and the emphasis on primary care, so it created primary care groups (PCGs). These enable groups of GPs and community nurses to commission and provide health services within cash-limited budgets for populations of around 100,000.

See Chapter 7 for the implementation of these reforms in Wales, Scotland and Northern Ireland

Figure 2.3

The organization of the NHS (April 1999)

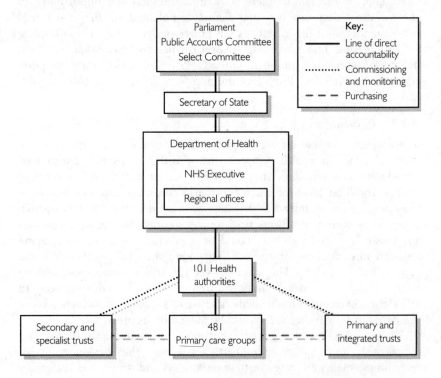

Emphasis on quality continues with the creation of two new bodies: the National Institute of Clinical Excellence and the Commission for Health Improvement. These were expounded on in June 1998 in the publication *A First Class Service – Quality in the new NHS*[43], which described how to enhance the setting, delivering and monitoring of standards.

See Chapter 10 for details

The government was anxious not to lose the impetus arising from the earlier *Health of the Nation* targets, and issued the green paper *Our Healthier Nation*[44] in February 1998, selecting four key issues. These regrouped the ones set in 1992, aiming to reduce deaths from:

- heart disease and stroke;
- cancer;
- suicide;
- accidents.

Initially no new money was promised for Labour's changes but by summer 1998, following the government's comprehensive spending review, extra funds were provided over a 3-year period on the condition that managers and clinicians in the NHS fulfilled their part of the bargain by securing better performance and in particular reducing hospital waiting lists. This had been a key target in Labour's election manifesto. The government's energy was palpable and the timetable for change correspondingly ambitious. Primary care's reorganization into primary care groups was to be done by 1 April 1999.

> PCGs seem to introduce another layer of management into the structure, as yet unacknowledged by the government

- 'Integrated care' to replace internal market.
- Health authorities to plan services for given populations in partnership with other public authorities.
- Primary Care Groups covering whole population to replace fundholding and to be responsible for purchasing services.
- Equitable allocation of funds.
- New National Institute of Clinical Excellence and Commission for Health Improvement to be set up.
- Curb on management costs to continue.

Box 2.6
The new NHS

CONCLUSION

This chapter has given the background to the creation of the NHS and the subsequent changes in its organization, together with brief details of some of the most significant legislative changes and reports. Fifty years after 5 July 1948 the NHS showed a remarkable ability to reinvent itself in response to changing government policies, health needs, medical advance and public expectations. Despite the continual changes, certain themes persist: attempts at improving responsiveness to patients, pressure on resources, the changing role of professionals, and political sensitivity. The following chapters examine these issues in more detail.

REFERENCES

1. The National Health Service Act, 1946. HMSO, London.
2. The National Health Service Reorganisation Act, 1973. HMSO, London.
3. DHSS (July 1980) *Health Services: Structure and Management*, Circular HC(80)8. HMSO, London.
4. The National Health Service and Community Care Act, 1990. HMSO, London.
5. *The new NHS; Modern – Dependable*. The Stationery Office, London 1997 (Cm 3807).
6. Ministry of Health (1945 & 1946) *Hospital Survey*. HMSO, London.

7. Ministry of Health, Consultative Council on Medical and Allied Services (1920) *Interim Report on the Future Provision of Medical and Allied Services* (Dawson report). HMSO, London.
8. *Social Insurance and Allied Services* (Beveridge report), 1942, HMSO, London (Cmnd 6404).
9. Ministry of Health and Department of Health for Scotland (1944) *A National Health Service*. HMSO, London (Cmnd 6502).
10. Op. cit., The National Health Service Act, 1946.
11. Ministry of Health (1962) *A Hospital Plan for England and Wales*. HMSO, London (Cmnd 1604).
12. DHSS and Welsh Office. Central Health Services Council (1969) *The Functions of the District General Hospital* (Bonham-Carter report). HMSO, London.
13. Ministry of Health (1956) *Report of the Committee of Enquiry into the Cost of the National Health Service* (Guillebaud report). HMSO, London (Cmnd 9663).
14. Medical Services Review Committee (1962) *A Review of the Medical Services in Great Britain* (Porritt report). Social Assay, London.
15. Ministry of Health. Central Health Services Council. Standing Medical Advisory Committee (1963) *The Field Work of the Family Doctor* (Gillie report). HMSO, London.
16. Ministry of Health. Central Health Services Council (1954) *The Internal Administration of Hospitals* (Bradbeer report). HMSO, London.
17. Ministry of Health and Scottish Home and Health Department (1966) *Report of the Committee on Senior Nursing Staff Structure* (Salmon report). HMSO, London.
18. Ministry of Health/DHSS (1967) *First report of the Joint Working Party on the Organisation of Medical Work in Hospitals* (Cogwheel report). HMSO, London.
19. Ministry of Health (1959) *Report of the Maternity Services Committee* (Cranbrook report). HMSO, London.
20. The Mental Health Act, 1959. HMSO, London.
21. Op. cit., The Porritt report.
22. Ministry of Health (1968) *The Administrative Structure of Medical and Related Services in England and Wales*. HMSO, London.
23. Committee on Local Authority and Allied Personal Social Services (1968) *Report of the Committee* (Seebohm report). HMSO, London (Cmnd 3703).
24. Royal Commission on Local Government in England (1966–69) *Report of the Royal Commission* (Redcliffe–Maud report). HMSO, London (Cmnd 4040).
25. DHSS (1970) *The Future Structure of the National Health Service*. HMSO, London. (This applied to England only.)
26. DHSS (1971) *National Health Service Reorganisation: Consultative Document*. DHSS, London.
27. Royal Commission on the National Health Service (1979) *Report of the Royal Commission*. HMSO, London (Cmnd 7615).
28. DHSS and Welsh Office (December 1979) *Patients First*. HMSO, London.
29. DHSS (July 1980) *Health Services Structure and Management*, Circular HC(80)8.
30. DHSS (October 1983) *The NHS Management Inquiry* (Griffiths report). DHSS, London.
31. DHSS (June 1984) *Health Services Management: Implementation of the NHS Management Inquiry*, Circular HC(84)13. DHSS, London.

32. DoH (January 1989) *Working for Patients*. HMSO, London (Cm 555).
33. DoH (November 1989) *Caring for People*. HMSO, London (Cm 849).
34. DoH (1986) *Primary Health Care* (discussion document). HMSO, London (Cmnd 9771).
35. DoH (November 1987) *Promoting Better Health: the Government's Programme for Improving Primary Health Care*. HMSO, London (Cm 249).
36. DoH (1988) *Community Care: Agenda for Action* (second Griffiths report). HMSO, London.
37. Commissioner for Public Appointments (1996) *Code of Practice for Public Appointment* (operational from 1 July 1996). HMSO, London.
38. DoH(1992) *The Health of the Nation*. HMSO, London (Cm 1986).
39. DoH (1996) *Choice and Opportunity*. HMSO, London.
40. The Primary Care Act, 1997. The Stationery Office, London.
41. DoH (1991) *The Patient's Charter*. HMSO, London.
42. Op. cit., *The new NHS*.
43. DoH (June 1998) *A First Class Service – Quality in the new NHS*. The Stationery Office, London.
44. DoH (February 1998) *Our Healthier Nation*. The Stationery Office, London.

3

CENTRAL GOVERNMENT AND THE NATIONAL HEALTH SERVICE

This chapter examines the role of ministers and civil servants in the Department of Health (DoH) and the NHS Executive (NHSE) and their relationships with the professional and managerial staff of the NHS. It also describes the history and background of the regional offices of the NHSE.

3.1 THE FUNCTIONS OF GOVERNMENT DEPARTMENTS

Governments need the legislative institutions of parliament and the administrative institutions of departments of state to make and implement their laws and policies, thereby to enable the balance of political power to influence the lives of the people. In the United Kingdom, each government department is led by a small team of ministers who are either elected Members of Parliament or members of the House of Lords. Supporting the Secretary of State, the head, are junior ministers and political advisors. Ministers are appointed by the Prime Minister, who determines how long they shall hold office and whether they shall be members of the Cabinet and any of its committees. When the Prime Minister changes or the government resigns, these political heads of the departments also change.

The permanent staff of the department, the civil servants, implement the political programmes of successive governments. They are required not to show or act on their own party political views but to serve each government of the day loyally. This requirement originated when the forerunners of today's departments were set up in the nineteenth century. There is built-in tension between the politicians and the civil servants. Ministers will want to make significant progress in implementing policies during their relatively short term of office, supported by their own party and their party's MPs. Civil servants, because of their more extended association with the department and their expert knowledge, may favour more gradual progress towards longer-term objectives and may wish to express constructive criticism. Overall the success of the relationship between the most senior civil servants and the ministers in the department will determine the department's perceived effectiveness. The Secretary of State's personality, style, and ability to assimilate a great deal of information quickly and accurately will be the keys to a positive working relationship.

Permanent secretaries head the civil servants in departments. In the case of the DoH there are two: one heading the DoH in London, the second (called the Chief Executive) in charge of the NHSE in Leeds. Permanent secretaries are responsible for the overall management and

As powers are devolved from Westminster and Whitehall to government institutions in Northern Ireland, Scotland, Wales and the English regions, the scope and remit of the central government will be modified. See Chapter 7

control of all aspects of the department's administration and for ensuring the ministers can fulfil their accountability to Parliament.

3.2 THE ROLE OF HEALTH MINISTERS

The Secretary of State's goals for their department may conflict with the priorities of the Cabinet. It is his or her function to argue specifically for the policies and funds the department requires. The Prime Minister and the Cabinet, on the other hand, will also expect the Secretary of State to take a wider political view, contributing and supporting the government on matters beyond their own department and to be prepared to be active in Parliament generally and within the party organization. The Secretary of State has to seek a balance between these demands which will, ideally, enable him or her not only to be successful in leading the direction of their own department but also to be an effective politician.

Because government departments have greatly expanded the scope of their activities, policy initiation and preparation increasingly have to be done by the civil servants and their professional advisors, leaving the ministers to pick out those initiatives they wish to be involved in and to be seen to champion. Career civil servants may work in several different departments for ministers of different complexions. As a result they may be more committed to matters of administration and procedure than policy, and the role of political advisors has developed as a counter-vailing party political or expert influence.

The NHS has seen how far-reaching the influence of outside advisors can be. Norman Fowler asked Roy Griffiths of Sainsbury's to examine the workings of the NHS: his report in 1983 led to the introduction of general management, which in turn prepared the ground for the even more fundamental reforms brought in by the National Health Service and Community Care Act, 1990. The use of advisors is often criticized by those who object to their ease of access to ministers and information and their lack of accountability.

3.3 ACCOUNTABILITY

What does it mean to say that the Secretary of State is constitutionally accountable to Parliament? Formally, he or she must see that the NHS is run in accordance with statute, in line with government policies, and that its operation is efficient. But such a generalization poses questions. It clearly is impossible for the Secretary of State to be held personally responsible for the actions of individual staff in the NHS and the line of accountability has been drawn more tightly. Accordingly, chief executives down the line are asked to declare that various things have been done. These declarations may not ensure that everything has in fact been done to plan but at least will allow named individuals to be held accountable if matters go wrong, and also enable the Secretary of State to make statements and answer questions in Parliament and in public.

As an elected Member of Parliament he or she is answerable to the

House of Commons and will be expected to reply to questions raised by other MPs. In addition he or she will be required to attend the Public Accounts Committee (PAC) to answer points raised by the Comptroller and Auditor General, who is an independent officer of Parliament, and any of the 15 MPs, drawn from all main parties, who make up the PAC. However the DoH Permanent Secretary and the NHSE Chief Executive (the second permanent secretary), can be asked to appear, as indeed can any of the NHS's accountable officers, the chief executives of health authorities and trusts.

Similarly all these people can be asked to appear before the Parliamentary Select Committee on Health, which examines aspects of the running of the NHS and provides critical assessments for the benefit of the House of Commons. Select committees give back-bench MPs a minor but influential role in the policy process. They have grown in importance as they have learned not to shirk from criticizing received views and that there are benefits in adopting cross-party opinions.

In addition to these bodies the Audit Commission undertakes the audit of health authorities (but not necessarily the NHS trusts) and issues reports on matters of concern. These reports are often critical of the status quo and are used as levers to assist policy changes.

Within the NHS the review process has steadily became more exacting. Following the 1982 reorganization regular ministerial reviews were set up. Initially each regional chairman was summoned to meet one of the ministers but in 1989 this process was developed to become a more detailed investigation of each region by the NHSME. Following a

Figure 3.1

Accountability in the NHS
(April 1999)

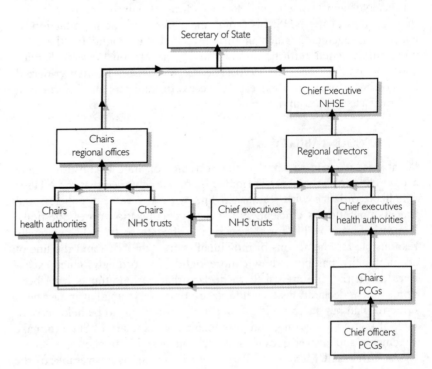

review an itemized letter was sent to the regional general manager; this was in effect a contract for the following year's work on which the success or otherwise of the region's performance could be judged. This process passed down the line to the health authorities.

This emphasis on setting objectives and evaluating performance has become more and more important. The 1997 Labour government took the matter even further in its proposal to set up a Commission for Health Improvement. As always, governments deploy carrot and stick inducements in their quest for better performance within the public sector.

See Chapter 10 for more details on standard setting and quality initiatives

3.4 THE DEPARTMENT OF HEALTH

When the Ministry of Health was first formed in 1919, it had responsibility for roads, national insurance, planning, environmental health and local government as well as the health services but, over the years, these other duties were transferred elsewhere. In 1951, local government housing passed to the new Ministry of Housing and Local Government and, with this, came the loss of a seat in the Cabinet and a considerable reduction of staff at the Ministry of Health.

The origins of the social security ministry go back even earlier, to 1916, when a Ministry of Pensions was set up. This was amalgamated with the Ministry of National Insurance, set up in 1944, and in 1966 these two joined the National Assistance Board to form the new Ministry of Social Security. In 1968, Richard Crossman, Lord President of the Council and Leader of the House of Commons, was involved with the Prime Minister, Harold Wilson, in planning the restructuring of certain government ministries that would further consolidate the total number of spending departments. The new Department of Health and Social Security (DHSS) was created in this way, with the seat on the Cabinet restored.

Enoch Powell was, as Minister of Health, a member of the Cabinet in 1962

The first Secretary of State for Social Services, as the head of the department was now called, was Richard Crossman himself. However, the merger did little to alter the organization of the two ministries since their functions and method of working were so different. Their workload steadily increased with the reforms of the health service in 1974 and significant changes in social security legislation. By the 1980s this had necessitated not only a Secretary of State but also two ministers of equal status accountable to him; one specializing in health and one in social security, each with a permanent secretary. By 1988, it was decided that any advantages of this linkage in one department were minimal, so the DHSS was split once more and given its own Secretary of State for Health. The first incumbent was Kenneth Clarke who, as Minister for Health, had supervised the general management changes in 1984–5.

3.4.1 The organization of the Department of Health

Following the merger of the health and social security ministries in 1968 the government decided to commission a review of the internal working of the health side of the DHSS. This was undertaken by McKinsey, helped by a team of civil servants. Their eight-volume report was published and implemented, without alteration, in 1972. Five main divisions were created: Services Development, Regional Liaison, Finance, Personnel and Works. Later in 1976 there was further discussion about the relationship of the DHSS to the NHS itself.

Seven years on, Griffiths as part of his management enquiry[1] criticized the lack of strategic direction within the Department and proposed a ministerially led Supervisory Board to oversee policy, and a Management Board accountable to it. This separation of strategy and policy implementation was reiterated in 1989 when the Supervisory Board was reconstituted as the Policy Board and the Management Board became the NHS Management Executive (NHSME). Soon after the implementation of the 1990 Act it was thought necessary to review the organization of the NHS at top level again, because of the wish to simplify the chain of command from Secretary of State down the line into the NHS. In October 1993 *Managing the New NHS*[2] was published, outlining a reorganized central executive and announcing the replacement of separate regional authorities by outposts of the NHS Executive. The recommendations were made into legislation in the Health Authorities Act, 1995, and implemented the following April.

The other significant proposal was to merge health authorities with family health service authorities, which arguably should have been undertaken as part of the 1990 Act

3.4.2 The Policy Board

Following Griffiths' strictures in 1983 about the internal operation of the DoH, the Supervisory Board was originally constituted with 14 members: three ministers, two RHA chairmen, the permanent secretary, the chief executive, the chief medical officer, the chief nursing officer (both appointed in a personal capacity), a leading clinician from the NHS and four people from major industries. The Board was explicitly charged not to concern itself with managerial issues but rather to produce advice for the Secretary of State (who took the chair) on the overall strategic balance of policies for the NHS, and to assess the effectiveness of the implementation of these policies. The Board needed to make sure that policies were compatible and did not have unintended results.

The Policy Board replaced the Supervisory Board in 1989 and its membership changed after the dissolution of the RHAs in 1996. The membership now includes the Secretary of State in the chair, with his full ministerial team, together with the Permanent Secretary, the Chief Executive and the Chief Medical and Nursing officers. In addition the eight regional chairmen also attend. The DoH stated in 1997 that the purpose of the Policy Board is 'to consider current NHS managerial issues'[3]. The NHS's perception of its overall importance is somewhat sceptical.

3.4.3 The NHS Executive

Griffiths recommended a Management Board to be accountable to the Secretary of State for implementing government policy. Effectively it had to bridge the gap between the public servants in the NHS and the civil servants in the DoH itself. From the beginning it had a different culture, which challenged the traditional civil service way of doing things. The first chairman, Victor Paige, left suddenly for reasons that have never been fully explained. The second chairman, Sir Len Peach, on secondment from IBM, was not asked to serve a second term although he had been popular within the NHS. There was marked change after 1988, with the appointment of Duncan Nichol, who was a career health service manager and as general manager of the Liverpool region had held a non-executive seat on the Management Board.

The Management Board's title changed to the NHS Management Executive (and in 1993 to NHSE). It was chaired by the Chief Executive, Nichol, himself. The NHSME had a membership of eleven, including another career NHS manager as Deputy Chief Executive, with particular responsibility for implementing the 1990 Act. The other members were directors of planning and operations, personnel, finance, information, estates and research and development. To these were added a nursing and a medical director, who were the DoH's deputy medical and nursing officers. Finally there was a director with responsibility for integrating primary and secondary care.

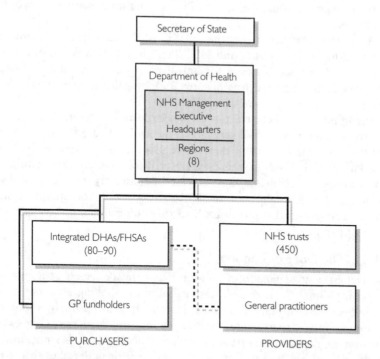

Figure 3.2

The NHS 1991

For the first time the chain of command continued from the Secretary of State down to the most junior member of the NHS staff. With this declared line of accountability came an emphasis on performance. It had been the case that the leading manager in a health authority would expect to hold his or her post for many years. This began to change after the introduction of general management and fixed-term contracts, which strengthened the ability of the government to command the NHS managers to do their bidding.

The implementation of the 1990 Act was a clear illustration of this. Despite the reservations that many people in the NHS had about the Act – most marked among clinical staff, less among managers – the changes were completely implemented within 5 years. The much closer relationship of the Chief Executive of the NHSE with the NHS had made this easier; a common culture facilitated the process.

The significance of the 1990 Act and the success with which it was implemented by the NHSE did much to enhance the NHSE's standing. The separation of duties between the DoH in London and the NHSE, necessitated by the decision toestablish the NHSE in Leeds in 1992, also helped, as did the setting up of eight regional offices in 1996 to replace the old regional health authorities.

Most organizations find their internal structures need to change from time to time, as their functions change. The Chief Executive, currently (1999) Sir Alan Langlands (another career NHS manager), is supported by six divisions: health care, research and development, human resources, planning, finance and performance, and nursing. In addition there are eight regional officers, facilitating the links between the centre and the NHS locally.

A notable absence from the NHSE is Estates, which became an agency along with Supplies and NHS Pensions. This was a result of the Thatcher government's desire to slim down government and, following the Next Steps initiative (see Section 3.6), transfer certain government functions to semi-autonomous agencies.

Shedding these discrete activities was expected to reduce significantly the overall numbers of civil servants in the DoH. There is little evidence that this happened (in 1998 there were 1741 civil servants in the DoH in London and 1762 in the NHSE) probably because the workload across the NHS as a whole has increased persistently. One consequence of increased accountability is more regulation, with the attendant staff input. Regional offices have been held to staffing limits of between 135 and 150 people.

3.4.4 The DoH in London

The Department of Health in London has its headquarters at Richmond House in Whitehall. It retains responsibility for looking after the needs of the Secretary of State and of Parliament. It is increasingly important to secure inter-departmental liaison to ensure that the policies of government departments are compatible. The DoH is also responsible for the overall policy direction of the NHS, and it undertakes this work through two internal groups: the public health group and the social care group. A third group within the DoH is concerned with departmental resources and services.

For the staff of the NHS, the work of the DoH in London may seem somewhat shadowy, but ensuring that government runs smoothly and that Parliament's needs are met are crucial statutory responsibilities.

3.4.5 Professional advice

Professional advice is a key input in the policy process and the DoH uses a wide range of medical and other professional experts to keep in touch with the latest views in the NHS and the latest developments in research and technology.

Previously there was a more formal advisory process. The National Health Service Act 1946 established the Central Health Services Council to advise the Minister on any matters relating to the NHS that were either referred to it or that it thought it should consider. Significant reports over the years included the 1954 Bradbeer report on administration[4], the 1959 Platt report on children in hospital[5] and the 1969 Bonham-Carter report on the functions of district general hospitals[6]. The Council was disbanded by the Health Service Act 1980. There are now standing advisory committees for nursing and midwifery, and for medicine. Members are appointed via nominations from professional organizations and similar bodies.

The Chief Medical Officer (CMO) has similar status to the Permanent Secretary at the DoH and the NHSE Chief Executive. He produces an annual report *On the Health of the Nation* which draws the government's attention to trends in sickness and hazards to health. While it is an independent report it may well be tempered by a perception as to what the government of the day will find acceptable. The CMO also has responsibilities to other departments including Social Security, the Home Office, and the Department for Education and Employment. In addition he advises the Ministry of Agriculture, Fisheries and Food and the Department for Environment, Transport and the Regions.

The Chief Nursing Officer heads nursing nationally; this is the single largest profession in the NHS. Most matters of patient care require the nursing perspective, because of nurses' responsibilities and experience in working with patients.

See Chapter 11 for more details on nursing

3.5 THE REGIONS

It is not possible to communicate directly with 100 health authorities, over 450 trusts and 481 primary care groups: they need an intermediate management level. A regional organization has existed in the NHS in various forms since 1948. Then, the NHS in England and Wales was divided into 14 regional hospital boards (RHBs) with, as the name implies, a responsibility for the largest component of the NHS, the hospitals. In 1959 one region (South West Metropolitan) was split into two, creating a new region known as Wessex, covering Hampshire, Dorset, most of Wiltshire and the Isle of Wight. After the 1974 reorganization, the RHBs became regional health authorities (RHAs) and their remit widened to include responsibility for overall planning of clinical services and employment of senior medical staff. They retained responsibility for planning and undertaking major capital works and allocating money to the area health authorities. The new RHAs were run by a chairman and members appointed by the Secretary of State.

During the 1980s the monitoring responsibilities of RHAs were further emphasized. The final change to RHAs prior to their abolition in 1996 occurred under the 1990 Act. As with the other authorities the Act altered, regions were reconstituted as boards of executive and non-executive directors. The chairman of the board and the five non-executive directors (who had to include a chairman of an FHSA and someone connected with the local medical school) were appointed by the Secretary of State. The role of the regions now emphasized more than ever the setting of performance criteria and the evaluation of results, as well as responsibility for ensuring that the major changes envisaged by the Act were being implemented satisfactorily.

However, regions did not seem to fit easily into the changes introduced by the 1990 Act. There was a danger they would make unnecessary work or interfere unduly in the freer market which was the hallmark of the 1990 changes. As a result, they were abolished by the

Figure 3.3

NHS Executive Regional Officer boundaries (from 1 April 1999). Source: NHSE

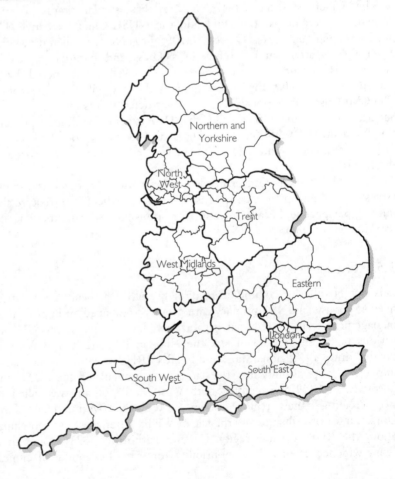

Health Authorities Act 1995 and replaced by eight regional offices of the NHSE. The only non-executive role remaining at regional level was the NHSE Chairman, who acts as a useful conduit between the chairmen of the health authorities and trusts and the Secretary of State and his or her ministers. The NHSE regional offices are staffed by a mixture of former NHS managers and career civil servants. They are all regarded as civil servants.

- Monitoring performance of health authorities.
- Monitoring performance of NHS trusts.
- Agreeing capital investment within financial limits.
- Managing research and development.
- Commissioning training and education.

Box 3.1

Main tasks of NHSE regional offices

A major factor in the organization of a regional level of management is constitutional devolution in the UK. The incoming 1997 Labour government took determined steps with the devolution of powers to Scotland, Wales and Northern Ireland, and many of the same issues arise within England itself, where economic and cultural differences between areas can be substantial. In the case of London, which had lacked a single planning authority since the Greater London Council's demise in 1985, the government introduced an elected mayor (1999). Working across several NHS regions' boundaries had made it harder to create suitably integrated health services for the capital's residents and workers. Accordingly it was decided in 1998 to reconfigure the four NHS regions covering London and South-east England into one regional office for the whole of London. It contains 16 health authorities, 69 NHS trusts and 4000 GPs. This altered the regional boundaries around London (Figure 3.3 and Table 3.1).

See Chapter 7

Despite these changes it is not yet clear how far regional government will be encouraged in England and what the consequences might be for the large public services such as health. On the one hand people within the NHS and many politicians would be against the absorption of the NHS into local government, but on the other hand such integration could make sense provided the regions were small enough to be sensitive to their population's needs and large enough to be economically viable. Integrating health services with local government services has been considered many times before, and is likely to continue to be discussed.

3.6 A CHANGE OF CULTURE

Before the 1980s there was a clear division between DoH civil servants, whose duty was to serve the government of the day, and the ministers of their department, and health service employees, whose focus of responsibility was to patients and local communities. Both were public servants but they saw their accountability in different ways. Following implementation

Table 3.1

NHS regions and health authorities, 1999

Region	Health authorities
Eastern (9)	Bedfordshire; Cambridge & Huntingdon; East Norfolk; East & North Hertfordshire; North Essex; North West Anglia; South Essex; Suffolk; West Hertfordshire
London (16)	Barking & Havering; Barnet; Brent & Harrow; Camden & Islington; Ealing, Hammersmith & Hounslow; East London & The City; Enfield & Haringey; Hillingdon; Kensington, Chelsea & Westminster; Redbridge & Waltham Forest; Bexley & Greenwich; Bromley; Croydon; Kingston & Richmond; Lambeth, Southwark & Lewisham; Merton, Sutton & Wandsworth
Northern & Yorkshire (13)	Bradford; Calderdale & Kirklees; County Durham; East Riding; Gateshead & South Tyneside; Leeds; Newcastle & North Tyneside; North Cumbria; North Yorkshire; Northumberland; Sunderland; Tees; Wakefield
North West (16)	Bury & Rochdale; East Lancashire; Liverpool; Manchester; Morecombe Bay; North Cheshire; North West Lancashire; St Helens & Knowsley; Salford & Trafford; Sefton; South Cheshire; South Lancashire; Stockport; West Pennine; Wigan & Bolton; Wirral
South East (15)	Berkshire; Brighton, Hove & East Sussex; Buckinghamshire; East Kent; East Surrey; Isle of Wight; Northamptonshire; North & Mid Hampshire; Oxfordshire; Portsmouth & South East Hampshire; Southampton & South West Hampshire; West Surrey; West Kent; West Sussex
South West (8)	Avon; Cornwall & the Isles of Scilly; Dorset; Gloucestershire; North and East Devon; Somerset; South and West Devon; Wiltshire
Trent (11)	Barnsley; Doncaster; Leicestershire; Lincolnshire; North Derbyshire; North Nottinghamshire; Nottingham; Rotherham; Sheffield; South Humber; South Derbyshire
West Midlands (13)	Birmingham; Coventry; Dudley; Hertfordshire; North Staffordshire; Sandwell; Shropshire; Solihull; South Staffordshire; Walsall; Warwickshire; Wolverhampton; Worcestershire

of the Griffiths proposals in the mid-1980s there has been a gradual culture change, which has affected both camps.

The reach of the civil service was curtailed by contracting out major functions under the Next Steps initiative in 1985. This enabled government to hold semi-autonomous agencies to account without having to manage them operationally. The officials who staffed these functions faced a major change of working conditions. Gone was the security they had automatically assumed: instead they were expected to focus much more clearly on the processes of government and on the outcomes of their particular field of operation. Into these new organizations came outsiders who had not gone through the traditional civil service training and promotion schemes, which had sustained a culture rooted in public school and Oxbridge values over many generations.

The DoH was no exception to these changes and the power of the NHSE provides a clear illustration of the new climate. At first it was conceived as the operational arm of the DoH, responsible for implementing government policy. It has developed in to the 'top office' of the NHS responsible in various ways for almost every aspect of the work.

The integration of NHS managers and civil servants within the NHSE has been beneficial. The NHSE Chief Executive himself is known personally to many of the other chief executives in the field and there is

NHS managers	Civil servants
Risk takers	Risk avoiders
NHS-centred	Minister-centred
Outcome-orientated	Process orientated
Manage their own careers	Careers are managed for them
Prefer verbal communications	Write everything down

Table 3.2

Cultural differences between NHS managers and civil servants

Source: based on Day, P. and Klein, R. (1997) *Steering but not rowing*. The Policy Press, Bristol

a greater sense of belonging to the same family. Yet within the DoH overall some tensions still cause problems (Table 3.2).

CONCLUSION

A perfect organization does not exist and there will continue to be adaptations in the role and functions of the DoH and the NHSE. *The new NHS* already referred to the need to review the role of regional offices. Whatever the arrangements the DoH and its executive will continue in their roles of devising policy, setting and monitoring performance standards, allocating resources which have been negotiated within public expenditure limits. They will also continue to ensure that the NHS as a whole remains accountable both to the government of the day and to the community at large.

1. DHSS (October 1983) *The NHS Management Inquiry* (Griffiths report). DHSS, London.
2. DoH (October 1993) *Managing the new NHS*. Department of Health, London.
3. DoH (1997) *The purpose, organisation, management and working of the National Health Service*. The Stationery Office, London.
4. Ministry of Health, Central Health Services Council (1954) *Report of the Committee on the Internal Administration of Hospitals* (Bradbeer report). HMSO, London.
5. Ministry of Health, Central Health Services Council (1959) *The Welfare of Children in Hospital* (Platt report). HMSO, London.
6. DHSS and Welsh Office, Central Health Services Council (1969) *The Functions of the District General Hospital* (Bonham-Carter report). HMSO, London.

4

HEALTH AUTHORITIES

Between 1948 and 1974 the three most important types of statutory health authorities were the hospital management committees, the local health authorities (part of local government) and the executive councils, which administered the contracts of family doctors, dentists, pharmacists and opticians. Many of these functions were united in 1974 under the new area health authorities (AHAs), and linked to the requirement to improve strategic planning and delivery of services. From 1982 to 1991 district health authorities replaced the AHAs. The administration of the four family practitioner services was transferred to independent committees in 1985, renamed family health services authorities (FHSAs). These were reunited with the health authorities again in 1996.

This chapter briefly recounts that history, particularly from the perspective of planning. Then there is an analysis of the reforms associated with the National Health Service and Community Care Act, 1990, which contained the statutory basis for the purchaser–provider split. Finally the chapter looks at the implications for health authorities of the Labour government's white paper *The new NHS*.

4.1 PLANNING SERVICES 1948–91

In the early days of the NHS, strategic planning was scarcely heard of: management's task was to control everyday matters and to solve immediate problems. Only in the 1960s was there a growing perception that the NHS needed to look ahead. The 1962 Hospital Plan was an important milestone because it set out an estimate of the required configuration of hospitals in the UK for the next 30 years. But it was limited because it made no attempt to assess future health needs or likely developments in medical sciences. What gradually became apparent was that a longer-term view would be required as well as the daily fire-fighting. The new health authorities were set up in 1974 on the assumption that it was necessary to divide the total population of over 50 million into smaller groups for the purpose of planning services. The intention was that operational matters should be left to local district management teams (DMTs) and that the area health authorities could then concentrate on forward planning and on creating the working relationships with other parts of the public services to facilitate the implementation of those plans.

This separation of functions did not work well. DMTs tended to clash with their AHAs on matters of strategic direction. The disputes could not to be resolved, so areas were abolished in 1982, giving districts responsibility for the planning, development and management of their health services in accordance with national and regional strategic guidelines, and for the provision of facilities. From April 1982 the new district management teams, with their own district health authorities, had to make integrated plans for the provision and development of primary care, general hospital services, maternity and child health services, for services for people with mental handicaps and mental illness and for elderly people, by then the largest single group requiring health care.

The functions of district health authorities were described in circular HC(81)6, May 1981[1]

From 1974 to 1991, although districts reflected the geographical distribution of the population, the main determinant was the number of patients who could be cared for at a single district general hospital (DGH), that is, a hospital capable of dealing with all the common types of specialist cases, including emergencies. The clinical catchment area of a DGH often reflected local patterns of health care dating back to the last century. To deploy expert staff effectively, it was assumed that all major specialties should have at least two consultants, so that a continuous service of high standard could be assured. The number of beds was generally set at 20–40 per consultant, which in turn could support a district population of a certain size, assuming 3.5 acute beds per 1000 resident population. Practical experience showed that a DGH would seldom be optimally effective with fewer than 400 beds. The traditional determinants of catchment areas had little to do with more modern administrative definitions of community boundaries. The majority of districts served a population of between 250,000 and 350,000. The district's resident population was the basis for its financial allocation from region.

The functions of the DGH were the subject of the Bonham-Carter report[2], published in 1969

This bottom-up manner of determining the size of a planning district was the very weakness that *Working for Patients*[3] had set out to eliminate. By defining the NHS around hospitals and secondary care, primary care received insufficient strategic attention.

See Chapter 8 for details of the financial allocation process

See Chapter 6 for full discussion of primary care

4.2   THE NEW PURCHASERS: DISTRICTS AFTER 1991

The National Health Service and Community Care Act 1990 changed the functions and constitution of districts. From 1 April 1991, the new health authorities, the 'purchasers', became responsible unequivocally for strategic planning, within which NHS trusts and GP services could provide services according to a clear framework. The first duty of a health authority therefore was to assess what the needs for health care were.

4.2.1   Needs assessment and priority-setting

No health authority can hope to have more than a subjective and selective view of needs without sound epidemiological research. Special pleading by doctors and other health professionals on the one hand, and public demand excited by sensationalizing media coverage on the other, tends to exaggerate and skew understanding of what is needed. The Director of Public Health, whose role was reformed by the Acheson report[4], became crucial to the health authority's planning effectiveness.

He or she is required to produce an independent annual report outlining the most important health priorities for the local health authority's population. From this the health authority produces its purchasing intentions, which also have to harmonize with government strategies and the views of others in the community – GPs, local politicians, social services and community representatives.

In practice, the impact and influence of the needs assessment process on the priorities and purchasing decisions of districts was limited[5], for a number of reasons. First, districts were under enormous time pressure to complete their annual contracting rounds. Many public health departments lagged behind because it takes time to carry out properly informed needs assessments. Second, health authorities had problems with the lack of epidemiological and medical information required to do proper needs assessments. The DoH sponsored research in this area to assist the process. Third, it was necessary to reconcile results of needs assessments with spending budgets to produce a set of actual purchasing priorities. Although a needs assessment may reveal a 'need' for medical care and treatment, it does not (and cannot) reveal anything about whether and how one particular need should be met in preference to another. Health authorities began to face the difficult task of agreeing priorities, or, as some would say, rationing.

4.2.2   Purchaser power

Immediately after April 1991, all interest concentrated on setting up the new NHS trusts (completed in 1996). The younger, more ambitious managers preferred to join these trusts rather than the health authorities. It was also feared that trusts, as providers, would continue to be able to dictate what services would be offered, irrespective of the health authorities' assessments. In the first year of the reforms, many providers did not pay much attention to their fundholder purchasers: providers merely assumed fundholders would fit in with their health authority's block contracts. By degrees, however, the power of the health authorities became more apparent, supported in due course by the government[6]. This power resided in the purchasers' potential to move contracts between providers. If a provider failed in some way it could be 'punished' by losing the contracts that would bring in funds to support that service. It has to be said that this power was often more notional than real, where alternative providers did not exist. In any case planning services by threat does not create a healthy environment; it encouraged purchasers and providers to behave badly on occasions. In a speech to the Royal College of Physicians[7], Brian Mawhinney, Minister for Health, said:

> *The purchaser–provider relationship cannot simply be restricted to formal negotiations... It has to be constant and ongoing. Both must realise that it is not a contest about who wins or loses in the contracting negotiation process. A dialogue needs to be developed in which purchasers and providers jointly work to achieve their objectives.*

The DoH sponsored the Clearing House of Health Outcomes at the University of Leeds and the production of *Effective Health Care Bulletins*, which drew together medical and economic effectiveness data on specific diseases. See details in Section 10.1

4.2.3 Contracting

Although the NHS had for many years contracted out a wide range of services, the 1990 Act greatly increased the significance and scope of this process. Contracts set out details of service, price, quality and timescale. Following the 1990 Act these contracts lacked the status of a legal document, and for this reason the original term 'service agreement' would have been preferable. Where purchaser and provider could not agree, the region acted as arbitrator. The process was not easy.

Block	A service e.g. accident and emergency services.
Cost and volume	A specific number of patient episodes at a specified price.
Cost per case	The cost of one specific patient or patient episode of care.

Box 4.1

Types of contract

Another problem arose with patients who could only be treated outside a health authority's normal contracts. These were known as 'extra contractual referrals' (ECRs). If the treatment was planned, permission could be sought beforehand and a price agreed, but often such cases were unforeseen emergencies and the health authority would have to pay the provider retrospectively. Although ECRs amounted to around only 3% of a health authority's contract activity, the administrative work they created was disproportionate. It took until 1998 to resolve the situation.

4.2.4 GP fundholding

The most significant change brought about by the 1990 Act was GP fundholding. This seems to have been a late addition to *Working for Patients*. In one important respect it never exactly fitted the framework of the purchaser–provider split, as GPs are both purchasers and providers. The idea of GP-based purchasing was originally proposed by Alan Maynard of York University, as a British version of the American health maintenance organization (HMO)[8], the American economist Alain Enthoven's preferred model. The scheme initially invited GP practices with over 11,000 patients to apply to hold and manage a budget designed to buy a limited range of in-patient, out-patient, day-case and diagnostic services for the patients on their lists. GP fundholders' budgets also covered pharmaceuticals prescribed by the practices and the costs of running the practice.

Although each of these budget elements was calculated separately, they were pooled, and savings in one could be used to spend more in another. The budget could not be used simply to increase GPs' own incomes nor to benefit the practice generally. Budgets were calculated to cover non-emergency care only and there was a limit of £5000 on the total amount a practice could spend on any one episode of care for a particular patient. Patients whose care cost more were paid for by the

See Chapter 14 on HMOs

health authority. Budgets for fundholders were deducted from the health authority's allocation.

Working for Patients argued that hospitals and their consultants needed a stronger (financial) incentive to look upon GPs as people whose confidence they must gain if patients were to be referred to them. The white paper also argued that GPs themselves needed stronger incentives to offer patients a choice of hospital.

In the first year of the scheme, 1991, around 7% of the population was covered, the qualifying list size having been reduced to 9000. Small practices with list sizes below that were allowed to combine with other practices in order to join the scheme. In the second year this doubled, and by the third year, list size having been reduced again to 7000, over 25% of the population was covered.

By 1997 around 60% of GPs had joined the scheme and a few had left it. The spread of fundholding was uneven, with a definite bias towards well-off suburban areas of the country. Other changes to the scheme were introduced as well as the reduction in qualifying list sizes. From April 1993 the range of services fundholders were allowed to buy was expanded to include community services, district nursing, health visiting and such other services as mental health counselling and services for people with learning disabilities. Terminal care, maternity and emergency treatment remained outside the scheme. The £5000 limit – designed to protect budgets from unexpectedly large claims – also remained.

Two controversial issues associated with fundholding were unresolved. The first concerned the basis for calculating fundholders' budgets. Health authority allocations (from which fundholders' budgets were deducted) were based on a formula reflecting each health authority's population, weighted for factors affecting the need for health care services (principally an age-standardized death rate as a proxy for need, known as the SMR, standardized mortality ratio). However, fundholder budgets were originally based on past referral patterns (often derived from data held by the GPs themselves). There was some evidence that many GPs had been successful in their negotiations with regions in securing larger budgets than their referral patterns suggested they needed. The political imperative to launch the scheme influenced regions not to argue too much over fundholders' budgets.

The second issue was fundholders' ability to secure better services for their patients than non-fundholders. Fundholders were not, in general, apologetic about this inequity. They argued that the whole point of fundholding was to improve services for patients, and that many of the improvements they secured – speedier laboratory test results, for example – became available to all the health authority's patients. The fact that many fundholders also secured shorter waiting times at hospital for their patients (queue jumping) tended to be less widely known.

Clearly, devolving budgets to GPs has empowered them to improve services for their patients. There is much evidence to show that fundholders caused hospital doctors to take a new interest in the demands of GPs and of their patients. The equity implications associated with fundholding were nevertheless important, although how important depends on a judgement about the value attached to the distribution of health care among local populations, compared with efficiency gains in total health care provision.

4.2.5 Variations on fundholding

As an alternative to single-practice fundholding, loose alliances of practices known as multifunds[9] were set up in some places, consisting of up to 70 GPs. These employed their own management staff (often recruited from health authorities). Multifunds claimed to possess extra purchasing leverage over providers. Multifunds also allowed GPs to act separately as individual practices if they wanted. The multifunds could make savings through economies of scale by reducing time spent on contracting.

One other development in fundholding – total fundholding – took place in 1994 in Bromsgrove, West Midlands. Four GP fundholder practices combined to take on the complete health care budget for the patients on their lists and responsibilities for national policies such as the waiting-times initiative and the *Patient's Charter*. Although this experiment was a local initiative, it received enthusiastic backing from the region and the DoH. A further idea, which in the event was not implemented, was 'practice-sensitive purchasing', where the health authority gave each practice an indicative budget within which they could purchase services. Unlike the other two variants, money would not change hands.

All these experiments helped to persuade the incoming 1997 Labour government that involving GPs in purchasing should be preserved even if, for political reasons, fundholding as a specific scheme had to be dropped (see Section 4.4).

4.3 JOINT COMMISSIONING

Health authorities were prompted to explore new models of purchasing, involving GPs more closely in purchasing decisions, partly by the fundholding initiative and partly by their dependence on GPs as general referral agents with the potential to upset the health authority's contracting arrangements. Health authorities had to involve FHSAs in this. As will be discussed in greater detail in Chapter 6, the two cultures surrounding these two bodies were substantially different. On the whole most health authorities had little time for FHSAs. The eventual amalgamation of health authorities and FHSAs in 1996 should have taken place in 1991. A great deal of time was wasted in that period, trying to make these two bodies work better together. GPs were mostly inclined to support health authorities, regarding the FHSAs merely as administrative functionaries in relation to the business aspects of their practices.

The relationships that health authorities had with the local authority social services departments were much more important. Throughout the lifetime of the NHS, the two had been trying to develop a satisfactory working partnership. Because of their different sources of funding – health from central government, social services via local government – it had always proved difficult to bring collaborative schemes to fruition.

But at least joint plans could be made, and around the country various joint commissioning initiatives began to flourish[10]. The advantages were obvious:

- seamless service for patient/client;
- avoidance of cost shunting between health and social services;
- better value for money;
- needs assessment free of bureaucratic barriers;
- promotion of innovative thinking.

Health authorities were not able to transfer actual funds to local authorities. Contrivances such as using cash-limited joint finance funds or laundering the money through third-party voluntary agencies were often set up to overcome the difficulty. These devices in turn tended to create more problems. The joint use of funds between the NHS and social services has yet to be satisfactorily achieved. Partnership schemes that build co-operation between agencies and across administrative boundaries may prove helpful in this.

It is a great help to joint commissioning if there are common boundaries. In 1974 not all health authorities were coterminous with local authorities. In 1982 even more of the new DHAs were not coterminous with their social services counties. Since 1996 unitary local authorities have replaced some of the two-tier counties and district authorities set up in 1974. The catchment areas of social services departments have become smaller and those of the health authorities larger. The consequences of this for planning and provision of services is one of the problems the Royal Commission on long-term care was asked to investigate in 1998. Conditions for effective joint commissioning are:

- common boundaries;
- established populations;
- similar levels of commitment;
- financial honesty;
- good relations with providers.

4.4   THE NEW NHS

Considerable effort was put into developing joint commissioning in the 1990s[11,12]. Would some of the lessons learned (see above) be applied in the future? *The new NHS*, published in December 1997, had an impact on this. After several years of experience in commissioning and purchasing, the two terms were no longer used synonymously. Commissioning was seen as the process of agreeing what was needed; purchasing

See Chapter 9 for the consequences of these difficulties for groups such as people with learning disabilities or mental illness

Under Section 28A of the NHS Act, 1977 health authorities can make payments for services but cannot transfer money in perpetuity

was the process of making service agreements (the preferred term to contracts). The new Secretary of State asked health authorities to produce Service and Financial frameworks (SFFs) and in particular to '...remove the worst aspects of the "Internal Market"'[13]. He set the commissioning agenda to:

- promote partnerships;
- ensure fairness;
- develop longer term collective agreements;
- improve financial management;
- involve the public;
- share information;
- reduce bureaucracy.

The new NHS pushed health authorities further away from direct purchasing, giving them the role of improving the health of their residents and ensuring effective outcomes. They were required to produce health improvement programmes covering a 3-year span and to do this with the full co-operation of GPs, other health care professionals, local authorities and the public.

The new arrangements required health authorities to ensure that national health strategies were implemented by providers, and that GPs' requirements for their patients were fulfilled by the NHS trust providers and indeed by GPs as providers. Their first major task was to set up the new primary care groups, which were Labour's way of capitalizing on the success of fundholding. At the most basic level PCGs are the agents of the health authority, in effect an advisory panel, but they can develop into free-standing bodies accountable to the health authority for the commissioning and provision of care for a specified population.

See Chapter 6 for a fuller discussion of primary care groups

Health authorities continue to be responsible for planning services in partnership with other agencies. Many of the impediments discussed above – financial, statutory, cultural and logistic – remain in the system. The market experiment introduced in 1991 effectively banned the word 'planning' in the particular NHS sense of ineffectual talking-shops. Fundholding altered the balance of power between general practice and hospitals. The waste inherent in a market system, and the new bureaucracy required to make it work, do not make it a more desirable alternative to the rational planning model that was attempted before. Whether the 'third way' produces more satisfactory results for patients remains to be seen. This will depend in some respects on the quality of management.

4.5   HEALTH AUTHORITY MEMBERSHIP

How do the corporate boards set up in 1991 differ from their predecessors? At health authority level, how do they function? Before 1974 members of hospital management committees represented a rather limited spectrum of local people and included hospital consultants from that vicinity, whose influence on the committee's decisions was considerable. In addition many hospitals had a house committee which was not statutory but was a legacy of pre-1948 days. Each HMC had several subcommittees to deal with finance, supplies, staffing, estates and so on. The committee process was elaborate and time-consuming for the chief officers. Executive councils were differently constituted with representative members from the four professions – medicine, dentistry, pharmacy and optical services. In local authorities there was a health committee but the independence of the medical officer of health was considerable.

In 1974 the new AHAs took over most of the local authority health functions but executive councils were reconstituted as family practitioner committees, answerable to the health authorities although they were effectively semi-autonomous. On the return of the Labour government in 1974, membership of health authorities was altered by the Secretary of State, Barbara Castle[14]. Substituting district health authorities (DHAs) for AHAs in 1982 gave each DHA one consultant, one nurse, one GP, one nominee from the region's medical school, one trade union member nominated from the local trades council, (usually) four local authority nominees and seven (occasionally more) generalist members. The total was not to exceed 19 members plus the chairman. The consultant and the GP were chosen by their peers. The nurse was not to be a member of staff of the same health DHA.

The membership of the DHA was a compromise: on the one hand democratic and on the other an example of patronage. Local authority members were nominees not representatives so did not have to maintain a political line, but this was not always understood by the members themselves. The professional members retained considerable influence which was used with an uneven sense of responsibility. Nevertheless, overall the membership usually demonstrated a cross-section of gender, age, geographical location, professional and political affiliations. As result it was unusual for DHAs and their predecessors, the AHAs, to be overtly political. Yet it was a large committee and, even with subcommittees, of which only the finance committee was statutory, decision-making was often difficult. The authority exercised by the chairman and, after 1984, the district general manager was important to progress.

The 1990 Act completely reconstituted health authorities and set up NHS trust boards, using the model of management boards for both. Health authorities are no longer a group of people appointed specifically as the local community's advocates. Instead there are five non-executive directors (sometimes called independent executives), up to five executive directors and a chairman. The criteria for selecting the new non-executives are more to do with business acumen and ability to make sense of complex issues than representing local interests. Despite this, many of the new non-executives still feel that they are there to do the best for their local communities; it is not always straightforward to satisfy government intentions and at the same time to honour the wishes of their local communities.

For the executive directors a similarly complex situation arises. As members of the corporate board they hold equal status, but in their separate functional roles they are subordinates of the chief executive. These tensions may explain why there have been difficulties with the manner in which some boards have conducted themselves. The new health authorities have had to ensure that there is a sensible separation of roles between the executive who were previously officers of the authority and the non-executives who should avoid interfering too closely in operational matters. The workload for non-executives can be heavy, and certainly exceeds the time indicated by the DoH during recruitment. The 1990 Act lays down that every health authority must have a chief executive and a director of finance and they must be on the board, as must be the director of public health. The remaining two places are a matter of choice and depend how the functional directorates are arranged. The tenure of executive directors is not prescribed, unlike their non-executive colleagues who can only serve two consecutive 4-year terms.

4.5.1   Corporate governance

The boards of health authorities and trusts are stewards of public money and advocates for the public interest. Following general concern about corporate governance voiced in the 1992 Cadbury report[15], and several procurement scandals in the NHS itself, the Secretary of State, Virginia Bottomley, issued a code of conduct in April 1994[16] covering accountability, probity and openness (Box 4.2).

Accountability	Everything done by those who work in the NHS must be able to stand the test of parliamentary scrutiny, public judgements on propriety and professional codes of conduct.
Probity	There should be an absolute standard of honesty in dealing with the assets of the NHS: integrity should be the hallmark of all personal conduct in decisions affecting patients, staff and suppliers' and in the use of information acquired in the course of NHS duties.
Openness	There should be sufficient transparency about NHS activities to promote confidence between the NHS authority or trust and its staff, patients and the public.

Box 4.2

Code of conduct for boards of authorities and trusts

This advice had to be reiterated as many health authorities found it difficult to make crucial decisions in public. They may have feared that media coverage would reduce complex issues to crude headlines, but as stewards of the common good, health authority members, both executive and non-executive, could not shirk this requirement.

CONCLUSION

A split between commissioning and providing continues for the time being. Health authorities are expected to make significant progress in improving the health of their populations. This was easier after the competitive market which they had had to manage was dropped. The government recognized that coherent planning across the public sector would achieve the desired results.

REFERENCES

1. DHSS (May 1981) *Membership of Health Authorities* Circular HC(81)6. HMSO, London.
2. DHSS and Welsh Office. Central Health Services Council (1969) *The Functions of the District General Hospital* (Bonham-Carter report). HMSO, London.
3. DoH (January 1989) *Working for Patients*. HMSO, London (Cm 555).
4. DoH (1988) *Public Health in England* (Acheson report). HMSO, London (Cm. 289).
5. Appleby, J. et al. (1994) Monitoring managed competition. In: *Evaluating the NHS Reforms* (ed. Robinson, R. & Le Grand, J.). Kings Fund, London.
6. Mawhinney, B. & Nichol, D. (1993) *Purchasing for Health: a framework for action*. NHS Executive, Leeds.
7. Ibid.
8. Maynard, A. (1985) Performance incentives in general practice. In: *Health, education and general practice* (ed. Teeling Smith, G.). Office of Health Economics, London.
9. Total Purchasing National Evaluation Team (1997) *Total Purchasing: a profile of national pilot projects*. Kings Fund, London.
10. DoH (1995) *Practical Guidance on Joint Commissioning for project leaders*, DoH, London.
11. Woolley, M. et al. (1995) *The Route to Total Care: joint commissioning of community care*. Institute of Health Service Management, London/Health Services Management Centre, Birmingham/Association of Directors of Social Services, London.
12. Shapiro, J. (1994) *Shared purchasing & collaborative commissioning within the NHS*. National Association of Health Authorities & Trusts, Birmingham/ Health Service Management Centre, Birmingham.
13. DoH (1997) NHS Executive letter to health authorities and trusts, 29th September.
14. DHSS (1974) *Democracy in the National Health Service: Membership of Health Authorities*. HMSO, London.
15. *Committee on the financial aspects of corporate governance* (December 1992) Report of the Committee (Cadbury report). Gee & Co., London.
16. DoH (1994) *Code of Conduct, Code of Accountability*, attached to Executive letter EL(94)40. DoH, London.

NHS TRUSTS

5

The new arrangements and organization of the purchasing part of the market introduced by the 1990 NHS and Community Care Act and the subsequent work of health authorities were covered in Chapter 4. This chapter examines the development of NHS trusts, which were also set up by the 1990 Act, as the other part of the market. The 1997 Labour government decided to retain the purchaser–provider split but removed the competitive elements that were central to the Conservative government's thinking. Before exploring these recent arrangements, trusts are discussed in their historical perspective.

5.1 HOSPITALS

As Chapter 2 showed, the history of hospital-based care can be traced back many centuries. But hospitals have become the most important element of health care in the twentieth century. This dominant position is now less certain as medical advances and economic pressures shift the principal setting of care back to the community.

The important role of most hospitals in the eighteenth and nineteenth centuries was not only, as Florence Nightingale put it, that: 'they should do the sick no harm'[1], but also to provide medical care and treatment to the poor. A large number of eighteenth-century hospitals were founded as charities for this purpose, while the rich employed their own private medical advisors. Many of these physicians and surgeons also provided their services to charitable hospitals for little or no remuneration. The origins of the duties and roles of today's hospital doctors are to be found to a great extent in the way hospitals organized themselves in the eighteenth century. For example St Thomas' Hospital in London specified in 1760 that its senior doctors should carry out a ward round twice a week, while assistant physicians had to attend wards three times a week, run out-patient clinics and generally fill in when their seniors were absent[2]. One hundred years later the total number of hospital beds in England and Wales exceeded 7500 and advances in scientific and medical knowledge were stimulating the creation of more hospitals.

Over time, hospitals (rather than the universities) also became centres for medical teaching and research, giving doctors a more central role in their management. The medical hierarchy increasingly reflected this rising status of hospital practice. Up to the First World War, existing hospitals expanded, cottage (community) hospitals flourished and doctors established new, specialist hospitals. By the Second World War, a greater variety of organizations and agencies was running, funding and maintaining a diversity of institutions. By 1939 there were about 3000 hospitals of all types in England and Wales in 1939, with about 500,000 beds. About 33% of hospitals were voluntary foundations, the rest were run by local authorities. A number of government and independent reports on the state of the country's health services (particularly the hospital sector) between 1900 and 1946 pointed to the need for improvements. The Nuffield Provincial Hospital Trust summary of the Hospital Survey[3] in 1946 revealed that many hospitals were over 50 years old, with quite a number being over a century old. The Nuffield report concluded that hospital services were failing to provide the public with the quality of care that was medically feasible.

Enormous cost pressures quickly became apparent following the establishment of the NHS in 1948. The 1955 Guillebaud report[4] could find little scope for efficiency improvements, pointing out that spending on the NHS had actually fallen as a share of national income, while the service had, at the same time, made enormous strides in the quality of provision of care. But the area again selected for criticism was the quality of hospital buildings. Guillebaud recommended trebling the capital allocation to the NHS – this was not accepted by the government.

It was not until the 1962 *Hospital Plan for England and Wales*[5] that a concerted attempt was made to improve the physical state of hospitals in the NHS. The Plan was ambitious, hoping to replace around a quarter of the then 2800 hospitals over a 13-year period. The Plan proposed a network of district general hospitals (DGHs) of around 600 to 800 beds serving populations of about 125,000. The services to be provided by DGHs would cover acute care as well as maternity care, with regional accident and emergency units being located in DGHs. In the event, the Plan was not fully implemented, although it did establish a new pattern

Figure 5.1

Numbers of psychiatric and non-psychiatric hospitals in England: 1980–1991

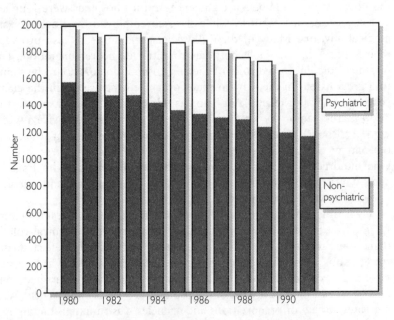

Source: adapted from NAHAT (1994) *NHS Handbook*, 9th edn. NAHAT, Birmingham

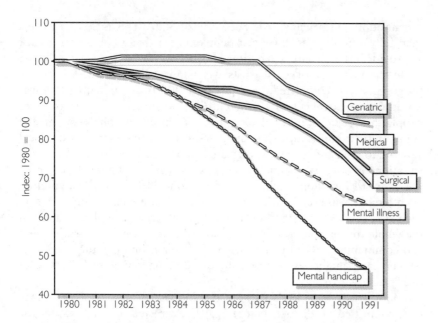

Figure 5.2

Beds in UK hospitals by type: changes in numbers between 1980 and 1991

Source: adapted from NAHAT (1994) *NHS Handbook*, 9th edn. NAHAT, Birmingham

of hospital services which largely survives. Figures 5.1 and 5.2 show how the numbers of hospitals and beds have changed in recent years. The NHS took over management of most private hospitals.

The introduction of the Griffiths general management approach in the mid-1980s created new management arrangements within districts. The reforms of the 1990 NHS and Community Care Act introduced further changes to NHS hospitals, disengaging them financially and managerially from their district health authorities. Before that Act, hospital and community units were clearly subordinate to the district, with unit general managers (UGMs) accountable to the district general manager (DGM). The Act altered that, making districts into purchasers and units into providers, in a more equal relationship. Abolishing directly managed units and giving trusts their own boards of management completed this separation.

5.2 SETTING UP NHS TRUSTS

The creation of independent trusts probably prompted more attention than any other element in the white paper *Working for Patients*. To opponents of the government, NHS trusts were clear evidence of privatization. Despite the Secretary of State's constant rejection of this claim, opponents of the trusts continued to stress this. In fact, trusts were, and are, semi-autonomous, non-governmental organizations which have taken on assets previously held by the state and for which they must make an annual repayment (although the timing can be varied at the discretion of the Department of Health). Managerially, all trusts are accountable to the Secretary of State; the NHS Executive's regional offices act as monitoring organizations on behalf of the Secretary of State. This makes trusts less than fully autonomous. But most people accept that a coherent network of providers is necessary in a national health system.

In the first year over 50 trusts were approved. Five years later the programme was completed, with just over 400 trusts. Initially there was no attempt to define trusts coherently; it was enough for a group of people based in a hospital or small group of hospitals or in the community to draw up a business submission and demonstrate local support to gain the Secretary of State's approval. This led to very wide variations in size, with some of the smallest having an annual budget of less than £15 million while the largest controlled over £150 million. Such a range was good if it reflected 'natural' differences in organization such as a small specialized hospital or a very large general hospital. On the whole the Secretary of State disallowed trusts that combined hospital and community services which, while they might improve the fluency of patient care, might also perpetuate the domination of secondary care over primary care.

Many trusts were set up by former individual units which together had comprised a district before 1991. Attracted by the scope for independence and the opportunity to get away from the supervision of the former boss (the district general manager) unit general managers worked with enthusiasm to establish their new organizations. It was notable that most trust chief executives came from units rather than DHAs. This gave the reforms the character of more youthful, innovative zeal. Certainly health authority chief executives (the title superseded that of DGM) felt initially that they were 'yesterday's men and women'. Although that gave impetus to the changes it scarcely improved relationships. Poor behaviour among managers was a noted characteristic of the early years and the competition required by the internal market exacerbated this. It was no coincidence that a theme of the new Labour government's approach after 1997 was to stress collaboration and co-operation instead of competition.

Most trusts comprised recognizable existing parts of local health care facilities. In a few cases the Secretary of State's disapproval of joint hospital and community trusts was overcome; this proved particularly important to a population with a relatively small general hospital. However, later on in the decade these hospitals again faced pressures (see below).

5.2.1   Ambulance trusts

Ambulance authorities were included in the trust reforms. The ambulance service before 1974 had been run by local health authorities. In 1974 the service was transferred to the new AHAs, with the exception of London, which had (and has) a service covering the capital as a whole, and the six metropolitan counties where the service was run by the appropriate RHA. During the 1970s and 1980s, the demand for ambulance transport rose with the growing numbers of patients, and also partly because of the worsening availability of rural public transport.

Year	Total	Emergency	Urgent	Planned
1987–88	20.29	1.85	1.12	17.30
1997–98	18.69	2.67	1.10	14.92

Table 5.1

Ambulance journeys (million)

Source: government statistics

There has been a continuing debate about whether the emergency and urgent ambulance service should be separated from other patient transport, particularly as it constitutes only 20% of the total number of journeys (Table 5.1). A DHSS working party[6] set up in 1980 under the chairmanship of Maurice Naylor, the outgoing administrator of the Trent Region, rejected the idea of a two-tiered service, with the possible exception of metropolitan areas, but suggested more could be done to create community transport for those in need, and that this might be a suitable project for collaboration with local authorities. The Naylor report was critical of the lack of good management and financial information, and recommended that the Steering Group on Health Services Information (the Körner Committee) should examine this. The Körner report on patient transport[7] was published in 1983, recommending a more comprehensive collection of operational statistics about patient transport.

The Naylor report had also emphasized the need for greater operational efficiency and, by 1990, the number of separate ambulance services in England had been reduced to 45, with nine in Wales and only one in Scotland. Training of ambulance personnel had gradually improved professional expertise, and this was a major issue in the long and damaging pay dispute in 1989. Months of industrial action failed to convince the government that ambulance staff deserved to be treated comparably with other emergency service personnel: firemen and the police. The separation of emergency work from the rest of the ambulance service is seen by some as the way to help improve the pay prospects of at least the more highly trained staff.

A National Audit Office report[8] in 1990 found that there was still room for increased efficiency through greater computerization, to achieve better work scheduling and revised response times. Traffic congestion is a major hazard and in London particularly there has been difficulty in reaching the standards for response time set by the *Patient's Charter*. This requires the ambulance to reach the patient within 14 minutes in urban areas and 19 minutes in rural areas, in 95% of emergency cases. These standards have been difficult to achieve even with the use of alternative transport such as helicopters and paramedical staff on motorcycles. Despite this an NHSE report[9] suggested in 1996 that the response time anywhere should ideally be only 8 minutes, this being the longest a patient suffering an acute emergency could be expected to survive unaided.

The 1990 NHS Act allowed ambulance services to apply for trust status and by 1994 all had become trusts. The number of ambulance trusts is gradually decreasing through mergers. Wales, Scotland and Northern Ireland each have a single trust. Some health authorities make service agreements with other services for non-urgent journeys, leaving the ambulance authorities to concentrate on emergencies.

5.3   THE FIRST FEW YEARS OF NHS TRUSTS

The liberal approach to the creation of trusts had some disadvantages. Having been set up with entrepreneurial intent, they were not always logically conceived to ensure smooth transition of care for patients. Then, because the new system required health authorities to make contracts with several trusts, this introduced an enormous increase in bureaucracy. In turn, each trust had to agree 30, 40 or more contracts with one or more health authorities. Also, the financial discipline exerted on NHS trusts is onerous. Although trusts have a new freedom to raise money for capital improvements, they cannot escape the disciplines of financial reality. Under the rules of self governance they have to make a 6% return on their assets and to operate within external financing limits (EFLs).

See Chapter 8 for details

Along with autonomy and freedom came responsibility and, in the context of the new health care market, uncertainty. If a trust did not secure sufficient contracts to maintain its organization, it could fail and have to be annexed to another trust. Thus health authorities could determine which trusts would have a future. In one case at least, a trust was destroyed by the reallocation of contracts. The government believed this sort of pressure introduced much needed discipline and enhanced efficiency through competition. But uncertainty could promote inefficiency.

What all this sacrificed was a systematic approach to planning health care facilities. This was particularly damaging for the hospital infrastructure. In particular, smaller general hospitals found themselves unable to provide a reasonable range of services at reasonable cost. For instance a maternity unit undertaking fewer than 3000 births a year would need only a small special care baby unit. Accordingly the cost per cot would be correspondingly greater because of the need to provide 24-hour specialized care even with a small workload. The options for smaller general hospitals were to scale down their scope and become a community hospital, restrict the services they provided, or accept becoming a satellite of a larger general hospital in another trust. After 1997 health authorities renewed the attempt to make better sense of the disposition of hospital facilities. A pattern of local, district, area and regional facilities (a model first outlined in the 1945 Hospital Survey) was considered a possible framework for planning. Meanwhile trust mergers continued at a steady rate.

To critics, trusts are no more than an ideological idea with limited potential for improving performance. Such critics would go further to say that setting up trusts was irrelevant to improving performance because greater financial efficiency and better patient communications have little to do with the organizational structure. Nevertheless, trusts have brought a new dynamism into health care management. At worst they may pay undue attention to public relations, at best they can renew the focus on responding to patients' needs effectively and efficiently.

5.4 TRUST MANAGEMENT

The boards managing each trust are similar to those running the health authorities. There are five non-executive directors appointed from nominations made by the community or from people responding to advertisements arranged by the NHSE's regional offices. They hold office for up to two consecutive terms of 4 years. In addition there is a chairman. On the executive side is the chief executive, the board's most senior appointment, and a finance director, a medical director and a head of nursing. These roles are specified; the one remaining board position can be held by a head of corporate affairs or human relations, or whoever is decided to make up a good executive team. Other people in the organization may carry the title 'director' without having board membership. The board is served by a secretary, who does not have executive powers. These boards are fundamentally different to their predecessors because the executive and non-executive members are corporately responsible for decisions. On occasions there may be a difficulty when the chief executive, who is the other executives' boss outside the board room, finds that his or her executive directors take a different view from him or her at the board room table. But overall the new boards have been an improvement, greatly facilitating effective decision-making.

> The majority of people of either gender in this role prefer to be called 'chairman'

Within the trust, the chief executive has freedom to organize the managerial structure according to his or her own judgement. Crucial to that organization is the involvement of doctors and nurses.

5.4.1 Doctors and nurses in management

The 1990 reforms brought about important changes for nurses and doctors in management. A risk from increasing doctors' involvement in management is to downgrade the professional status of the nurses and therapists with whom they collaborate. Many nurses feel that they have suffered a further diminution of their status following on that caused by the introduction of general management in 1984. In most trusts the nursing director does not manage the majority of the workforce directly. Each trust must have a nursing organization capable of deploying nurses effectively, in line with the standards laid down locally by purchasers and nationally by the United Kingdom Central Council for Nursing, Midwifery and Health Visiting (UKCC). Within the trust, therefore, nurses are usually grouped in relation to clinical practice so as to maximize their expertise in the various specialities: medicine, surgery, gynaecology, paediatrics and so on. Nurses also have a role in quality assurance, using their knowledge of patient care to raise standards.

> See Chapter 11 for further details of nursing

Attempts to involve doctors in decision-making were brought into new focus in 1990. Only spasmodic progress had been made in this before, through the 'Cogwheel' system of clinical committees[10] and through membership of management teams and of the health authorities themselves. Doctors were forced to behave more conscientiously as the key managers of health care resources. *Working for Patients* stressed that they must be properly accountable for the consequences of their clinical decisions. They could no longer treat patients with little regard for the financial and other resource consequences. Two measures were suggested: medical audit, to look more closely at outcomes, and the creation of clinical directors, to head multidisciplinary teams in each main speciality.

There may be over a dozen such clinical directorates within one large trust, accountable to the trust chief executive for the proper management of patient care within allocated resources[11]. This managerial responsibility also includes the requirement to achieve agreement to protocols for increasing the effectiveness of the clinical care of patients. Allocating control of this to doctors is unwelcome to those other professions who have long sought to free themselves from being seen as the servants of doctors and have demanded a more equal partnership. Some clinical directors insist upon complete control of the staff within their directorate. This may produce tight management, but it can also decrease the mobility of staff within a hospital. Mobility is desirable for training and developing experience, and also makes the best use of limited resources. Most clinical directors do not have the time to undertake the full managerial function. Because of their clinical workload they need support from a business manager. However, clinical directorates can provide small teams with incentives to bring about change and introduce new ideas, particularly if they release resources for the directorate itself to redeploy.

The clinical director could become even more crucial with the increasing emphasis on the need to demonstrate the effectiveness of clinical interventions. *The new NHS* called this 'clinical governance' and the issue was highlighted in 1998 when revelations were made about poor clinical outcomes for children undergoing heart surgery at the United Bristol Hospitals, and other examples of poor clinical practice in relation to cervical screening were exposed.

See Chapter 10 for details on evidence-based medicine and effectiveness

CONCLUSION

In some ways the creation of NHS trusts revived the smaller, more focused type of health service delivery organization that was a feature of the pre-NHS voluntary hospitals. Many people within trusts feel that they have more incentives to be successful than when they were working in units as part of the monolithic district health authority structure. Critics are still concerned that the separation of the provider from the purchaser leads not only to increased bureaucracy but also to less accountability as each party blames the other for shortcomings in the system. Trusts can claim that the health authority has given them inadequate resources. Health authorities can retort that trusts are inefficient. Whatever the grounds for the accusations, the split of functions is likely to continue. However, trusts are likely to change in one important area, primary care. The next chapter examines the implications for trusts of primary care groups.

REFERENCES

1. Nightingale, F. (1863) *Notes on Hospitals,* 3rd edn. Longman Green, London.
2. Pater, J. (1981) *The Making of the National Health Service.* Kings Fund, London.
3. Ministry of Health (1945 & 1946) *Hospital Survey.* HMSO, London.
4. Ministry of Health (1956) *Report of the Committee into the Cost of the National Health Service* (Guillebaud report). HMSO, London.
5. Ministry of Health (1962) *A Hospital Plan for England and Wales.* HMSO, London. (Cmnd 1604) HMSO.
6. DHSS (1980) *Report on Patients' Transport Services* (Naylor report). HMSO, London.
7. DHSS (January 1983) *Steering Group on Health Services Information, Working Group G, Interim report* (a Körner committee report). HMSO, London.
8. National Audit Office (July 1990) *National Health Service – Patient Transport Services.* HMSO, London (Cm 565).
9. DoH (1996) *Review of Ambulance performance standards.* NHS Executive, Leeds.
10. Ministry of Health/DHSS (1967, 1972, 1974) *Joint report on the Organisation of Medical Work in Hospitals* (Cogwheel reports). HMSO, London.
11. Dixon, M. et al. (1990) *Models of Clinical Management.* Institute of Health Services Management, London.

6

PRIMARY CARE

Primary care is the NHS's term for the services provided by doctors, nurses, dentists and other professional staff at the person's first point of contact with health care

Community care comprises the primary care services provided to the person in their own home

See also Section 9.4 for a detailed discussion of primary care services

Primary care is the term used in the NHS to describe the cluster of services provided by doctors, nurses, dentists and other professional staff at the patient's first point of contact with health care. Community care is a little different, because it usually means providing primary care services to the person in their own home.

General practice in the UK is a unique phenomenon. In most other countries doctors are specialists who have access to hospitals to investigate and treat their own patients. In the UK most GPs work from their own surgeries or health authority owned health centres. A very few GPs have direct admitting rights to their own beds in community hospitals, and some may also hold contracts with the local trust to enable them to work as clinical assistants to a hospital consultant.

This chapter explores the history of primary care and explains the innovations to the organization and delivery of primary care set out in *The new NHS* in 1998.

6.1   GENERAL PRACTICE UP TO 1996

Doctors worked in the community as generalists until the nineteenth century, when the development of hospitals encouraged increasing medical specialization. The professional status of general practice declined as that of hospital medicine rose, although the public's image of the GP as family friend and counsellor remained strong. Older people still recall, accurately or otherwise, the days when the family GP seemed to be constantly available and on call, locums (temporary deputies) were unheard of, a request for a home visit was not contested by the GP's receptionist but willingly accepted. GPs may claim a less rosy picture of the past, and draw attention to the gradual decline in their professional status. They believe their earning power fell after the establishment of the NHS. By the mid-1960s, GPs were so dissatisfied that only a major initiative by the Minister of Health, Kenneth Robinson, saved the NHS from GPs' mass resignations. Since then, GPs feel general practice has become the recognized worthwhile alternative to hospital medicine. In terms of earning power, the GP can now reach his or her optimum salary much sooner than a hospital doctor, who may require up to 15 years training to reach consultant status.

The organization of general practice was haphazard during the first part of the twentieth century. In 1920, the Dawson Report[1], still quoted with approval by today's advocates of state-controlled medical care, proposed that GPs should work from health centres, which would be centres offering the range of primary health care services. The 1945

Labour government upheld this idea. In some counties good progress was made in setting up health centres. Elsewhere, GPs showed reluctance to operate from state-owned premises, fearing that this would compromise their independence. This view is now so prevalent that health authorities have sold off many health centres to the GPs who practise in them. The idea of an integrated, multi-disciplinary primary health care team is as strong as ever, and is at the heart of the most recent reforms in general practice.

See also Section 6.3 on the organization of general practice

The 1946 NHS Act missed the opportunity to integrate the management of the three separate parts of the health services. It established administrative bodies called Executive Councils to administer the contracts of GPs, retail pharmaceutical services, opticians and general dental practitioners. GPs regarded this separation from the hospital service as necessary to their professional autonomy: they strenuously opposed being made employees of the NHS. The principle of being contracted with, rather than employed by, a health authority has remained crucial to most GPs. However, the 1997 NHS (Primary Care) Act allows GPs to be employed on a salaried basis by an NHS trust. This has already proved useful in those areas having difficulty in finding GPs to practise or for those GPs who do not want to enter the considerable business commitment as a principal in a general practice.

6.1.1 Family Practitioner Committees

Executive Councils were renamed Family Practitioner Committees (FPCs) in 1974. They were usually coterminous with Area Health Authorities and thus with the non-metropolitan county or metropolitan district council boundaries. There was less encouragement for joint working with the disbanding of the AHAs in 1982, because the FPCs' boundaries did not match those of the health district. In 1974, of the 90 FPCs in England, 60 related to one or two districts, 17 to three districts, seven to four districts and, in six instances, the FPCs had to cope with five or more districts. This uneven organizational basis emphasized the separate position of FPCs in relation to districts, and there were few efforts to overcome the administrative obstacles in order to work together to improve primary care.

The membership of FPCs included equal numbers of professional and lay people. Of the 15 lay members, one had to be a nurse, four each came from health and local authorities and the rest from the local community. A survey published in 1985 demonstrated that middle-class people, lawyers, accountants, company directors, teachers and personnel experts, predominated over those from other backgrounds. Drawing recruits from a relatively narrow social band is typical of the public services, and is a function of the relative ease with which those individuals can arrange time off work to undertake these duties. There were eight doctors, who could include GPs working in the FPC's own area, three dentists, two pharmacists and two opticians. The professional members of the FPCs probably shared many of the social values of the lay representatives, so the criticism that FPCs were dominated by professional interests was difficult to refute. The strict procedural rules for patients wanting to make complaints, for instance, illustrate this. FPCs were repeatedly and justifiably criticized for being insensitive to their consumers. This explains the considerable emphasis on consumers' needs found in the subsequent reforms.

Chapter 13 discusses the complaints procedure in more detail

6.1.2   Family Health Services Authorities

From 1974 to 1982 FPCs were an administrative division of the AHAs, although the retention of their own committee enabled them to preserve their belief in their much-guarded autonomy. Following the disbanding of the areas, they became accountable to a designated district. But from 1 April 1985 they became wholly independent under the Health and Social Security Act, 1984. The membership categories remained the same until their reconstitution as Family Health Services Authorities (FHSAs) in 1990.

Although the mix of lay and professional elements was retained, each new authority has only 11 members: five lay, one GP, one community nurse, one pharmacist, one dentist and the general manager, all appointed by the regional health authority (RHA) plus a chairman appointed by the Secretary of State. The new FHSAs were accountable to the RHA. Many of the new general managers of FHSAs were recruited from the mainstream of health services management. The status of these appointments ended some years of frustration among FPC chief officers who had been allocated lower rank than their counterparts in the rest of the NHS. With additional responsibilities created by the 1990 reforms and the GP contract, the FHSA chief executives could attain similar salaries to colleagues in trusts and health authorities.

The opportunity to amalgamate FHSAs with health authorities was not taken as part of the 1991 reforms, probably because it was felt that progress towards a more primary care led NHS would be jeopardized if FHSAs were absorbed into the health authorities. Even if this reason was valid, five years were spent in the two authorities finding it difficult to work together not only, in many cases, because of different boundaries, but also because of different cultures. In order to overcome the difficulties in many parts of the country non-statutory health commissions were set up to ease the path to the statutory merger of HAs and FHSAs in April 1996.

All four professions with HA-administered contracts have local representative committees at which they can record their views on the way the HA is operating. When new contracts for GPs and dentists were being negotiated and implemented, this 'safety valve' was particularly valuable. One of the more important aspects of the FHSAs' work was to monitor GPs' drug expenditure. They aimed to reduce drug expenditure in general practice by means of indicative drug budgets. The regions set an overall drug budget based on assumptions about average prescribing costs. HAs allocate this money in turn to each practice, not each GP. The aim is to place drug expenditure under pressure without going so far as to fix a cash limit for it. Patients are not denied the drugs they need (although some dissident GPs said that any control on their prescribing practice would, in fact, do that). The information regarding prescribing and its cost by each practice and each GP or according to each main type of drug, provided by the Prescription Pricing Authority's prescription analysis and cost tabulation (PACT), is clearly important to the FHSAs and the GPs themselves in this context.

See also Section 6.5

6.1.3   Standards in general practice

At the start of the NHS the GP was more likely to work alone, and even in a group practice could not rely on the support of other clinical staff in the same way as now. District nurses, midwives and health visitors were employed by the local authority and in some counties many of the surgeries were publicly owned. Advances in team-working were most likely to take place in health centres. There was a growing awareness that collaboration between professionals needed to improve if patients' needs were to be met effectively. From the 1980s onwards the importance of primary care attracted greater attention, resulting in the National Health Service and Community Care Act 1990 and the 1990 new GP contract.

The rising status of general medical practice has been steady since its low point in the early 1960s. Numbers of GPs increased, working hours were reduced, training was improved and practice conditions modernized. Despite this, some public dissatisfactions remained, and the 1990 contract was a response to these. There was a strong feeling that GPs were less interested in their patients' needs than they had been and were increasingly reluctant to visit patients at home. It was a common experience for a patient on one GP's list always to be seen by other doctors, not even partners, but locums or deputies who were sometimes hospital junior doctors earning extra money and certainly not trained in general practice. From the NHS itself, DHAs were critical of GPs' ability to run effective primary care health programmes; they cited the public's use of districts' own child health departments and family planning clinics as evidence that general practice was failing to be the single reliable provider of comprehensive family care that the GPs claimed.

See Section 6.1.7

6.1.4   Primary Health Care

In response to these criticisms the government issued a green paper entitled *Primary Health Care – An Agenda for Discussion*[2] in April 1986. It concentrated on increasing the overall standard of general practice through introducing a payments system that would give incentives to GPs who were more available to their patients, who increased their range of preventive work and who reached certain target outcomes in such services as vaccination and cervical screening. The government said that patients should have more information about GP services and should be allowed to choose or change their GP more easily. It suggested consumer opinion could be voiced through patient participation groups. The FPCs themselves were asked to spend more time clarifying their role with districts and to be more cost conscious. These broad recommendations formed the basis of the subsequent reforms, which influenced the new GP contract.

The green paper also covered other aspects of primary health care. It said that dental services could be improved to encourage continuity of care and preventive work. Allowing doctors and dentists to advertise their work was seen as a way of improving public awareness. The removal of the subsidy on spectacle frames was more overtly political, guaranteed to offend those wanting the NHS to be free of all direct charges to patients.

6.1.5   *Promoting Better Health*

Eighteen months later the government issued a more definitive white paper, *Promoting Better Health*[3]. The proposals built on the responses to the green paper and deliberately focused on three main objectives: improving general standards of primary care, giving the consumers greater choice and increasing the emphasis on health promotion. The government said these objectives could be met by enhancing consumer power, by stimulating some degree of competition between GPs and by offering new financial incentives to GPs to co-operate with these policies.

Doctors' pay is discussed more fully in Chapter 11

The white paper was greeted with enthusiasm because it appeared to place primary care in a more favoured position, demoting acute care from the limelight it had long monopolized. Nevertheless, the GPs' negotiators soon decided that the white paper was a threat to their autonomy. The relationship between the doctors' union, the British Medical Association (BMA), and the government, always uneasy, deteriorated rapidly. Despite this, the government pressed on with both *Working for Patients* and the new GP contract, which incorporated many of the ideas in *Promoting Better Health*. These simultaneous initiatives became confused in the minds of the public and GPs. A poll at the time found that only one in five members of the public had a clear idea about the point or the substance of these reforms. The white paper's proposed reforms to FPCs were implemented in the 1990 Act.

6.1.6   Prescription charges

Prescribed medicines were free when the NHS commenced in 1948. Charges were first introduced in 1951, abolished in 1965 and then reintroduced in 1968, since when they have been increased virtually annually. Charges have raised increasing amounts of money, despite a rising proportion of exemptions. Around 85% of people receiving prescriptions do not pay. Charges covered only 6.5% of the gross cost of all drugs and prescribing fees (1997). There is little unambiguous evidence that charging for prescriptions has had much impact on demand by those in need. It has been suggested that a more effective way to reduce 'frivolous' prescribing would be to charge the doctor for writing a prescription rather than the patient for presenting it. *The new NHS* places additional controls on drug expenditure by including drug costs in a cash limited budget. It remains to be seen whether prescribing costs will reduce as a result.

6.1.7 The 1990 GP contract

The GP contract's origins go back to the 1987 white paper *Promoting Better Health*, which emphasized the importance of health promotion and consumer choice. It requires general practices to publish a directory of services so that patients can be better informed. GPs must give personal details, age, gender, special interests and deputizing arrangements. There is compulsory retirement of GPs at 70. The contract itself specifies minimum standards of medical care. GPs have to be available for patients 26 hours per week, over 5 days, and to accept 24-hour responsibility for their patients. This means that deputies are only acting as agents of the GP, who, therefore, has to be confident of the ability of the deputy to look after his or her patients to a proper standard. To facilitate their continuous responsibility, GPs are expected to live reasonably near their patients, even if the practice is in an inner city area. Each practice is expected to publish an annual report describing the facilities, premises and staffing levels, together with detailed statistics on prescribing practice and hospital referral rates.

The new contract changed other things. GPs were allowed to behave competitively. Advertising, for long ruled unethical, was permitted. Larger practices (or combinations of smaller practices) were encouraged to become fundholders. GPs, like hospital doctors, were obliged to undertake a systematic review of their clinical practice and its effect on patients. Each HA was required to set up a Medical Audit Advisory Group with a membership not exceeding a dozen people, of whom one should be a consultant and one a public health doctor. A report had to be made to the HA annually.

Promoting Better Health contained proposals for managing family practitioner services more effectively, in line with the overhaul of the rest of the NHS following the introduction of general management in 1985. FPCs, and then the FHSAs, were expected to set objectives, allocate resources and monitor and evaluate results in the same way as DHAs did for the rest of the NHS. This required a much more explicit relationship with general practitioners, and it needed such measures as indicative prescribing budgets, proper GP practice budgets, medical audit and more sophisticated information systems to monitor GPs' prescribing habits and hospital referral rates. This level of scrutiny was greeted with nervousness by many GPs, particularly when it was linked to the specific conditions to be written into their new contract which the BMA worked out with the Department of Health from March 1988 to May 1989. When the BMA negotiators had agreed the terms, the general membership rejected the agreement. Despite this, the then Secretary of State, Kenneth Clarke, fixed the final contract with some minor amendments for implementation from 1 April 1990[4]. As with many of these battles with the doctors in the past, the experience of the new arrangements was not as bad as they predicted, although there was undoubtedly a considerable increase in the administration GPs had to undertake.

In retrospect it is clear that the open-ended cost of GP services could not be allowed to continue, especially as DHAs had always had to work within a cash limit, whatever the needs of patients. Scrutiny of prescribing practice and referral patterns had shown variations which revealed unnecessary and wasteful clinical interventions. Medical audit was long overdue. Under their new contract, GPs lost some of their independence and became more closely scrutinized by their FHSAs. Examination of their efficiency and effectiveness was now more in the public eye than before. For instance, vaccination rates were published by some FHSAs, showing which practices were not meeting the targets.

6.2   PRIMARY CARE GROUPS

In 1997 the incoming Labour government wanted to capitalize on the perceived success of fundholding while at the same time, rejecting the philosophy that underpinned it. Primary care groups (PCGs) were the chosen way forward, as set out in the white paper *The new NHS*. It proposed that all GPs should join a PCG, which would normally cover a population of around 100,000 (in fact the range is 50,000–250,000). GPs can stay within their own practices. These new groups were influenced by the experiments in locality commissioning and total fundholding.

PCGs are clinically led by GPs and community nurses, and are responsible for contributing to the health improvement plans drawn up by health authorities. To achieve this PCGs have to demonstrate that they have taken into account the views of their patients, other agencies (in particular the social services departments) and local people more generally. The main functions of PGCs are to:

- improve health and addressing health inequalities;
- develop primary care and community services;
- commission a range of hospital services.

As with the fundholding scheme, PCGs combine commissioning, purchasing and providing functions, and in this respect have acquired those responsibilities of the DHAs which were removed by the 1990 Act. A major innovation is that the funding of general practice is totally cash limited, the money being allocated by the regional offices via health authorities. These new financial arrangements have caused anxiety to those GPs who worry about how to maintain their premises and staffing levels if resourcing patient treatments has to take precedence. PGC membership is as follows:

- 4–7 GPs;
- 1–2 practice/community nurses;
- 1 social services nominee;

Joint commissioning and total fundholding are discussed in Chapter 4

- 1 lay member;
- 1 HA non-executive director;
- PGC Chief Executive (*ex officio*).

Realizing that the introduction of PCGs would take time and that there was not a common starting point, the government proposed a four-stage approach. At level one PCGs just provide the HA with professional advice, much as local medical and GP committees already do. At level two PCGs take devolved responsibility for managing budgets for health care in their areas, acting as the HA's agent. More ambitious PCGs can go to level three and become free-standing trusts accountable to the HA for commissioning health care and being held accountable for the results. At level four, to which few yet aspire, a new primary care NHS trust takes on full responsibility for commissioning health care in line with their given population according to service agreements made with the HA and with secondary and specialist care trusts. Level four trusts will presumably make the present community care trusts redundant. They will be managed, like other trusts, by a board with eleven members: a chairman, five non-executives and five executives. The budget for such a trust is likely to be around £60 million per annum[5].

The timetable for introducing the PCGs was tight, all GPs in England and Wales to be so organized by April 1999. HAs were given the responsibility for achieving this[6], but by this date many PCGs still did not have chief executives in post. Scotland and Northern Ireland were given a year's grace.

6.3 THE ORGANIZATION OF GENERAL PRACTICE

The organization of general practice has changed considerably. GPs have increasingly grouped together not only to share the burden of constantly being on call, but also to benefit from the advantages of a larger organization which can command attached staff, better administrative support and more modern premises. In 1967 there were 4406 GPs in single-handed practice, but by 1996 this had declined to 2863 (30% of total practices in England and Wales). Practices with six or more doctors had grown from 736 in 1967 to 1180 (11%) in 1996. Over the same period the total number of GPs in England and Wales has increased from 20,260 to 28,900, reducing the number of patients on each doctor's list; the average is now under 2000. In theory, the smaller the list, the more time the doctor can spend with each patient. But this has to be set against the amount of time the GP spends at work; the average length of the GP's working week has shortened substantially, much as it has for other workers in the last 20 years. Indeed, the GPs' contract now stipulates that they only have to be available for patients for 26 hours a week, and this can include travelling time. The aim is to continue to reduce list size but this depends on sufficient trainees entering general practice.

A typical GP surgery comprises a group of doctors, most of them fully trained and therefore holding principal status, with one or two

part-timers or trainees. Attached to this practice will be other professional workers, particularly nurses. A district nurse, trained for work in
the community, may be employed by the practice or she/he may be
employed by an NHS trust. Similarly, the health visitor, a specialist
nurse who works with children and mothers and the elderly, will also
usually be employed by a trust. Both these categories of staff have
become increasingly independent, expecting to work *with* rather than *for*
GP colleagues. The practice nurse is more directly under the direction of
the GPs, providing a nursing service at the surgery. This nurse usually
works from a treatment room, undertaking relatively minor procedures
such as dressings or taking specimens, and testing those that do not need
sophisticated analysis at the hospital pathology laboratory.

Some practices do a great deal more to provide comprehensive
primary care for their local community. This was one of the main
reasons for establishing health centres, but large practices within their
own premises have also developed the concept of primary care, offering
a base for a range of associated services including social work,
chiropody, occupational therapy and physiotherapy. Space is sometimes
made available to provide counselling support for patients with problems
related to bereavement and to those who are suffering from the effects
of alcohol or drug misuse.

The larger the practice and the more services it offers, the more it
needs to be well organized. All but the smallest practices now have a
practice manager. This was encouraged by the former FPCs, partly
because it allowed GPs to concentrate on clinical rather than administrative matters, and partly because it ensured that the administration was
conducted in a manner that allowed FPCs more easily to collect the data
they needed to calculate GPs' pay. Some practice managers are people
on their second careers, often originally from the armed services and
industry, who encountered much less difficulty entering GP practices
than they did the more closed management hierarchies of hospitals and
health authorities.

Each practice generates a great deal of administrative work. Some
GPs still use the small old-fashioned envelope patient record which was
standardized over 70 years ago. They claim that a modern A4-size
record would be difficult to handle when doing home visits. But the
disadvantages of the small record are obvious if the patient has had more
than a minimum number of investigations and the envelope is stuffed
full of correspondence and laboratory or X-ray reports, all necessary to
ensure a properly documented patient history. At the other extreme,
experiments are proceeding using a single credit card format compu-
terized record, which can hold all significant data for the average patient.
The patients can then carry the card themselves. In 1984, the DHSS
encouraged the introduction of computers into general practice, essentially to force doctors to maintain accurate lists of current patients.

Fundholding encouraged major advances in the use of computers in
general practice as designated funds were allocated for this purpose in
the fundholding agreement. This has improved information accuracy.

For instance, in the past, most lists were inflated by counting patients who had died or moved but whose names still appeared. This came to light when the lists were used for calling up women for routine cervical smears. Computerization of practice records has advanced considerably over recent years and has provided important information about GPs' prescribing and referral patterns.

Most practices have an appointment system managed by the receptionists. There has been considerable criticism of the extent to which these staff make an initial assessment of the patient's request and decide whether and when the patient should come to the surgery or receive a home visit from the GP. The effectiveness of their gate-keeping, or the reluctance of GPs, as well as the greater mobility of patients anyway, is responsible for the number of home visits steadily declining. The range of facilities at the surgery allows patients to be treated more effectively there than at home. A GP can obviously see far more patients if they come to the surgery than if he or she has to make many home visits.

General practice acts as an important filter, caring for those patients who do not need the more expensive resources of the hospital. There are over 325 million GP consultations a year in the UK (1996), many of which would probably be dealt with by a specialist in other countries and would result in many more referrals to hospital. Moreover, the GP who is aware of the patient's home and family context is better able to understand their overall health needs, instead of treating the symptoms in isolation. In highly specialist-dominated health care systems, the patient is at greater risk of being misdiagnosed. Though the cost of family health services is large – £8.9 billion in 1996 in England – a more specialized service, with greater hospital emphasis, would be even more costly. This is one of the reasons other countries spend more on their health services: they provide more services and beds in hospitals.

Three other professional services contribute to primary health care: general dentistry, dispensing pharmacy and optical services.

6.4 GENERAL DENTISTRY

Dentists opt to work as general practitioners, or in the community, especially with children and the disabled, or as hospital specialists in oral surgery or orthodontic remedial work. Before the NHS was founded, the general state of dental health was poor, and, although dental benefits were available under the National Health Insurance Scheme to 13 million of the working population, only about 6 million made claims. The division of the profession into three main areas of activity encouraged standards to improve. For instance, the 1944 Education Act provided for free dental inspection for all children in state schools, and enlarged the scope of the School Medical Service which, though it had been founded as long ago as 1907, had failed to diagnose and treat sufficient numbers of children needing attention. General dental practitioners have always worked from their own premises. They had no continuing

See Chapter 12 for more details

responsibility for their patients in between courses of treatment until this became a feature of the 1990 contract.

Increasingly dental practitioners have chosen to withdraw from the NHS and successive governments have not found ways to reverse this. Charges for NHS dental treatment were first introduced in 1951. These charges have become substantial; perhaps there is not more protest at the erosion of the NHS dental service because people have come to assume they will always have to pay. Dental health has improved over the years but this is still influenced by social deprivation. It is a matter of continuing concern that charges for dental services deter some of those in the most need from seeking essential dental treatment.

The Dental Practice Board is responsible for assessing the fee for approved treatments and it pays general dental practitioners direct. Information is provided to health authorities on a regular basis. Community trusts also provide a community dental service. This is particularly useful in screening school age children, and in treating people who do not or cannot have dental treatment elsewhere, such as those in financial need or those with disability.

6.5   PHARMACEUTICAL SERVICES

Pharmacists work in a variety of settings, retail, hospital or in commercial manufacturing and research. In 1996 there were around 12,300 dispensing chemist and appliance contractors in the UK, 8% more than a decade earlier. The HAs are responsible for regulating only the retail pharmacists, who dispense and sell medicines to the public over the counter. Some GPs, particularly in rural areas, also supply the drugs they prescribe. In theory, GPs can prescribe only drugs or appliances (but not foods or toiletries) that will, in their opinion, benefit the health of their patients. The pharmacist, more popularly called the chemist, supplies the prescribed drugs on receipt of the doctor's prescription. The pharmacist purchases drugs from a wholesaler or direct from the manufacturer and is reimbursed by the health authority. At the end of each month the pharmacist sends the prescription forms to the Prescription Pricing Authority (PPA) and it calculates the costs of the ingredients according to the Drug Tariff – a list of approved drugs issued by the Department of Health. For each prescription, the PPA also calculates the on-cost allowance for the pharmacist's overhead expenses and profits, the dispensing fee and an allowance for containers. The health authority is then notified of the amount to be paid to the pharmacist for the month's prescriptions. In addition, information on prescribing and dispensing is sent to the GPs themselves and to the health authorities and the NHSE.

The PPA came into existence in 1974 to continue the work that had been carried out since 1948 by the Joint Pricing Committee and, before that, by the Joint Pricing Bureaux under the National Insurance Scheme. Its main offices for England are in Newcastle-upon-Tyne, and there are eight other offices in the north of England, each handling the prescriptions from a particular part of the country. In 1996 they handled 485 million prescriptions which represented 9.9 prescription items per head of the population compared to 7.3 items 10 years earlier. The other parts of the UK have their own local offices. The PPA has eight members, one nominated by HAs, one doctor, one pharmacist and the rest of the non-executives are provided by the DoH in the same manner as for other health authorities and trusts.

The information prepared by the PPA has become more detailed and timely with the introduction of PACT (prescribing analysis and cost tabulation). This new scheme was started in 1988; it not only made monthly reports to the FHSAs but also provided the GPs themselves with quarterly and (from 1991) monthly information to help them monitor their own prescribing. These arrangements continue. PACT provides three types of report: it shows an individual practice's costs against the average in the HA and the national average, and gives the number of items prescribed and the average costs of items in that practice; it allocates the prescribing data into six major therapeutic groups; it can give a breakdown of costs for each GP (this is only done on request, and may be asked for if a practice or a GP is showing persistently higher than average prescribing costs).

A pharmacist wishing to set up as a retail chemist must register his or her premises in accordance with the Medicines Act, 1968, and this is done through the mediation of the Pharmaceutical Society of Great Britain. HAs attempt to regulate the distribution of pharmacies and offer inducements where there is no easily accessible service. Chemists have to apply to the HA for a contract, which specifies terms and conditions. These include opening hours and participation in the out-of-hours rota. As businesses, chemists' shops can succeed only if they also sell toiletries and other goods as well as proprietary non-prescribed drugs and preparations.

Two agencies have been set up to regulate medicines and appliances. The Medicines Control Agency (MCA) is responsible for ensuring that medicines are safe, effective and up to standard. They work closely with the European Medicines Evaluation Agency. The MCA also has an inspectorate to help the process of regulation. It is financed by fees charged to the pharmaceutical industry. The Medical Devices Agency was set up by the DoH in 1994 and is responsible for regulating and advising on any product used with patients other than drugs. The equipment ranges from walking frames to syringes. It too works closely with European colleagues.

6.6 OPTICAL SERVICES

The fourth professional service regulated by HAs is provided by opticians. At the time of the introduction of the NHS, there were several groups testing sight and supplying spectacles, and they possessed various professional qualifications. In order to regularize the situation, it was decided to place all sight-testing in the hospital sector under specialist

Ophthalmic medical practitioners	Medically qualified doctor and eye specialists who test sight and prescribe lenses
Ophthalmic opticians or optometrists	Test sight and prescribe and dispense lenses and other optical appliances
Dispensing opticians	Supply frames, dispense lenses and fit contact lenses

Table 6.1

The different services undertaken by opticians

doctors (called ophthalmologists) while the dispensing of spectacles was allowed outside hospitals. But, because hospitals seemed unlikely to be able to cope, Supplementary Service was set up by the 1946 National Health Service Act. It allowed ophthalmic opticians to continue testing sight as well as dispensing spectacles. They were placed under NHS contracts, administered through the Executive Councils (later FPCs and then FHSAs). The National Health Service Act, 1968, removed the word 'supplementary' and the name changed to General Ophthalmic Service (GOS).

Most of the work is done in the community, although orthoptists, who treat squints and other malfunctions of the eye, mainly work in eye departments in hospitals. An optician does not have a list of patients like a general medical practitioner but is paid a separate fee for each item of service under the terms of his or her contract with the HA. Since the National Health Service Act, 1984, the NHS no longer pays for spectacle frames and only partially subsidizes the cost of lenses, although children and other high risk groups are exempt from charges. The increase in charges was a prelude to the introduction of charges for sight-testing and dental treatment brought in under the Health and Medicines Act in 1988. In 1999 the Secretary of State announced the removal of charges for eye testing. Some 65% of the population over 16 wear glasses and this percentage increases with age.

All four professions with HA contracts have local representative committees at which they can record their views on the way the HA is operating. When new contracts for GPs and dentists were being negotiated and implemented, this 'safety valve' was particularly valuable.

CONCLUSION

The 1990s have brought significant changes to the provision and organization of a range of NHS primary care services. Many of these resulted from the 1990 Act and the 1990 GP and dentists' contracts. The changes stem from a fundamental belief that primary care needed to be enhanced, not only because it was likely to offer more cost effective ways of providing care than hospital services (a hope yet to be reliably proven) but also because it was felt that the patient's interests would be better served. The guiding principle has to be that the patient should be seen at the right time in the right place for the right reason by the right person.

1. Ministry of Health, Consultative Council on Medical and Allied Services (1920) *Interim Report on the Future of Medical and Allied Services* (Dawson report). HMSO, London.
2. DHSS (1986) *Primary Health Care: An Agenda for Discussion.* HMSO, London (Cmnd 9771).
3. DHSS (1987) *Promoting Better Health: the Government's Programme for Improving Primary Health Care.* HMSO, London (Cm 249).
4. DoH (1989) *General Practice in the National Health Service: The 1990 Contract.* HMSO, London.
5. DoH (February 1999) *Letter from Minister of State to Chairman and Chief Executives, Primary Care Trusts.* DoH, London.
6. DoH (August 1998) *Health Circular HSC 1998/139.* NHS Executive, Leeds.

7

THE NHS IN SCOTLAND, WALES AND NORTHERN IRELAND

The general principles governing the NHS are the same throughout the United Kingdom, and the reforms following *Working for Patients* have applied throughout the UK (although a year later in Scotland and Northern Ireland). It is incorrect to assume that the way health services are organized in Wales, Scotland and Northern Ireland is exactly the same as in England. Despite the differences, the general principles of the NHS can be expected to remain in place[1] even in the context of devolution of certain powers to the individual nations (see also Chapter 15). This chapter outlines the more important variations between the four countries.

Spending per head of population varies considerably between the countries of the UK (see Table 7.1), with Scotland spending 25% more than England. This is partly accounted for by higher staffing levels.

Table 7.1

UK spending per capita on health services, 1996/97, £

England	656
Wales	769
Northern Ireland	811
Scotland	822

Source: Office of Health Economics (1997) *Compendium of Health Statistics*. OHE, London

7.1 SCOTLAND

Scotland became part of the UK 300 years ago but retains many of its own traditions, which are reflected in its constitutional and legal framework. Geographically it comprises two distinct areas: the sparsely populated Highlands and Islands and the densely populated and industrial Lowlands. It has a population of 5.1 million. The policies devised by Parliament in London have to be tailored to fit Scotland's circumstances. The legislation that originally created the Scottish Health Service was the National Health Service (Scotland) Act, 1947, passed on 21 May 1947, which established an organization based on the same tripartite principle as in England and Wales. The hospital and specialist services were administered by five Regional Hospital Boards: Northern, North-Eastern, Eastern, South-Eastern and Western with 65 Boards of Management, analogous to the Hospital Management Committees in England and Wales. Family practitioner services were administered by 25 executive councils, and there were 55 local authorities employing a medical officer of health with a responsibility for community and environmental health services. The Secretary of State for Scotland was responsible for the whole of the NHS in Scotland, with support from civil servants in the Scottish Home and Health Department.

In December 1968, after extensive consultations with a wide range of interested parties both within and outside the NHS, the Secretary of State for Scotland published a green paper containing suggestions for reorganizing the service, *Administrative Reorganisation of the Scottish Health Services*[2]. It met with a wide measure of support which enabled the Secretary of State to proceed with the publication of a white paper in July 1971, entitled *Reorganisation of the Scottish Health Services*[3] containing the government's proposals for legislation to institute the reorganization.

The National Health Service (Scotland) Bill was introduced in Parliament in January 1972 and received Royal Assent on 9 August 1972. The appointed day for the first reorganization of the NHS in Scotland was 1 April 1974, as it was in England and Wales, so there remained just under 2 years for preparations to implement the new arrangements. Under the National Health Service (Scotland) Act, 1972, amended and consolidated by the National Health Service (Scotland) Act, 1978, health boards were created for each area of Scotland, to act as the single authority for administering the three branches of the former tripartite structure.

Two new bodies, without precedents in the pre-1974 structure, were created at national level – the Scottish Health Service Planning Council and the Common Services Agency. These were not precisely mirrored in England, their functions being shared by the DHSS and the regional health authorities, although in Wales there was also a Common Services Agency. Provision was made for professional advice to be available both nationally and locally through consultative committees, but no specific bodies were established to pursue collaboration between the local and health authorities in the same way as the Joint Consultative Committees in England and Wales. There were bodies for representing the views of users of the health services in each district, called Local Health Councils, similar to the Community Health Councils across the border. The 1972 Act also established an ombudsman for Scotland, who started work on 1 October 1973.

The reorganization of local government created new local authorities in Scotland which came into being on 15 May 1975, that is, just over a year after the NHS reorganization and the new local authorities in England and Wales. There were nine regional authorities, divided into 56 districts, and three Island Councils created by the Local Government (Scotland) Act, 1973, whose boundaries closely followed the health board boundaries, the main difference being that the Strathclyde region contained four health boards. This Act also provided for local community councils within the districts – a feature absent from the arrangements in England and Wales.

7.1.1 Health boards

The 15 health boards in Scotland were directly responsible to the

Secretary of State for Scotland for the planning and provision of integrated health services in their areas; 10 of the 15 areas were divided into districts. Each board had a chairman appointed by the Secretary of State and between 14 and 22 members appointed from nominations put forward by regional and district local government authorities, trade unions, the health care professions, the universities and a variety of other organizations. The health boards were mainly concerned with major policy matters and the broad allocation of resources, delegating authority to manage the service to four senior officers of the board – the chief administrative medical officer, the chief area nursing officer, the treasurer and the secretary – who together constituted the area executive group. These officers had both individual professional and team responsibilities in a similar way to the area team of officers of the AHAs in England and Wales. The chief administrative dental officer and the chief administrative pharmaceutical officer joined the Area Executive Group for the discussion of items relevant to their responsibilities. The team had to present advice and information to the board to help it to establish policy and priorities. Health boards were encouraged to set up area programme planning committees, similar to the English district health care planning teams. Most boards created such committees for the main groups of users.

Chapters 4 and 9 discuss joint planning

In each of the districts, the district administrator, district nursing officer, district medical officer and district finance officer constituted the district executive group and they were jointly accountable (unlike in England) to the area executive group for a number of functions as well as being officers of the health board. Another important difference was that in Scotland there were no GP or hospital consultant representatives directly involved in the district management arrangements. This was because there had always been a much stronger tradition of medical administrators in Scotland. Medical superintendents had not dwindled as they had done south of the border. Clinicians were used to working with administrative medical colleagues.

7.1.2 Further reorganization

In *The structure and management of the NHS in Scotland*, issued in 1979[4], health boards were asked to review their management arrangements. Originally reforms were intended to coincide with the English *Patients First* changes in 1982 but in fact they took longer. Eventually the Secretary of State for Scotland announced on 10 November 1983 that all districts would be scrapped, leaving health boards (Figure 7.1) with subordinate units only. The size of units varied considerably.

The National Health Service and Community Care Act 1990 applied to the whole of the UK; Part II refers particularly to Scotland. There was little enthusiasm for creating trusts. As Scotland had never had separate authorities for family health services, the structure was that much simpler. There were now 15 health boards and, by April 1998, 47 NHS trusts.

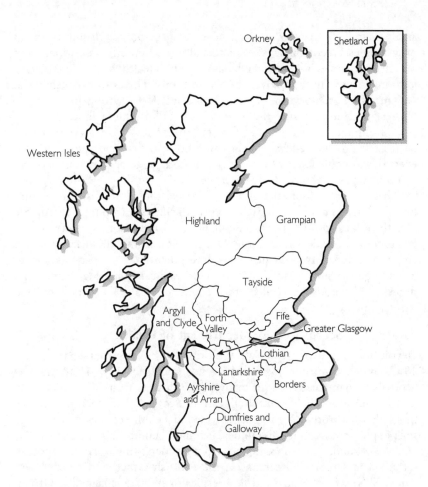

Figure 7.1

Scottish health boards

7.1.3 *Designed to care*

In December 1997, the Scottish Office and the Department of Health issued a white paper *Designed to care*[5]. The structure proposed is less confusing than the English model, with clearer lines of accountability. At the head of the NHS is the Management Executive responsible for policy, national strategy and performance management. The 15 health boards are accountable to it. Health boards are responsible for agreeing 5-year health improvement programmes with trusts in partnership with other agencies. Primary care trusts (PCTs) replace the idea of primary care groups in England, with the unequivocal responsibility for planning and provision of all primary care including mental health services. These trusts incorporate groups of GP practices called local health care co-operatives (based on natural geographical communities and membership is voluntary), as well as hospitals. The PCTs supersede fundholders, who had not been as numerous as in England, covering only 50% of the population. To balance the primary care trusts, acute secondary care trusts continue but are subject to major review. This has already been undertaken in Glasgow, where a number of acute providers have been amalgamated. Both types of trust have to agree on health improvement programmes, recognizing the importance of smooth transition from primary to secondary care and back again. Health boards establish a joint investment fund to cover these transitions. This is to make sure that patients do not block the system by being in the wrong place at the wrong time and to ensure the optimum use of hospital facilities.

The number of trusts is likely to fall to about 28. They are managed by trust teams headed by a chairman who also sits *ex officio* as a non-executive on the local health board. This arrangement assists a closer relationship between the board and the trust.

There are also four special health boards: the all-Scottish Ambulance Board (a trust until 31 March 1999), the State Hospitals Board, the Health Education Board for Scotland and the Scottish Council for Postgraduate Medical Education. As elsewhere in the UK there is strong emphasis on quality both in terms of responsiveness to patients and to provide guidance to practitioners on new medical technologies including drugs. This body is called the Scottish Health Technology and Assessment Centre.

7.1.4 The Scottish Office Department of Health

Devolution of power from Westminster was an important part of the 1997 Labour government's policy agenda and from April 1999 the new Scottish Parliament took over many health powers from Westminster. In health education and financial allocation, Scotland had been in advance of England. In other areas, such as mental health services and services for people with learning disabilities, it trailed behind England.

In Scotland, the supreme government department is the Scottish Office. The senior civil servant in the Scottish Office is the Permanent Under-Secretary of State, and he presides over the Management Group. There is a Chief Executive for the NHS in Scotland. Until the Scottish Parliament became operational the Secretary of State for Scotland was, through the form of the NHS legislation, personally accountable to the Westminster Parliament for the Scottish health services in the same way as the Secretary of State for Health and the Secretary of State for Wales were for the NHS in England and Wales.

The 1972 Act created the Scottish Health Service Planning Council, which was partly derived from the former Scottish Health Services Council, an influential body that advised the Secretary of State on shaping policy for health service provision in Scotland. Like the Central Health Services Council, its counterpart in England and Wales, it was made up of representatives from all the major professional groups with an interest in the health services. The Planning Council was created to ensure that effective strategies could be devised and implemented to improve Scottish health service provision on an integrated basis, in a context of limited resources, with the fullest participation from the health authorities.

The Council prepared a report, published in December 1980 with the Secretary of State's blessing, entitled *Priorities for Health Care in*

Before 1974 some chairmen of hospital management committees were *ex officio* members of their regional hospital boards

Scotland[6] and guidance issued in December 1997 required corporate contracts to be drawn up with objectives for the key issues:

- mental health;
- cancer;
- coronary heart disease/stroke;
- tackling inequalities;
- improving health;
- developing primary care;
- promoting care in the community;
- reshaping hospital services;
- organizational development following *Designed to care*.

Three other tasks were added to this: reducing waiting times, managing peak emergencies and developing health improvement programmes together with other agencies.

Health indicators show a worse picture in Scotland than elsewhere in the UK, particularly for heart disease, where the incidence is among the worst in the world. Life expectancy at birth is 72.6 for men and 78.0 for women (1998 figures), shorter than in England and Wales. Health education is therefore another priority area and the Health Education Board for Scotland provides information and training for members of the public, for specific groups and for health professionals. It aims to collaborate with other agencies to increase effectiveness. Deprivation is a major cause of bad health and considerable attempts have been made in Scotland to ensure that resources are fairly and appropriately allocated. In the 1970s a formula similar to the English RAWP (Resources Allocation Working Party) was introduced, known as SHARE (Scottish Health Authorities Revenue Equalisation). *Designed to care* signalled that this would be reviewed with the intention of distributing funds in a way '...which is more objective and needs based with the aim of promoting equitable access to health care...' (para 102).

Outside the Scottish DoH is the Common Services Agency (CSA), whose management committee is responsible for providing a wide range of services to government departments and also includes representatives from health boards. In 1985 the Scottish Health Management Efficiency Group (SCOTMEG) was set up to undertake a national programme of efficiency reviews and to monitor the progress of the CSA and the health boards in implementing their recommendations. They first studied the hotel services and then began to scrutinize clinical work. They were helped by the Clinical Resource Use Group, set up in 1987 to disseminate good practice. SCOTMEG was disbanded in the early 1990s.

Scotland has maintained a strong tradition of medical education to very high standards for centuries, and its four university medical schools (Edinburgh, Glasgow, Aberdeen and Dundee) produce one-fifth of all medical graduates in the UK. The professional bodies have grown up independently of those in England and have achieved notable prominence. The Royal College of Physicians (Edinburgh), the Royal College of

Surgeons (Edinburgh) and the Royal College of Physicians and Surgeons (Glasgow) are the oldest; the Scottish Radiological Society, the Scottish Committee for Community Medicine and Scottish members of the Royal Colleges of General Practitioners, Obstetricians and Gynaecologists and Pathologists, and the Faculties of Anaesthetists and of Community Medicine, join the older Royal Colleges in being recognized professional groups contributing advice through the National Medical Consultative Committee to the Planning Council. The BMA is also active in Scotland, and its Scottish General Medical Services Committee contributes to the National Medical Consultative Committee. The Scottish Junior Staffs Group Council is a body similar to the Hospital Junior Staffs Group Council for England and Wales, while hospital consultants are represented through the Scottish Committee for Hospital Medical Services.

Collaboration between medical schools and the health boards is formalized through four University Liaison Committees. In the field of postgraduate medicine, the Scottish Council for Postgraduate Medical Education was founded in May 1970 to promote the ongoing development of medical practitioners through extensive programmes of teaching and refresher courses.

There are a number of other professional and administrative bodies with important duties in the Scottish National Health Service, which are similar in constitution and objectives to those bodies described in the chapters relating to England and Wales. They include the Scottish Health Advisory Service, the Scottish Medical Practices Committee, the Scottish Tribunal, the Mental Welfare Commission and the Scottish National Board for Nurses, Midwives and Health Visitors. In addition, the mental health services are governed by the provisions of the Mental Health (Scotland) Act, 1984, and social work, probation and after-care services are covered by the Social Work (Scotland) Act, 1968 as amended.

Although the Scottish Parliament at first has little scope to increase public expenditure, it can influence the distribution of resources. The NHS in Scotland faces the challenge of tackling poor health with even more rigour.

7.2   WALES

The laws of Wales are generally much closer to England's than are those of Scotland or Northern Ireland. Arrangements for health care are similarly more alike. Although the provisions of the National Health Service and Community Care Act 1990 applied to Wales, organizationally there are differences. Up to 1974 there were a Welsh Hospital Board, local hospital management committees, and executive councils as in England. Thereafter, the Welsh Office was allocated both departmental and regional responsibilities with a Health and Social Services Department under the overall responsibility of the Secretary of State for Wales. This minister was responsible to Parliament in Westminster for many functions in addition to health, which has led to periodic criticisms. The Royal Commission noted in 1979 that the Welsh Office was too remote from health authorities and their problems[7]. However, a regional authority as well as the area tier would have been excessive, given that the whole population of Wales is only 2.85 million (similar to that of a small region in England). Communication within Wales has always been difficult, with the industrialized south separated from the rest of the country by mountains and relatively poor road and rail services.

In 1982, the eight area health authorities became nine district health authorities. Except in Glamorgan, the most populated county, the new DHAs were coterminous with county councils. FPCs (later FHSAs) and community health councils continued. A reduction to five health authorities occurred in 1996 (see Figure 7.2).

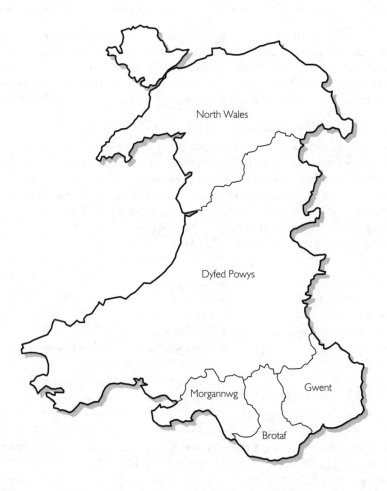

Figure 7.2

Welsh health authorities

Within the Welsh Office the managerial approach is similar to the English DoH although the principality does not necessarily formulate and implement policy in parallel with England. Sometimes it is ahead (health promotion policies), sometimes it lags behind (implementation of the internal market).

There is a Health Policy Board, and an Executive Committee comprising the Director of the NHS in Wales, the civil servants who head divisions (see Box 7.1), and some of the professional heads of departments, including the chief medical and nursing officers, that meet fortnightly.

Box 7.1

Health divisions in Wales, 1998

- Health Financial Management.
- Primary and Community Health.
- Health Strategy.
- Health Services and Management.
- Public Health.

In addition there is a separate Health Professional Group which provides advice on medical, nursing, scientific, pharmaceutical and environmental issues. The Welsh Planning Forum, set up in 1988, was disbanded by the 1990 Act, which reduced some of the need for central planning. Nevertheless there is a strong central influence on health policies.

7.2.1   Health promotion

Professional review panels have been developing practical advice on how to achieve these aims, and the Welsh Health Promotion Authority (later retitled Health Promotion Wales), headed by a chairman, executive director and a small management board, initiated what has been described as the largest campaign of its kind in Europe, Heartbeat Wales. It started in 1985, aiming to reduce heart disease. In 1997, 15 health gain targets were issued (Box 7.2).

Box 7.2

Health Gain Targets, Wales, 1997

- Lung cancer
- Breast cancer
- Cervical cancer
- Heart disease
- Stroke
- Accidents
- Suicides
- Low birth weight

- Back pain
- Arthritis
- Mental health
- Smoking
- Consumption of fruit and vegetables
- Consumption of alcohol
- Dental caries (tooth decay)

Source: Welsh Office (DGM(97)50)

These were endorsed in May 1998 with the publication of *Better Health, Better Wales*[8], which recognized explicitly that health in Wales showed marked variations due to the wide range of social, economic, and environmental factors. This is an important acknowledgement of the link between deprivation and health, which the previous Conservative government had always been unwilling to accept directly, from the reluctant publication of the Black report in 1980 onwards.

With the increased devolution of authority to Wales there is greater emphasis on Wales-only initiatives such as an all-Wales corporate plan for health aimed at tackling aspects of poor health particular to Wales. Life expectancy is about one year less than in England, and the death rates from heart disease are 18% higher; cancer death rates are 10% higher.

As part of the 1997 Labour government's devolution proposals, Wales gained its own National Assembly in 1999 with the responsibility, among other things, for running the NHS in Wales. Accordingly, Health Promotion Wales and the Welsh Health Common Services Authority, which in the past has had separate divisions for capital and the estate, supplies, manpower, information technology, prescription pricing and for artificial limbs and appliances, will be included together with the Welsh National Board for Nursing, Midwifery and Health Visiting in the Assembly's remit.

7.2.2 *Putting Patients First*

In January 1998 the Secretary of State for Wales presented the white paper *Putting Patients First*[9] to Parliament. It specified that the Welsh Assembly's Health Department is headed by a Director who, as Accounting Officer, continues to be accountable to the UK Parliament and its Public Accounts Committee. The five health authorities are accountable to the Assembly and continue to be required to undertake needs assessment and strategic planning, confirmed in health improvement programmes in co-operation with other public services. This is made more difficult by the rearrangement of Welsh local government into 22 unitary authorities during 1996–8.

The HA and trust chairmen and non-executive board members are appointed by the Assembly and the executive board members are appointed by the authorities and trusts themselves, with the Assembly's health officials acting as assessors.

The trusts are being reconfigured to give more coherence, reducing from 30 to 15 (including an all-Wales ambulance trust). They employ 54,000 staff. Unlike Scotland and England many of the trusts are responsible for the whole range of care. HAs are advised by local health groups (LHGs), but retain strategic responsibility for the health of the population through health improvement plans. LHGs are expected to work within those plans. Setting up LHGs was an attempt to bring commissioning to the grass roots. To encourage this they are given budgets, at first on an indicative basis. Part of this allocation is ring-fenced to provide resources for a new primary care development fund which allows GP practices to maintain or develop services. Previously the rules attached to GP funding restricted this to fundholders.

There is a tension between trust reconfiguration and the creation of LHGs. Unlike England and Scotland, LHGs are not well-placed to provide community services along the lines of the English primary care groups. Coterminosity with local authorities is regarded as important. In Cardiff's case the LHG catchment area will be very large, so to overcome this primary care partnerships can be set up covering smaller populations. The bureaucracy that these new arrangements create could be as cumbersome as those they replace.

In due course budgets will be subdivided on a practice basis. Transition from local health group to fully fledged trust is not permitted for the time-being, pending further experience. Local health groups are coterminous with local government unitary authorities to facilitate joint working, and to overcome the difficulty of local government authorities' catchment areas becoming smaller while health authorities' have expanded.

In 1991, the Welsh Office published a document aimed at making the best use of staff (Box 7.3).

Box 7.3

PEOPLE: Personnel principles for NHS Wales

Performance Management
Equality of Opportunity
Open Communication
Planning Ahead
Local Emphasis
Efficiency and Effectiveness

In 1993 'Towards 2000' aimed at safeguarding non-medical education. An NHS Wales staff college was established in 1995, responsible for management development throughout the NHS in Wales, including executive and non-executive staff and clinicians involved in management.

7.3   NORTHERN IRELAND

During the the first 50 years of the NHS, Northern Ireland has experienced periods of considerable legislative autonomy, with its own Parliament at Stormont. Political instability caused this to be replaced by direct rule from Westminster for over 20 years, until a new, directly elected Assembly was introduced in 1998. The organization of health services in Northern Ireland is least like that in England; the most significant element is full integration of social services and health services management since 1973.

The health services and local government arrangements were changed when direct rule was introduced. County councils were abolished and replaced with 26 district councils with greatly reduced powers. Housing was taken over by a new statutory authority, the Northern Ireland Housing Executive; education became the responsibility of five education and library boards. The health and welfare services were integrated under four health and social service boards[10] (Figure 7.3), accountable to the Secretary of State for Northern Ireland, who appoints their chairmen and vice-chairmen. The boards had a mixed membership: 30% were district council nominees, 30% were from the health professions and the remainder from voluntary and other lay bodies. The

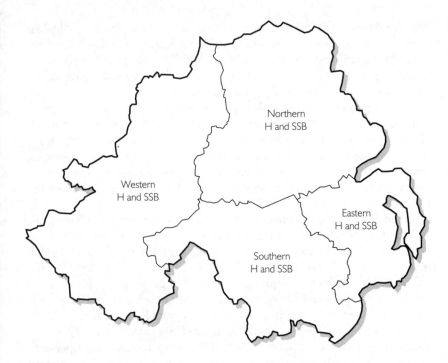

Figure 7.3

Northern Ireland health and social
services boards

Northern
H and SSB

Western
H and SSB

Eastern
H and SSB

Southern
H and SSB

boards were geographical, as their names suggest: Eastern, Northern,
Western and Southern were responsible for 17 districts, covering populations from 43,000 in Omagh to 250,000 in North and West Belfast and
coterminous with one or more district councils.

When the new service started in 1973 the two partners – health and
social services – perceived themselves to be unequal. Social services staff
felt vulnerable, anxious that their funds might be eroded by health
service demands. But these initial anxieties disappeared and many would
now maintain that the Northern Ireland model is much better for
patients and clients particularly given the intractable problems of joint
working in the rest of the UK. It is also much easier to provide seamless
care for such groups as those with mental illnesses and elderly people.
However, the need for stronger commitment to preparing joint plans
with housing and education persists.

The introduction of general management was more gradual in
Northern Ireland. It was established at board level in 1985 and in
Districts in 1990. Similarly the introduction of the internal market and
fundholding was slower than in the rest of the UK, the Royal Victoria
Hospital in Belfast becoming the first trust in 1993. By 1996 there were
20 trusts covering the province, serving the population of 1.65 million.
Fifty-three per cent of the population was covered by fundholding. In
common with the rest of the UK trusts and fundholding were superseded
in 1999.

The Northern Ireland Department of Health and Social Service is
also responsible for social security, the Child Support Agency and the

Benefits Agency. The overall expenditure is nearly £5 billion, which is over 50% of the total public expenditure in Northern Ireland. Expenditure on health and social services in 1997/8 was £1164 million on hospital, community and personal social services, £380 million on family health services and £60 million on centralized services such as research and development, training and health promotion. A number of agencies provide specialist services: health promotion, blood transfusion, medical physics, nursing and postgraduate medical education. Within the DHSS there are three core groups, responsible for the allocation of resources, for policy and an executive. These in turn are advised by five professional groups who have a specific remit for advising the Northern Ireland Office overall.

As in Scotland and Wales, certain functions are not provided by the boards directly, but are undertaken centrally through a Central Services Agency. In Northern Ireland this body contracts with independent general practitioners and supervises the dental, pharmaceutical and optical services. The Agency is also responsible for prescription pricing, for certain personnel duties concerning hospital consultants and registrars, for supplies, support services, advisory services and legal matters.

Consumer interests in Northern Ireland are represented by health and social services councils set up in 1991. They monitor the operation of the local services and provide advice on improvements. The Eastern Council has 30 members, the remaining three have 24 members, 40% of whom are district council nominees, 30% voluntary body nominees and the remainder, appointed by the DHSS, have a general background.

Northern Ireland spends more per head on health and social services than England and Wales. This is not only a response to the health consequences of its prolonged sectarian and political problems but also simply a result of more professional staff and more beds per head of population. Despite this, health indicators show an unsatisfactory picture. Northern Ireland has the UK's highest death rates from respiratory disease and a rising death rate from cancer. Two strategic documents, *Health and Well-being into the Next Millennium*[11] and *Well into 2000*[12] set out ways to help combat these problems.

The 1997 government's NHS reforms were a little delayed in Northern Ireland while the new Assembly was set up. A consultative document *Fit for the Future*[13] (significantly not a white paper) was issued in May 1998. It reflected some of the differences that already exist between Northern Ireland and the rest of the UK and interestingly provided two options. Model A envisaged little change other than strengthening the strategic role of health and social service boards, establishing primary care groups and reconfiguring some trusts. Model B was more radical, while also recalling the integrated commissioning and providing authorities that preceded the 1990 Act (Box 7.4).

The future organization of health and social services in Northern Ireland relies on the ability of the new Assembly to grasp fundamental issues of distribution of funds and facilities. To date such decisions have often been compromised by central rule from Westminster. Difficult

One region	Strategic planning, common services, public health, regulation and inspection
Six to eight local care agencies	Commissioning and providing services for populations of 200–300,000
Primary care partnerships	For commissioning and providing local care within framework provided by Local Care Agencies for populations of 25–30,000

Box 7.4

Fit for the Future *Model B*

decisions have forced managers to grapple with the political aspects of planning and delivering services role.

CONCLUSION

The differences in the organizations of the health service in the four countries of the UK arise from their different constitutional and political traditions. They also reflect demographic and geographical differences, which show how progress can be made in achieving such key goals as joint planning and service integration. In terms of health outcomes, comparisons with other countries certainly help to judge how effective a health service is. Epidemiological and health service statistics enable the effectiveness of the four services to be assessed. This data needs to be analysed in relation to various other health and performance indicators. Looking at the NHS overall, despite its distinctive achievements, fundamental differences in standards of health care and of patient care still persist in the UK itself.

REFERENCES

1. Hazell, R. and Jervis, P. (1998) *Devolution and Health*. The Nuffield Trust, London.
2. Scottish Home and Health Department (1968) *Administrative Reorganisation of the Scottish Health Services*. HMSO, Edinburgh.
3. Scottish Home and Health Department (1971) *Reorganisation of the Scottish Health Services*. HMSO, Edinburgh (Cmnd 4734).
4. Scottish Home and Health Department (1979) *Structure and Management of the NHS in Scotland*. HMSO, Edinburgh.
5. The Scottish Office, Department of Health (December 1997) *Designed to care – Reviewing the National Health Service in Scotland*. The Stationery Office, Edinburgh (Cm 3811).
6. Scottish Home and Health Department, Scottish Planning Council (1980) *Priorities for Health Care in Scotland*. HMSO, Edinburgh.
7. *Royal Commission on the National Health Service* (1979) HMSO, London (Cmnd 7615).
8. Welsh Office, NHS Wales (1998) *Better Health Better Wales*. The Stationery Office, Cardiff.
9. Welsh Office, NHS Wales (1998) *Putting Patients First*. The Stationery Office, Cardiff (Cm 3841).
10. *The Health and Personal Social Services (Northern Ireland) Order 1972*, DHSS, Northern Ireland.

11. DHSS Northern Ireland (1996) *Health and Well-being into the Next Millennium*. The Stationery Office, Belfast.
12. DHSS Northern Ireland (1997) *Well into 2000. A Positive Agenda for Health and Well-being*. The Stationery Office, Belfast.
13. DHSS Northern Ireland (1989) *Fit for the Future – a consultation document*. The Stationery Office, Belfast.

Financing the National Health Service 8

In its first year of existence, the NHS spent around £440 million. In 1998, its 50th year, this had risen to over £42,000 million – a massive increase. Allowing for inflation, the NHS is spending nearly 3.5 times more than it did in 1948. And yet, in comparison with most industrialized countries, the NHS is not only inexpensive (some would argue too cheap) but represents good value for money. This chapter is concerned with three basic questions: Where does the money to pay for the NHS come from? What does it cost to run the service? What are the implications of this system?

8.1 Sources of funding

Money for the NHS is derived from three main sources (see Figure 8.1): central government tax revenues, national insurance contributions and other sources such as charges to patients. By and large, general taxation has been and remains the primary source of funds for the NHS. Before 1974, community health services were funded from local authority rates and the rate support grant from central government; thereafter these came within the health authorities' budgets.

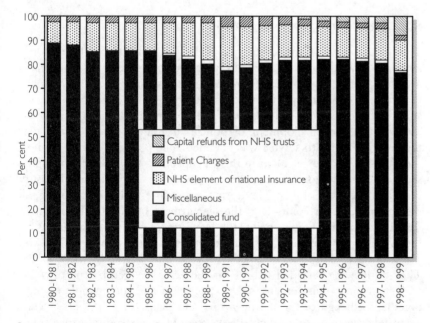

Figure 8.1

UK NHS: sources of funding

Source: statistics compiled from DoH (1995, 1997) *Government expenditure plans 1996/97 and 1998/99*, (Cm 3212 and 3912). HMSO, London

There is a popular misconception that the national insurance contribution is the main source of NHS funds but, as can be seen, national taxation provides most of the money. Most national insurance contributions are paid by employers and employees within the Pay As You Earn system (PAYE). Direct payments by patients themselves were not part of the original plan for the NHS but were introduced in 1951. There has always been opposition to charges, despite exemption arrangements. Charges for prescriptions, dental examinations, sight tests and spectacles have markedly influenced who uses these NHS services and when and how often they present themselves, with consequences for their health. Charging for doctors' prescription medicines began in 1951, was abolished in 1965 and then reintroduced in 1968, although pregnant women, mothers, children, some elderly people and patients with some chronic conditions have always been exempt. By 1997, 85% (388 million) of all prescriptions were exempted[1], which may partly explain why the successive increases in prescription charges have been well above the rate of inflation. Prescription charges income represents only 6.5% of the gross cost of all drugs and dispensing fees (1998). Patients also pay for private beds in NHS hospitals and this money is simply counted as income for the trust; until 1991 individual hospitals were not allowed to make a profit on these services, which were subject to fixed pricing by the Department of Health.

Because the main source of funding for the NHS is general taxation and because the tax structure (at least for direct taxes) is mildly progressive, this means that the financing of the NHS is also mildly progressive; that is, it is inequitable – in favour of the poor[2].

See also section 6.1.6

8.2 HOW THE GOVERNMENT PAYS

The major source of money for the NHS, the consolidated fund, is not automatically administered year by year, but is traditionally only made available after an intricate process of negotiation within central government departments. Until 1997 the process was as follows. Discussions between senior officials in the Department of Health and the Treasury on the development of policies lies at the heart of the way money for the health service was obtained. The public spending team of the Treasury is a key element in this: it supervises expenditure through a series of consultations during the year with the department, Treasury ministers and the Cabinet. The normal procedure is that each spring, all the spending departments (e.g. the Department of Health, Department for Education and Employment, the Department of Trade and Industry, the Ministry of Defence) submit preliminary returns to the Treasury. These are prepared in accordance with guidelines agreed by the Cabinet. They outline the revalued figures for the years covered by the previous plan, with proposals for any new expenditure and for possible savings, together with figures for the new year and plans for a further 2 years. They take account of Cabinet discussions of the medium-term economic outlook and of their priorities, as well as of detailed economic assumptions provided by the Treasury. In preparing them, the departmental officials confer with their Ministers in order to work out their proposals for the continuation of existing policies and the development of new ones. This process is not always straightforward since there may well be disagreement about what current policy actually is. Departmental officials then have detailed discussions with officials from the spending team in order to agree on statistical assumptions and their effect on the projected future cost of existing policies.

The departmental principal finance officers, although officials of their own departments, need to foster the closest relations with the Treasury in order that they may give their own department an accurate picture of the proposals that are likely to be successful with the Treasury, and those that will need persuasion to be acceptable. They need to be in a position to assess the likely balance of demands for new spending between competing departments and to get as much as they reasonably can for their own departments.

The next stage of the process involves the Treasury ministers. Together with Treasury officials they study the implications of its expenditure proposals in the light of their assessment of the economic climate and the government's overall macroeconomic strategy. They have to decide whether the proposals could actually be paid for within the overall spending limit set by the Treasury. The Chancellor of the Exchequer's view is presented to the Cabinet, and he may find that increased spending will be possible in some areas, but more often he suggests that some cuts in the projections of individual departments will have to be made or that increases in one department have to be matched by decreases in another. The Cabinet discusses these points, and individual ministers have to try to persuade their colleagues over the precedence of their claims for resources. Much may depend on whether the Prime Minister (who chairs Cabinet meetings) is in favour of certain policies rather than others. He or she will have already had confidential meetings with the Chancellor, and his or her own mind may be made up before the Cabinet meets. Nevertheless, the discussions continue from June to November after which the Cabinet's decisions are revealed in the Chancellor's Autumn Statement. Subsequently, spending plans are embodied in the white paper on public expenditure, which is published early the following year as a series of departmental reports. It is also debated for 2 days in the House of Commons, but this is usually a formality and few if any amendments are made to it. This is, however, an area where MPs could exert more influence over future government policy, if they chose to play a more active part, particularly in Select Committees. The plans are set out in a form in which Parliament actually votes the money for the year ahead.

Once Parliament has agreed to the allocations for each department, through the annual 'votes', its involvement is temporarily ended. Later in the financial year that the vote covers, departments may, through their ministers, come back for more money. The Treasury puts forward requests for supplementary allocations after discussion with the departments, and Parliament agrees to allow the additional money. Parliament is subsequently involved in the scrutiny of departmental spending through the work of the Comptroller and Auditor General and the investigations of the Public Accounts Committee.

This public expenditure system is not only an administrative process essential for the everyday conduct of the nation's major public services but also a means of putting into effect the political choices of the government of the day. With the election in 1997 of the first Labour government for 18 years, the traditional cycle was interrupted in favour of the comprehensive spending review (CSR). Like many new governments before, the new administration embarked on a review of all government spending, with a view to meeting its manifesto commitments. The CSR reported in the summer of 1998, with health and education receiving large increases in funding relative to other departments. In the 1997/8 expenditure round, the government broadly stuck to the previous Conservative administration's spending plans, but this did not preclude some additional funding for the NHS and some other departments. The CSR departed from the yearly cycle and instead adopted a 3-yearly public spending round.

8.3   DISTRIBUTING THE FUNDS

When the Department of Health finally receives notification (usually in late December) of its allocation for the following financial year beginning in April, it is able to pass money on to the regions (and subsequently on to local health care purchasers) in accordance with their previously agreed budgets based on a population-based formula. Following the reorganization of regions in England, allocations are now formally made directly to health authorities and, prior to the phased abolition of the fundholding scheme, then split between health authorities and GP fundholders. However, following the white paper *The new NHS*[3] and the introduction of primary care groups (PCGs) in 1999 as the new local purchasing organization embracing all GP practices and taking on the majority of the purchasing decisions of their local health authorities, allocations now flow to PCGs via health authorities.

From 1975 to 1991 historical imbalances began to be corrected through RAWP, named after the report of the Resource Allocation Working Party[4], which suggested that each region should have a target allocation based on a formula that took into account its population's age structure and factors that affected the need for health care – chiefly (as a proxy for morbidity) death rates standardized for age, known as standardized mortality ratios (SMRs). A similar formula was also applied to the distribution of capital money (see Section 8.4). This enabled health authorities to anticipate their likely future financial allocations and thereby enhance their ability to plan strategically. But eliminating geographical inequities takes time. It takes a long time for significant funds to be made available for deprived areas and for that extra spending power to show up as improved health care. In the past, regions have relied on the growth element in their annual allocations from the DoH when trying to obey the RAWP criteria for distributing money to their health authorities' according to relative need. They had difficulties in those years when the money first had to be used to meet shortfalls in mainstream revenue budgets arising from the DoH's failure to compensate fully for the effects of inflation.

8.3.1   Regions

Under the 1990 Act RAWP was scrapped, and replaced with a very similar formula under which health authorities were expected to work on the basis of budgets calculated from the size of their resident populations weighted to reflect relative need for health care. The progress of regions towards their RAWP targets between 1975 and 1991 was generally consistent but slow. By 1991, however, most regions were within 1 or 2% of their target allocations. It is important to point out that over this period (and, indeed, after 1991) the formula for distributing funds to regions was not consistently applied: every year ministers and the DoH exercised considerable discretion over the actual allocations each region received and hence the speed with which each region moved towards its target. The most notable example of this was the protection received by the Thames regions covering London, which have consistently received a greater share of funds than the formula strictly would allow. Traditionally, London has been over-provided with health services in comparison with the rest of the country and compared with the need for services suggested by the distribution formula. However, ministers and the DoH felt that moving money out of London as quickly as the distribution formula prescribed would disrupt services too much. Therefore the pace of change was deliberately slowed down.

Since 1991, the weighted capitation formula has undergone a number of changes in attempts to reflect more accurately different areas' differential need for health care. Although population size and demographic structure remain key determinants of the share of the total budget each area receives, socioeconomic factors have also been introduced as extra weights alongside mortality proxies for morbidity.

8.3.2   Fundholders

While some money is retained to fund regions themselves (plus any services purchased by regions on behalf of health authorities) the bulk of the funds were, before April 1999, allocated directly to health authorities. In turn, they have been responsible for setting budgets for their local GP fundholders. Generally, health authorities did not use the national weighted capitation formula for allocations to fundholders, but constructed budgets based on fundholders' historic use of hospital and other services. Part of the difficulty of employing the weighted capitation formula has been technical – GPs do not operate in discrete areas (unlike health authorities) which can be easily matched with census and other data necessary to compute weighted capitations. Concern over potential allocation inequalities between fundholders and non-fundholders (whose services were purchased by health authorities) led most health authorities to explore the possibilities of devising a funding formula which reflected that used at national level. To an extent this work was overtaken by the phased abolition of fundholding and the creation of PCGs.

8.3.3   Primary care groups

Primary care groups now control most of the health care budget, and their budget allocations are determined in a similar way to the previous weighted capitation formulae. It is of fundamental importance that PCGs receive one unified stream of cash limited funds to cover hospital and community health services, family health service prescribing and general medical services. This unification enables PCGs to decide on the general pattern of their health care spending without the virement problems previously created by having separate budgets. However, it also means that the previously 'open ended' prescribing budget (and that part of the general medical services budget which was also open ended) are now firmly cash limited.

8.3.4   Joint finance

Although most public sector purchasers' revenue comes from the Exchequer via the Department of Health, they do have other sources of income, one of the most important being joint finance. The local authorities' shortage of resources had meant that patients no longer requiring NHS hospital care nevertheless remained in hospital because social services departments were unable to pay for accommodating them in the community. Until 1976 health authorities were not authorized to transfer money to the local authorities, but in that year the rules changed, in return for a commitment to set up specifically agreed new services that would benefit both sets of authorities[5].

However, with continuing pressure on budgets in the 1980s, authorities became unwilling to commit future funds in this way and joint finance ceased to be a useful vehicle for achieving flexible improvements in community care. A DHSS working party[6] in 1985 and the Audit Commission[7] in 1986 underlined the difficulties, and the second Griffiths report[8] in 1988 advocated a simpler system by assigning to one or other authority the lead responsibility for a care group. *Caring for People*[9] accepted this principle but the administration of joint finance became further complicated by the new system under the 1990 Act; in this, social services departments have to construct 'care packages' for individual clients, and may ask the health authorities to contribute financially.

8.3.5   Special sources

Another special source of funds is the earmarked sums governments provide as incentives to encourage prompt local implementation of national policies. These are taken from the national NHS budget and are not distributed within the weighted capitation formula. Health authorities have in the past received these payments for such initiatives as the public education campaign about AIDS, tackling waiting times and lists, but also to underpin managerial action, for example to speed the introduction of the 1990 Act and the 1999 changes.

Local sources provide funds too. Trusts or 'free monies' are accrued from public donations in support of special local projects such as the purchase of a scanner or amenities for patients and staff. With the creation of trust hospitals, these funds were transferred from health authorities to the hospitals and community units.

While the main source of income for trusts comes via their formally negotiated contracts with purchasers, a small proportion – on average around 1–2% – is obtained from 'extra contractual referrals' (ECRs). These include patients admitted to casualty departments as emergencies at trusts which are not located in the patient's district of residence, and patients referred by their GPs to trusts which do not have a contract in place with the patient's 'home' authority. Emergency ECRs attract an automatic payment from their home district; permission to treat elective ECRs, on the other hand, has to be negotiated with the the home district – who may refuse the referral if they consider a patient would receive adequate care under an existing contract. Following *The new NHS*, a new process has been put in place to deal with ECRs. First, health authorities are now encouraged to set up special contracts to deal with the bulk of their existing ECRs. Second, any referrals not covered in this way – known as 'out of area treatments' (OATs) – are funded retrospectively. This avoids some of the bureaucracy of the old ECR system by adjusting health authority budgets for the year following the OAT. It is similar in may ways to the system that was in place before the internal market.

8.3.6 Providers

The providers of health care – NHS trusts and others in the voluntary and private sectors – are at the end of this financial distribution chain. Public sector purchasers (PCGs and, for certain services, health authorities, the DoH itself and the regions) are responsible for commissioning health care for their local populations. They are free to buy care from whomsoever they please and are not restricted to public sector providers. However, almost all the money voted by Parliament to the NHS does in fact find its way to trusts via the commissioning system. Although *The new NHS* set out plans for abolishing the internal market – and hence its associated market-type mechanisms such as contracts – commissioners retained the process of agreeing what are essentially contractual agreements with their chosen providers. Such service agreements detail the service to be provided and the price to be paid. However, *The new NHS* encouraged commissioners to enter long-term agreements with providers as part of its aim to improve integrated care and draw providers back into a shared responsibility for appropriate service usage. Historically, a typical NHS trust received most of its income from its local health authority, with the remainder made up from contracts with neighbouring health authorities, GP fundholders

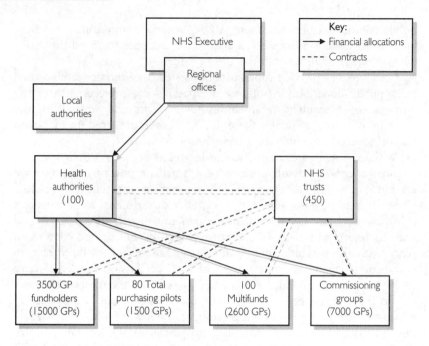

Figure 8.2

Financing and accountability
arrangements before *The new NHS*

and other sources such as private patients and non-health care related income such as charges for car parks, in-hospital cafes, etc. The introduction of PCGs as the main purchasing organization in the NHS means that trusts receive most of their income from this organizational group.

Figures 8.2 and 8.3 summarize the key responsibilities and flows of

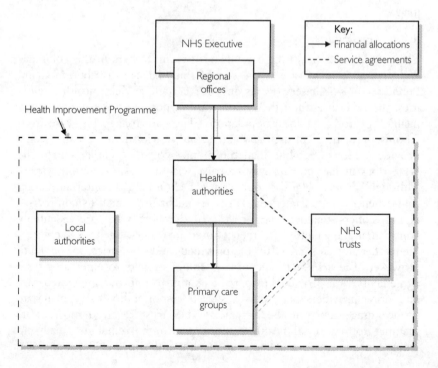

Figure 8.3

Financing and accountability
arrangements after *The new NHS*

funds before and after the changes brought about in 1997 by the white paper *The new NHS*.

8.4 CAPITAL AND REVENUE

Traditionally, NHS expenditure is divided into two categories – capital and revenue. Capital expenditure purchases assets which generate benefits over more than one year. Examples of such assets in the NHS include land purchased for building, the erection of new buildings, the extension of old buildings and the adaptation of existing buildings for health purposes, and the cost of initial equipment, furniture and stores for these buildings. These costs are incurred in relation to hospitals, clinics, health centres and for offices of administrative bodies such as the health authorities themselves. Revenue expenditure, on the other hand, covers the costs of services in the current year. These include the remuneration of medical, nursing, paramedical and other professional staff; the remuneration of managers, accountants, storekeepers, cooks, domestics, porters, engineers and maintenance staff; the cost of goods and services needed to provide residential care for patients and accommodation for staff; the cost of drugs, appliances, fuel and the repair of equipment and maintenance of buildings. These lists of items are not exhaustive but simply indicate how health service costs have been classified.

The reason for making a distinction between capital and revenue expenditure may not be immediately clear. In private sector organizations it is essential for the calculation of the annual profit margin, where profit is the income derived from a given level of expenditure. This calculation is obviously difficult to transfer to the accounts of the NHS, where the 'income' is not obtained in monetary terms. There are, however, four reasons why the capital/revenue distinction is made in the financing of the NHS.

First, a decision on spending priorities must involve some analysis of whether the expenditure is part of a commitment made in the past (e.g. staffing a hospital built many years ago) or expenditure which will require funding over future periods (e.g. the maintenance of a new operating theatre installed during the current year). Second, in order to analyse trends of expenditure over several years it is wise to separate out those items which represent the cost of maintaining existing services from items for new services for which large sums of money are required at the very start. If this distinction is not made, there is a danger that total expenditure patterns over a period of several years will not reflect the fact that expensive projects were started in some years and not in others. Taking an example over 10 years, it can be seen from Figure 8.4 that a project was started in year 3 and another in year 7. Assuming for simplicity's sake that these two projects were new wings of an existing hospital and that the building work was completed in one year, it can be seen that each new wing requires revenue expenditure for running costs in all subsequent years. If only the bottom line (total expenditure) were

Figure 8.4

Capital and current expenditure

Years	£ million – excluding inflation									
	1	2	3	4	5	6	7	8	9	10
Current expenditure: original hospital premises	5	5	5	5	5	5	5	5	5	5
Current expenditure: first new wing			1	1	1	1	1	1	1	1
Current expenditure: second new wing							1	1	1	1
Total Current Expenditure	**5**	**5**	**6**	**6**	**6**	**6**	**7**	**7**	**7**	**7**
Capital expenditure: first new wing		5								
Capital expenditure: second new wing						5				
Total Capital Expenditure		**5**				**5**				
Total Capital and Current Expenditure	**5**	**10**	**6**	**6**	**6**	**11**	**7**	**7**	**7**	**7**

taken, this would give a distorted picture for analysis of the increased costs over that period.

Third, it is necessary to make the capital/revenue distinction in order to compare NHS regions and also to compare expenditure on the NHS and other government departments. Capital expenditure almost always involves large sums of money and, if the distinction is not made, public expenditure is difficult to plan. Capital projects which were necessary for the adequate maintenance of existing assets (e.g. replacing worn-out equipment) might otherwise not obtain sufficient priority, bearing in mind the scarce resources available to the public sector. Fourth, in judging the timing of expenditure, current items represent a continuing financial commitment which cannot normally be significantly reduced. Capital commitments on the other hand can be brought forward or postponed, depending on a government's over-all economic strategy. In practical terms, this means that there is normally no possibility of deciding that hospital sheets should not be laundered or that nurses should not be paid, whereas building a new hospital can be delayed for 1 or 2 years if the government wishes to save that money in the current year.

The rigid application of the distinction between capital and revenue expenditure has, in the past, been criticized for discouraging local managers from using their discretion to finance services in a flexible and economic way. It also used to be the rule that all unspent money had to be returned at the end of the financial year, thus penalizing those authorities who, through wise financial management, had been able to achieve economies. They found that their underspending could result in a reduced financial allocation for the following year. However, these anomalies have been recognized.

8.4.1 Capital charges

Following *Working for Patients*, capital was redefined as an asset which would cost £1000 or more to replace[10]. Before 1991, capital expenditure in the NHS had always been considered as buying fully depreciated assets, so that once a new building was acquired, it was treated as having no financial value. The value of equipment was not amortized over a period, with the result that when it came to be renewed there was no existing money ready to pay for it.

In a service funded annually by taxation the argument for treating capital money in this way is that if each health authority had to set aside all the funds it expected to need for its future capital purchases, a considerable sum of money would have to be held in reserve and could not be used meanwhile for legitimate recurring expenditure. The effect of this nationally would be to freeze large sums of public money, which could otherwise be put to immediate use. *Working for Patients* challenged the old assumptions. It encouraged trusts to value their capital stock at current prices and to make efficient use of all their capital assets. For instance, land should no longer be left unused if its sale could benefit the trust. Trusts have been required to maintain asset registers which include all equipment with a value of over £1000. Depreciation was calculated on ordinary accounting principles but based on the current value of the capital assets. Interest charges were calculated on the current value of those capital assets. Land and property values were calculated with the assistance of the District Valuer. For depreciation purposes the government expected that the life of a building would not exceed 100 years, an interesting judgement given the number of hospitals that still occupy buildings considerably older than this.

8.4.2 Distributing capital

Under the old RAWP scheme capital money was distributed to regions on a similar basis as revenue. However, the need for, say, new hospitals or maintenance or, to a lesser extent, equipment in hospitals, does not follow the exact pattern of the need for services provided from the revenue budget. Capital is required more sporadically: an area may need considerable capital investment over a short period of time, after which its need for capital will be low for some years. Therefore, the distribution of capital below the level of regions has been based much less on rigid formulae and more on bids and negotiations reflecting long-term plans to renew or replace buildings and equipment. In the past, every region received a long list of capital schemes put up by its health authorities. Most major building works took years to be realized as they were fought for through the evaluations and option appraisal process. Depending on the scale of the scheme, approval was given by regions, or the Department of Health or, for very large projects, the Treasury.

Following the 1990 Act, several changes occurred in the way capital was distributed in the NHS, but a number of issues remained unresolved.

Relatively small-scale capital investment (new equipment, upgrading the estate and buildings, etc.) became the responsibility of trusts and had to be funded from their own internally generated income (received largely from health authorities) and/or external borrowing (mainly from the DoH which offered loans at low interest rates). Trusts needed to plan their capital investments and make sure that they had sufficient income streams over the years to pay associated capital charges (see Section 8.4.1). There is some evidence to suggest that the introduction of capital charges significantly reduced the number of potential capital works, because trusts had had difficulty guaranteeing that future streams of income would cover the charges. The DoH set a limit on the amount of internally generated income and borrowings each trust could devote to capital investment by establishing an external financing limit each year. To the extent that trusts use internally generated income for capital projects the old distinction between capital and revenue no longer applied.

In December 1997, responsibility for making recommendations to ministers on the prioritization of major capital schemes (including those funded from private finance sources, see below) was given to the new Capital Prioritization Advisory Group (CPAG). The group considers schemes costing over £25 million, and prioritizes bids broadly on the basis of health service need.

8.4.3 The Private Finance Initiative

A significant new approach to the funding of capital schemes in the NHS was introduced in 1995. Faced with the explicit need to invest in the capital infrastructure of the NHS, but constrained by macroeconomic policies which required curbs on public spending, the then Chancellor, Kenneth Clarke, put forward the idea of private investment in the public sector[11]. The Private Finance Initiative (PFI) aimed to encourage private consortia of bankers, builders and design and build organizations to provide finance, building and estates expertise to the NHS (and other public sector organizations). In effect, the private sector provided long-term loans to the NHS, which then entered a contractual obligation to repay these loans over an agreed period (up to 60 years in some cases).

The PFI was slow to start in the NHS mainly due to legal problems concerning the powers of trusts to enter into PFI agreements and uncertainties surrounding the sharing of risk. A review of the PFI in 1997 led to the NHS (Private Finance) Act in the same year[12], which resolved the legal difficulties. The review also prioritized stalled PFI schemes, and recommended that 15 major schemes (totalling £1.2 billion) should go ahead. These schemes included major new district general hospitals in Norwich, Dartford and Gravesham and Carlisle. In 1998, private finance provided around 17% of the total capital allocation (£1.9 billion) in England. By 1999/2000, the PFI was expected to contribute over a quarter of the total capital expenditure in the NHS. Figure 8.5 shows trends in the sources of capital funding for the NHS. The Labour government has been criticized by its supporters for continuing the PFI,

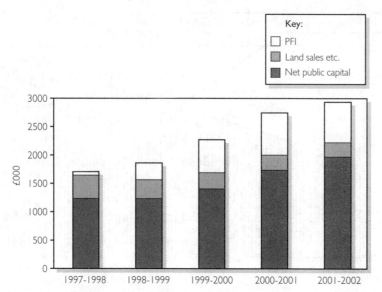

Figure 8.5

Planned gross capital spending:
English NHS

Source: statistics compiled from DoH (1995, 1997) *Government expenditure plans 1996/97 and 1998/99*, (Cm 3212 and 3912). HMSO, London

but in reply the government has maintained that building improvements are so urgent that it would be foolish to rule out this access to capital.

8.5   THE COST OF THE NHS

Over the years the amount of money spent on the NHS has risen substantially. There are three ways of looking at the increase (Figure 8.6). First the rise in the actual cash totals, from around £0.5 billion in

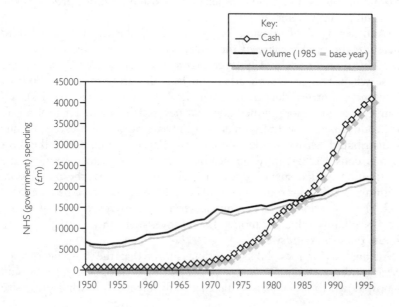

Figure 8.6

Cash and volume net spending on the UK NHS

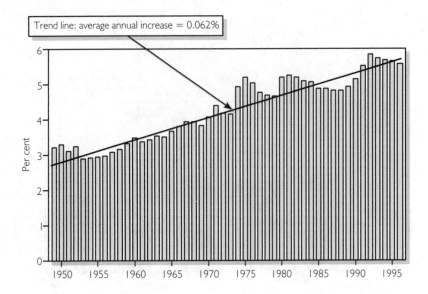

Figure 8.7

Total net UK NHS spending as a percentage of GDP

Trend line: average annual increase = 0.062%

1949 to over £42 billion in 1998; but these amounts are misleading because inflation has reduced the purchasing power of the NHS budget over that period. Recalculating the figures at a constant value shows the true size of the increase. The Treasury traditionally uses a measure of general inflation in the economy as a whole – the gross domestic product (GDP) deflator – in order to measure 'real' changes in public expenditure. This provides an indication of the opportunity cost of the NHS to the rest of the economy. However, the NHS is not a typical consumer, and the prices of the goods and services it buys – doctors, nurses, drugs, etc. – have tended to rise faster than the GDP deflator. Using NHS-specific measures of inflation to deflate the cash allocations produces real expenditure in 'volume' terms.

Another way of looking at spending is illustrated by the third measure: the NHS's share of the GDP, which has risen from under 4% in 1949 to about 6% in 1998 (see Figure 8.7). These trends make more sense when compared with others, such as the proportion of GDP that different countries devote to their health services (Figure 8.8). Of course, spending more money does not necessarily buy better health care or produce better health. Nor does it indicate how health care spending is distributed across whole populations. For example, while the USA spends considerably more on health care than any other country, the distribution of that spending is extremely uneven across the population. Within the UK the resources allocated to the NHS can also be compared with the allocations to other public services (see Figure 8.9). Whether the UK obtains value for money for its investment in the NHS is not a simple question to answer.

An analysis of total NHS spending shows that the hospital sector's share started at about 51%, rose to around 67% in the early 1970s, and is now down to 54%. This is meant to fall further, following successive

Some measures to promote efficiency are discussed in Chapter 10

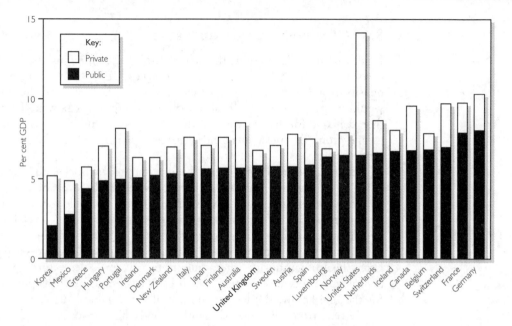

Source: compiled using material from the *Organisation for Economic Co-operation and Development Health Database 1997*, OECD, Paris

governments' intentions to give greater priority to community care and family health services. The number of NHS hospitals has declined from 2441 (1959) to around 1500 (1998) and beds have similarly been cut back from 455,100 to 205,000 over that period. Yet, since 1975 the proportion of the budget spent on direct care and treatment as opposed to preventive and supporting services has climbed to 67% of the total hospital spending. Another significant area of spending within the NHS is pharmaceutical medicines. Spending on drugs has been one of the fastest growing areas within the NHS. The number of prescription items issued has grown from around 4 per head of population in the early 1950s to around 9 in 1998. Spending on drugs now constitutes around 12% (£4.5 billion in 1998) of the total expenditure on the NHS.

Figure 8.8

Total health care spending as a percentage of GDP: international comparisons: 1995

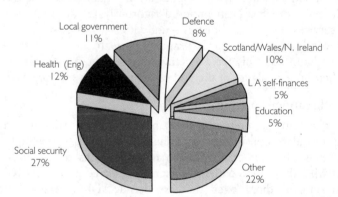

Figure 8.9

1998–99 share of public spending

Source: statistics compiled from DoH (1997) *Government expenditure plans 1998/1999*, (Cm 3912). HMSO, London

8.6   CONTROLLING EXPENDITURE

Health services throughout the world display a continuous rise in their costs. Ironically, in 1944 Sir William Beveridge's proposals for a comprehensive health service assumed that improving the health of the nation would reduce demand for health services, whereas it is now understood that demand for health care is virtually infinite and there is thus no escape from the permanent need to set priorities and, ultimately, to ration access.

Different health care systems have attempted to tackle the issue of rising costs in different ways. In the NHS, each level of authority monitors the planned and actual spending of the one below it within the overall constraint of fixed global budgets set at national level by the Treasury. The DoH sets guidelines for the regions and they in turn watch how health authorities keep within the limits they have set them. Each health authority then monitors its providers through the contracting process. The more detail each level builds into its guidelines for the one below, the less freedom it allows for local discretion. With the retreat from the internal market, and the introduction of PCGs, monitoring of providers has become less tied to a contractual/market model and has moved back towards more traditional management control within the context of nationally imposed performance and monitoring frameworks (see Chapter 10). Overall, however, this system of global budgets has acted as an extremely effective constraint on total expenditure to the extent that while the chief concern in most other countries is cost containment, in the UK it is widely thought that too little is spent.

8.6.1   Budgets

Budgets serve three main functions in commercial organizations: planning, control and costing. In the NHS these functions traditionally had a low priority, but since 1974 the parallels with business have become stronger. Business planning and the systematic approach to controlling expenditure that it implies are now accepted. The discipline of cash limits too has been imposed rigorously in the NHS and other public services. Health authorities – and latterly, PCGs – are notified of their revenue allocations for a year and have to manage within these whatever happens. This has sometimes forced them to cut services to make their books balance at the end of the financial year each March.

8.6.2   Treatment pricing

In other countries, alternative systems have been tried in order to constrain escalating health care spending. In the USA for example, there have been sophisticated attempts to help clinicians to understand the costs of what they do to patients. Diagnostic-related groups (DRGs) have been developed there over the last decade. DRGs classify patients according to a predetermined list of nearly 500 separate conditions, which have been costed to enable the doctor to check the actual cost of his treatment of that condition with an average and, importantly, given the concern of medical insurers about spiralling costs, to provide a check on excessive care given to patients. The disadvantage of the system is its own high administrative cost; every procedure in the USA needs to be priced for billing purposes, thus requiring the inclusion of an administrative overhead. Moreover, a problem known as 'DRG creep' has reportedly occurred whereby doctors have classified patients in DRG categories attracting higher payments from insurers than warranted by a patient's actual condition, age etc. The National Casemix Office in the UK has been actively working on a British version of DRGs – health related groupings (HRGs). So far (1998) there is no national system, although trusts have in some cases used a DRG/HRG type of classification for some of their services[13].

The National Casemix Office was set up as part of the Department of Health Resource Management Initiative. It acts as an information source on casemix measures and as a centre for the development of measures such as DRGs and HRGs

Since the NHS reforms of 1990, the system of global budgets at national level as a way of controlling expenditure still remains. At a local level, and in the general framework of the health improvement programme which sets out the long-term health strategy for both purchasers and providers, purchasers exert some financial control pressure on providers through their service agreements which specify budgets and activity levels. Under the internal market, expenditure control within trusts was derived partly from market imperatives (if costs and hence prices are not controlled then there is the risk of losing business) and partly through external controls such as accounts audited by the Audit Commission and DoH set controls such as external financing limits. But balancing the books can prove difficult. In 1996/7, for example, nearly one-third of all trusts failed to achieve break-even on their income and expenditure, and over half failed to make their required financial return (to cover debt repayments to the Exchequer, etc). The abolition of the internal market, but the retention of the separation between purchasers of care and providers, introduced by *The new NHS* white paper, has not removed the purchaser's ultimate market sanction to take their business elsewhere, but it has been relegated in the list of possible actions that can be taken in order to keep trusts on track financially.

The Audit Commission also carries out value for money investigations, see Chapter 10

8.7 PRIVATE HEALTH CARE

In August 1975 the DHSS published a consultative document called *The Separation of Private Practice from the National Health Service*[14], which set out proposals to reduce the number of pay beds in NHS hospitals and to control developments in private practice, in line with the Labour party's stated commitment to the electorate. The proposals met with fierce opposition, particularly from hospital doctors who had already been in dispute with the government in 1974/75. Nevertheless, the Health Services Act, 1976, enabled the Secretary of State to promote the separation of facilities available for private practice from NHS premises, and a quarter of the 4000 beds available in the NHS were withdrawn. A new health services board monitored and authorized private hospitals and nursing homes to ensure that the interests of the NHS and its patients were not disadvantaged. With the change of government the Board and the other provisions were repealed by the Health Services Act, 1980. It has since become easier for a patient to change from NHS to private status even during the course of one particular treatment, and managers cannot ensure that there is no manipulation of the system to benefit private patients.

From the patients' point of view, however, private health care ensures that treatment will be obtained from a chosen consultant in accommodation which will probably be private and that little or no waiting will be required. By 1996, around 13.6% of the population had insurance cover to allow them access to private care if they should wish it[15]. However, up to 30% of all treatments (such as hip operations) in certain areas (such as London) are carried out privately. Clearly this raises implications for NHS financing, and also for the controls currently in place to enforce consultants' NHS contracts[16].

With the introduction of the internal market and the explicit possibility of public sector purchasers commissioning care from private sector providers, there were suggestions that the private sector would expand considerably at the expense of NHS health care providers. In fact, for a variety of reasons, this did not happen. For example, private health care provision is unevenly spread across the country and in many areas is virtually non-existent. For NHS purchasers, however, local provision of health care to their local populations was an important factor in deciding where they placed contracts. Cost, or price, was not the only criterion used.

CONCLUSION

How societies pay for their health care is not simply an accounting matter but is bound up intricately with the way societies view health, health care, the rights of the individual and the role of governments. In the UK, political decisions taken at the inception of the NHS have meant that health care is funded largely on a whole population basis out of general taxation. Over the years there have been some fluctuations in sources of finance but these have been minor. Even with the radical reforms of the 1990 Act the method of funding the NHS was left unchanged, reflecting recognition of the broadly held view that health care is a special service which for ethical, social and political reasons should not be treated purely as a commodity to be traded in an unregulated market. The internal financing arrangements within health care systems – how purchasers receive their allocations, how hospitals are reimbursed and so on – are also more than a straightforward question of accounting. Allocation methods and payment systems can be powerful forces for change, whether by ensuring a degree of equity in provision or promoting changes through incentives in the way providers operate, the level of services they produce or whom they serve. And it is at this level that the 1990 reforms of the NHS had their biggest impact. The

Within this figure there are marked differences. Wales and Scotland have only 4% insurance holders compared with England's 10%

Full-time consultants in the NHS work to a contract held by their trust of 10/11ths of a full working week. The remaining 1/11th allows them to work privately if they wish – a hangover from the inception of the NHS when the then Minister of Health Aneurin Bevan negotiated this deal with the BMA to persuade consultants to join the service. However, if private work increases this will start to raise conflicts (if they don't exist already in some areas) between the consultants and their NHS employers, who may well be in direct competition with the private hospitals for whom their consultants also work

NHS budget has been the most important factor in containing costs – an issue many other countries have struggled to deal with.

The changes brought about by *The new NHS* white paper again have left unchanged the funding sources for the NHS, acknowledging that the advantages of paying for health care from taxation outweigh its disadvantages or the benefits to be gained from alternative forms of financing. Similarly, while the white paper introduced new organizational structures such as primary care groups, how money finds its way down the system essentially adheres to existing criteria, which attempt to match funding with the need for health care. Moreover, the abolition of the internal market, but the retention of the separation between commissioners and providers of care, means that the flow of funds to providers will still be controlled by purchasers (as opposed to an automatic budget allocated to providers). The promotion of longer-term agreements between commissioners and providers, the new strategic framework and a renewed focus on partnership with shared responsibility together with the continued emphasis on value for money and the control of expenditure, make the management of the NHS even more demanding than before. It remains to be seen whether these efforts *will* improve the health of the nation.

REFERENCES

1. Office of Health Economics (1998) *Compendium of Health Statistics*. OHE, London.
2. For a useful summary of the evidence, see, for example: Propper, C. (1998) *Who pays for and who gets health care?: Equity in the finance and delivery of health care in the United Kingdom*. Nuffield Occasional Papers: Health Economics Series No 5. The Nuffield Trust, London.
3. Department of Health (1997) *The new NHS*. The Stationery Office, London (Cm 3807).
4. DHSS Resource Allocation Working Party (1976) *Sharing Resources for Health in England* (RAWP Report). HMSO, London.
5. DHSS (1976) *Joint Care Planning: Health and Local Authorities*, Circular HC(76)16. DHSS, London.
6. DHSS (July, 1985) *Progress in Partnership*. HMSO, London.
7. Audit Commission (December, 1986) *Making a Reality of Community Care*. Audit Commission, London.
8. DoH (1988) *Community Care: Agenda for Action* (second Griffiths report). HMSO, London.
9. DoH (1989) *Caring for People*. HMSO, London (Cm 849).
10. DoH (1989) *Working for Patients. Working Paper 5. Capital Charges*, para. 2.2. HMSO, London.
11. HM Treasury (1995) *Private Opportunity, Public Benefit*. HMSO, London.
12. National Health Service (Private Finance) Act 1997, Chapter 56. The Stationery Office, London.
13. NAHAT (1994) *Developments in Contracting: A National Survey of Purchasers and Providers*. NAHAT, Birmingham.
14. DHSS (1975) *The Separation of Private Practice from the National Health Service*. HMSO, London.

15. Office of Health Economics (1995) *Compendium of Health Statistics*. OHE, London.
16. See for example Yates, J. (1995) *Private Eye, Heart and Hip*. Churchill Livingstone, London.

SERVICES FOR PATIENTS

9

The National Health Service was created to provide:

a comprehensive health service designed to secure improvement in the physical and mental health of the people ... and the prevention, diagnosis and treatment of illness[1].

Has this grand intention been satisfied? This chapter looks at the evidence from services for various groups of patients and clients. It starts with a historical account of how these services have been planned within the NHS and the renewed emphasis on planning partnerships heralded by the 1997 Labour government.

9.1 PLANNING IN THE NHS

Planning in the NHS has passed through several stages (Box 9.1).

1946–62	Little or no strategic planning.
1962–69	Emphasis on hospital planning.
1969–74	Rational planning underpinning reorganisation proposals.
1974–82	Area planning and resulting bureaucracy.
1982–90	Return to district planning.
	Development of community care.
1990–97	Internal market in lieu of formal planning.
	Tension between patient demands and population needs.
	Emphasis on targets and sanctions.
1997	Renewed acceptance of systematic planning.

Box 9.1

Planning in the NHS

Chapter 2 showed that a compelling case for nationally organized health services emerged from the recognition that health care was ill co-ordinated and inadequate. Substantial demands arising from the Second World War, and long before, could not be met properly. The creation of the NHS in 1948 was expected to pave the way for better planned services in the future. For the 1945 Labour government, the NHS was the principal foundation of its overall concept of the new welfare state. However, rising expenditure soon became a major problem, and in 1953 the Guillebaud Committee was set up to examine the financing of the service. Its report, in 1956[2], exonerated the NHS from the accusation of wasteful use of resources. So the Conservative government was forced to introduce plans for the more systematic use of NHS resources.

9.1.1 The 1962 Hospital Plan

One result was the publication, in 1962, of *A Hospital Plan for England and Wales* (the 1962 Plan), which might be said to be the first major attempt to plan in the NHS. This concern has become an unavoidable discipline, and was central to the subsequent reorganizations. The 1962 Plan showed that although capital expenditure had risen from £8.7 million in 1949/50 to over £31 million in 1962/63, overall national direction was lacking. The capital schemes were largely *ad hoc* solutions to local problems.

The moment has therefore come to take a comprehensive view of the hospital service as it is today and to draw the outlines of the service which we mean to create[3].

The 1962 Plan reviewed the existing provision of beds, suggesting norms for each major care group, and translated these into specific targets for each region and within each region for each hospital management committee. It must be emphasized that the 1962 Plan was only about hospitals and beds. It briefly acknowledged care in the community and accepted that the development of hospital services must be complementary to developments in preventive and domiciliary care. Local health authorities were asked to review their services in conjunction with hospital authorities, but no consultative machinery was suggested, and the overriding impression given by the 1962 Plan was that only hospital development really mattered.

This focus was understandable. The state of many hospitals was shameful. Over 45% of them had been built before 1891 and some 21% before 1861; many were old workhouses, now often used for geriatric patients. These buildings had mostly been constructed following the 1834 Poor Law Amendment Act. Emergency medical service (EMS) hospitals, in comparison, built at the beginning of the Second World War, had a more flexible, single-storey design. With changes in illness patterns, the time had come to convert some of the special hospitals to more appropriate uses. Infectious diseases hospitals and sanitoria could quite easily be adapted, although they were often remotely situated. The 1962 Plan envisaged a gradual reorganization, in order to build up a central district general hospital and reduce the number of small and outlying hospitals. A yearly review of progress was intended to assess changes of circumstance and the availability of capital resources. The 1962 Plan was relatively well received at the time. The process of centralization and the 'bigger-is-better' movement was in tune with the 1960s spirit of optimism and expansion.

The 1962 Plan and the subsequent 1969 Bonham-Carter report[4] concentrated on the district general hospital as the focus of hospital care. The term 'district general hospital' was first used by the Ministry of Health Building Note No. 3, in 1961, to describe a large hospital with between 400 and 800 beds, capable of providing a full range of diagnostic and treatment facilities in all the major specialities and some, at least, of the sub-specialities. In 1966, the review of the 1962 Plan curbed some of the initial optimism and modified the original plans, but the basic philosophy was endorsed by the Bonham-Carter report, which described the functions of the district general hospital. The logic of its conclusions would have resulted in some district general hospitals becoming very large indeed, with possibly up to 1500 beds. This has never found much support, as it is believed that such large institutions do not work well and are bound to be impersonal. A consultation paper issued in May 1980 by the Minister for Health, Gerard Vaughan, entitled *The Future Pattern of Hospital Provision in England*[5], put the brake on building district general hospitals because of their escalating cost. During the 1970s, attempts had been made to standardize the designs using three different systems entitled Best Buy, Harness and Nucleus, which were intended to cut the design cost and, in the case of Harness and Nucleus, to permit phased construction. Costly monoliths such as the Royal Liverpool Hospital had frightened the DHSS and health authorities alike. The paper proposed that district general hospitals should not normally exceed 600 beds and that smaller hospitals should be retained wherever 'sensible and practicable'.

The 1945/46 Hospital Survey[6] had originally outlined the need for four levels of hospital provision at local, district, area and regional levels. Unfortunately despite the 1962 Plan, a systematic approach to hospital provision overall was not implemented. Instead hospital development has been characterized by grand plans which have then been modified and by florid local campaigns to protect much loved if sometimes inefficient units. So supporters of local or community hospitals have had to use action politics rather than rational planning to preserve their units. Similarly, medium-sized district general hospitals (of which there are 30 in England with under 300 beds, serving more remote communities) have found that their future has had to rely on becoming a distant satellite of a much larger hospital. Setting up NHS trusts made matters worse as it established competition rather than co-operation between hospitals, as each tried to maximize its earnings and expand its business against a background of declining bed numbers, brought about by faster throughput and increased emphasis on non-hospital treatment.

9.2   PLANNING PROCEDURES, POLICIES AND PRIORITIES

Throughout the 1960s it was becoming apparent that systematic planning could not take place in a vacuum. The needs of all patients had to be reviewed in co-operation with other branches of the NHS, particularly local health authorities and family doctors. The tripartite separation was proving a serious impediment to effective planning.

The Ministry of Health had published a local authority planning document in 1963 entitled *Health and Welfare – the Development of Community Care*[7], but it was much less directive than the 1962 Plan, because local authorities were more autonomous than Regional Hospital

Boards. The 1974 reorganization of the NHS was, therefore, not founded on much experience of systematic planning. Hospital management committees had been content to run hospitals on a day-to-day basis; they had few ideas about what was needed in the future. For most administrators, plans still meant bricks and mortar only. The 1974 reorganization tried to change this by differentiating between two types of administration: one concerned with operational management (mostly in the districts) and the other concerned with planning (mostly at the AHAs). Because this broad classification was too crude and simplistic, it never worked in practice, and was a key reason for the abolition of AHAs in 1982.

However, because planning was made an obligatory function, the DHSS did try to provide advice on procedures and policies. First the policies. *Priorities for Health and Personal Social Services in England* (known as the Priorities document) was published in 1976[8]. Its aim was to make the priorities of the government more explicit while acknowledging the ever-present constraints, and to state that planning was a 'co-operative enterprise', involving the various tiers of the DHSS and NHS as well as local authorities and voluntary bodies. Only through this form of extended discussion could choices be made. Barbara Castle, the Secretary of State, emphasized that 'choice is never easy, but choose we must'. The document was anchored on the assumption that, if authorities were given more of the facts, they would decide upon priorities more effectively. Studies of policy implementation suggest that so simple a model of rational planning was out of touch with reality. *The Way Forward*, in 1977[9], was less specific about rates of growth of services and more vague about time-scales, while encouraging a continuing debate on priorities. Nevertheless, the general focus on planning remained. AHAs began to provide guidelines for their districts, collating district plans and developing fruitful relationships with local authorities, particularly social services departments.

One intended encouragement to the authorities to plan was the DHSS's changes to the rules for allocating resources to them. The adoption of the recommendations of the Resource Allocation Working Party report (RAWP)[10] in 1976 required RHAs to think much more carefully about how they were spending their money. Those RHAs expecting to gain under RAWP clearly were encouraged, but the losers, particularly the London regions, had to examine their services with even greater rigour if the planned cuts were not to have a devastating effect.

Joint financing was first introduced in 1976[11]; it provided earmarked money for schemes jointly agreed between health authorities and social services departments. In the following year a further DHSS circular outlined in some detail the arrangements for joint financing of both capital and revenue schemes[12]. This initiative made a substantial difference to relationships between health authorities and local government. No longer did co-operation rely almost entirely on good faith as there was now extra money, destined for agreed schemes. Initial caution on the part of the authorities meant that not all of them made

See Chapter 8 for details of RAWP

use of the joint finance funds they were offered. In 1979 and 1983 further amendments were made to overcome these problems, particularly by extending the period over which schemes could be financed from this special allocation.

The detailed arrangements are described in Chapter 8

Another policy initiative of the 1970s was *Prevention and Health: Everybody's Business*, in 1976[13]. Health promotion had never been made an explicit priority in plans, thus ignoring a key goal of the 1946 NHS Act. This was despite considerable improvments in the health of the nation. As the document pointed out, the death rate from tuberculosis and the other main infectious diseases had been substantially reduced. But these gains had unmasked other health problems which needed to be tackled, and the document called for discussion on the remaining and emerging problem areas. Although promoting good health is cost effective overall many of the factors contributing to ill health – poverty, unemployment, environmental pollution, working conditions – are beyond the remit of health authorities, their response has often been lukewarm.

The history of health service planning is a story of optimistic intentions tempered by caution. The 1976 Priorities document, remarkable for its detailed plans, was trimmed a year later by *The Way Forward*. The concern that hospitals were taking too much of the available resources continued through the 1980s. Two early contributions were *Care in Action*[14] and *Care in the Community*[15], both published in 1981. Although *Care in Action* was released before the 1982 reorganization, it was addressed to the chairmen and members of the new district health authorities. The pamphlet, described as a handbook of policies and priorities, aimed to help the DHAs to take local initiatives, make local decisions and shoulder local responsibility. Local decision-making was the general theme of the 1982 reorganization, a reaction against the results of the top-heavy 1974 formula. A separate (and shorter) preface was addressed to chairmen and members of social services committees, emphasizing the responsibility of DHAs to collaborate with social services committees and departments. *Care in Action* differed from the 1976 Priorities document in its focus on the range of options for health provision. The importance of the potential contribution from the voluntary and private sectors was underlined. This theme of partnership was to be developed more strongly in later documents. *Care in Action* also stressed the need for greater efficiency so that more patients could be seen for the same financial outlay.

9.2.1 Care in the Community

Community care was believed by many to be not only a more humane alternative to institutional care but also as a cheaper option (this belief was unsubstantiated). *Care in the Community* stated strongly that most people needing long-term care would prefer to remain at home as long as possible, a view well supported by current opinion, but also fuelled by the less altruistic view that it would be cheaper to reduce the capital costs and a substantial proportion of the revenue costs of running these buildings. Voluntary organizations were seen as being able to play an important part in contributing services to support the community. In 1983, the circular confirming the principles of *Care in the Community* allowed health authorities to extend the joint financing arrangements to voluntary bodies as well as social services departments. The circular went further by recommending that control of long-stay hospitals could be transferred to local authorities in order to accelerate the discharge of people from health authority administered institutional care. These two DHSS initiatives, however, neglected the crucial message of the Working Group on Inequalities in Health, in 1980 (Black report)[16], which called for a frank recognition of the links between standards of health and social class. It declared the pressing need for significant targeted funds, over many years, to reverse fundamentally some of the greatest deprivation.

Following the 1982 reorganization, planning took a new direction. The comprehensive overview of the service, relying on national norms for each care group, had proved inflationary, encouraging an over-provision of facilities and manpower which had become increasingly embarrassing to the government. Looking back over the Priorities document, *Care in Action* and other advice of the middle and late 1970s, it was plain that everything had become a priority. Realism now demanded less idealistic plans, particularly as the national economy had not improved as expected. The report of the NHS Management Inquiry (Griffiths report)[17] argued for making decisions more quickly and ensuring that they were implemented. This meant tackling the over-elaborate planning process that had been fostered since 1974 and was, by the mid-1980s, proving counterproductive. There was increasing emphasis on partnership, outcomes and decision-making. Efficiency means doing the same for less or doing more for the same. Partnership means getting voluntary bodies and the private sector to contribute to health care. Outcomes were provided in the health targets set by *The Health of the Nation*[18].

9.2.2   Planning teams

The 1974 reorganization created the first serious attempt to plan on a multi-disciplinary basis. Prior to this, most disciplines did not bother to plan rationally or, if they did, failed to take all interests into account. Health Care Planning Teams (HCPTs) were set up in 1974 to draw together professionals concerned with particular groups of clients or patients. The idea was that each team should examine the existing level of service and make recommendations to the District Management Team (DMT) for improvements. The teams were formally approved by the AHA, but, in practice, membership and scope were decided and arranged by DMTs to whom HCPTs reported. In 1977, HCPTs changed their title to District Planning Teams (DPTs) but their function remained the same. The 1974 reorganization also created Joint Consultative Committees (JCCs) within each area, made up of members of county or metropolitan district councils and health authorities. These committees were serviced by the Area Team of Officers. Due to the workload of implementing the reorganization, these planning teams were slow to get under way. In March 1975, the DHSS published a comprehensive handbook called *Guide to Planning in the National Health Service*[19], which set out the detailed tasks to be performed at each level in the structure and explained the concepts of annual and strategic planning. The Guide was implemented in 1976 by a publication called the *NHS Planning System*[20].

A key to effective planning has always been collaboration with local authorities but this was always problematic. There were political, cultural and financial obstacles. Governments attempted to overcome these with a stream of reports, circulars and directions. In 1977 the DHSS required health and local authorities, with the advice of the JCC, to set up Joint Care Planning Teams (JCPTs). Unlike the non-executive JCC, these new teams were to be made up of officers of the respective authorities and included, wherever appropriate, officers from housing, social and health services. The JCPTs could also include nominees from voluntary organizations and consumer groups. Because they crossed the health and local authority boundary these teams could only be advisory, not executive. Each JCPT advised its JCC, which in turn made proposals to its respective authorities. In some cases joint financing was very slow because the AHA or social services committees might reject the proposals conducted under the auspices of this system. Both JCPTs and DPTs needed information to do their work effectively, but found it was not always available in a useful form. This contributed to the complete review of NHS information undertaken by the Körner Committee[21].

Thus an elaborate infrastructure was established. The NHS Planning System endorsed the 1972 proposals for an annual planning cycle which, modelled on the public expenditure parliamentary system (see Section 8.2), prepared and processed plans at certain times of the year, allowing district plans, for instance, to arrive at the region in time (it was thought) to influence budget allocations for the following financial year, and also to give an indication of other developments requiring regional involvement. The advent of RAWP made the system of bidding for funds less significant because it proposed a formula for the allocation of resources. In the event, RAWP proved slow to implement at district level. As a result of the 1990 Act, it was abandoned before equity of allocation had been achieved. This goal returned in Labour's proposals.

See Chapter 8 for full details

As early as 1979, *Patients First* had acknowledged that the new planning system was not fulfilling its role. Its introduction had varied between regions, some of them enthusiastically producing their own versions of the system. By 1982 there was serious anxiety. The system seemed to encourage self-perpetuating talking shops, and not all districts and regions were committed to making it work properly. Accordingly, the Department of Health introduced a revised planning system. This was necessary in any case, following the abolition of AHAs. The revised system designated the DHA as the basic planning unit for health care and asked them to supply 5-year strategic plans, with annual operational plans derived from them. The advice also suggested annual reviews, but argued for less consultation because this was now deemed too time-consuming. District members succeeded to the AHA places on JCCs. District JCPTs continued. Where there were overlapping boundaries, the District JCPT provided a forum for co-ordinating policies and practices between different social services departments.

The 5-year strategic plan was meant to give a concise summary of 'perceived needs, policies and goals' and to include references to capital and manpower costs. In practice, the traditional split between strategic plans and operational plans continued to cause difficulties. In so far as planning is deciding how tomorrow should be different from today (strategy), the chosen means of achieving that difference (operation) determines what to do. Strategies tended to become compromised by events, and some regions amalgamated the strategic and operational elements of each year's plan. This did not remove the need for districts to make clear their overall direction in their annual plans, which had to be in line with national and regional policies. The system of annual reviews was introduced in 1982 (see Chapter 3) to ensure that districts were conforming. First, the Secretary of State reviewed each region, and then, in turn, the regions reviewed the districts.

9.3   PLANNING FOR COMMISSIONING, PURCHASING AND PROVIDING

The introduction of market competition following the 1990 Act did not remove the need for planning, either at national or local level even though the process lost currency. In due course purchasing became separated from commissioning, acknowledging that commissioning was about strategic direction while purchasing was the process of agreeing contracts. This separation of functions was useful in that it respected GP fundholders' right to decide what their patients needed. Theoretically this should always have been within the context of HAs' plans but HAs only interfered with fundholders' purchasing intentions when they might substantially destabilize health provisions. In fact the power of fundholding GPs has made the HAs much more responsive to their wishes.

See Chapters 5 and 6

Under the 1990 Act NHS trusts are required to produce annual business plans which detail their financial futures, articulate their mission and set out their schemes for service provision and capital investment. Together with projected income streams, this provides the NHS Executive with the core information on which to base decisions about each trust's external financing limit (EFL, see Chapter 8). But these plans must be aligned with the HAs plans and intentions.

HAs are also required to produce an Annual Report prepared by their Director of Public Health. This independent report highlights where the health of the district is giving cause for concern. For instance, heart disease rates or death rates from a particular form of cancer may be higher than average, or infectious disease incidence may be related to a lower than average rate of immunization. The HA can use this report to formulate the priorities their commissioning plans should address. But HAs also have to work with government policies and priorities, which have become increasingly emphatic. Strategic direction from the centre has not declined as the market evolved. Indeed, this could be said to have fatally weakened the market concept by limiting managers' scope for successful trading. Planning regained some of its former value when the competitive ethos of the market was repudiated in 1997.

Under the provisions of *The new NHS*, health authorities are required to produce a health improvement programme jointly agreed with NHS trusts, primary care groups and with social services. The white paper stressed that building planning partnerships and monitoring performance were both crucial. The greater emphasis on accountability implies even more stringent monitoring, to ensure planning works through appraising needs, formulating plans, implementing plans and monitoring of results. Planning systems cannot guarantee results. The gap between intention and achievement can be difficult to bridge in any large organization pursuing complex goals.

The importance of trying to agree compatible plans between health care and social care has been a recurrent theme. During the 1980s report after report stressed the need to work together, culminating in the 1989 white paper *Caring for People*[22]. Seven years later in *The new NHS* the Labour government urged the NHS to work in partnership 'by breaking down organisational barriers and forging stronger links with Local Authorities [so that] the needs of patients will be put at the centre of the care process.'[23]

9.3.1 Community care

In the 1980s the DHSS set up a working party to make sense of the planning muddle by clarifying health and social services responsibilities. Its report, *Planning in Partnership*[24], was published in 1982 but made little impact. The Audit Commission's report *Making a Reality of Community Care*[25] was more outspoken. It castigated all the authorities in detail for their poor performance. For instance, there had been little overall increase in the support given to elderly people requiring home helps or meals on wheels. These simple services are widely recognized as effective in enabling elderly people to live at home rather than needing hospital or residential care.

The Audit Commission examined the more fundamental issue of the rundown of hospitals for the mentally ill and those with learning disabilities. Patients were too often discharged without adequate community support and left dependent and vulnerable. This short-sightedness and inhumanity fuelled regrets that the closure of the larger institutions had been encouraged. These clearly had provided a relatively better quality of life, despite their size and dilapidation, than the isolated existence that many discharged patients were now forced into. The costs of making community provision for them fell on the social security system in particular, an important factor in persuading the government that the problem would need to be addressed. The money released by closing down large institutions was meant to be used to better effect in the community, but this needed special allocations to bridge the period of transition and then better organization of community support. Landlords could abuse the system by charging excessive rents because the social security payments had no upper limits for individuals in private accommodation. Payments were subsequently fixed according to the individual's degree of physical dependency and their personal financial position.

The Audit Commission drew attention to the confusion about which agency should be in charge of what services, and strongly urged that lead responsibility should be unambiguously assigned, in order to stop the 'passing the buck' it believed to be rife. The government's response was to turn to Sir Roy Griffiths again, whose first report on the organization of the management of the NHS it regarded as such a success. Griffiths' second report, *Community Care; Agenda for Action*[26], appeared in March 1988 and was far less radical than his first. He did not really offer solutions to the problems but rearranged them by introducing arbitrary new definitions of health care and social care. He said more attention should be paid to the individual and less to the organization, and to making voluntary or private care equally available alongside statutory provision. The state was not to interfere as much as it had done; rather it should adopt an enabling role, fully in line with the government's overall philosophy. However, clear direction was needed, from a minister with particular responsibility for formulating objectives and monitoring results. Griffiths favoured transferring the management of community care to local authority social services departments, and it may have been this, as well as his rather vague financial proposals, which delayed the government's response.

Eventually, the white paper *Caring for People: Community Care in the Next Decade and Beyond*[27] was published in November 1989. It presented a new concept of case management, whereby each person requiring care is assessed, often by a multi-disciplinary process, prior to the preparation of their individual care package. Clients' own views were to be taken into account, but they would no longer receive payments from the social security office. Instead, the money was to be administered by social services departments, who were to use means tests to establish client eligibility and provide a more sensitive and economical use of funds. One of the government's concerns had been the huge growth in payments from the Exchequer via the social security system into private and voluntary nursing and residential care over the previous decade – a subsidy estimated at over £1 billion[28]. The doctrine of separating purchasing and providing, central to *Working for Patients*, was also prominent here: social services departments were encouraged to give up their direct management of residential accommodation and to buy what they needed from the independent sector. To ensure standards were maintained in this 'arm's length' arrangement, they were required to set up inspection and regulation systems along the lines of those used by health authorities in relation to private nursing homes.

As the Audit Commission recommended, the white paper allocated lead responsibility to social services departments, who took on the prime responsibility for people with learning disability, while using health service staff in a specialist role. The problems of patients discharged from long-stay mental illness hospitals were acknowledged, and a new grant was introduced to enable social services departments to improve community services in advance of patients being discharged.

The main criticism of the white paper was the lack of convincing financial detail. Some feared that social services departments might run out of money before the end of the year and, to avoid this, would accept lower standards. The 1990 Act, which implemented the new arrangements, did not clarify this. Subsequent statements by ministers and the DoH implied that in assessing clients' needs, social services departments should be aware of the limits to their budgets. Finance, not need, was the ultimate constraint on care. *Caring for Patients* was finally implemented in 1992, with the means testing element only being felt by patients and their carers in 1994 when local authorities started to charge for services previously provided at no cost. However, the criteria to be used in deciding what was a HA responsibility and what was social services' had to be negotiated locally and this led to anomalies.

Increasingly, elderly people and their relatives have become aware that they are now expected to pay for their care in old age, if they can afford to. This betrayal (as many see it) of the fundamental NHS principle that care should be free at the point of need has fuelled a significant political debate which the 1997 Labour government attempted to defuse by setting up a Royal Commission.

The remainder of this chapter discusses each care group in more detail, examining policy intentions and what has been achieved through the implementation of these policies.

The Royal Commission on the Elderly was announced in December 1997, chaired by Sir Stewart Sutherland. It reported in March 1999

9.4 PRIMARY CARE

Primary care covers both clients and patients. It refers to the work undertaken by general practitioners and other community staff in maintaining health and supporting the ill when out of hospital. First, the maintenance of health. This is supported on a national basis through such public health measures as clean air regulations, proper sewerage systems, environmental health inspection and through occupational health services and systematic surveillance of babies and children. All children can be immunized against infectious diseases, although this is not obligatory. The environmental health services, rather surprisingly, have never been formally integrated with the NHS, except that the Director of Public Health often acts as the named officer responsible to local authorities for giving medical advice. He or she will sometimes also act as the local authority's agent in implementing such regulations as those governing the transfer of someone with an infectious disease to a hospital for treatment.

It is difficult to define the proper limits on the extent of the functions

See Chapter 6 for the organization of primary care

of the health service. No one would suggest that the NHS should try to tackle bad housing or unemployment, even though both are proven contributory causes of ill-health. The public health programme of the last 150 years is a success story. In the UK, clean water is now universally available and cholera totally eliminated. Similarly, enteric fevers such as typhoid are rare. A century ago four babies in every ten did not survive childhood and maternal mortality was common. Now there are fewer than 50 maternal deaths per year. The infant mortality rate (deaths per thousand live births) is 6.0 (1996) – it was about double that in 1976 and three times higher in 1960. Immunization programmes have controlled many infectious diseases, and smallpox has been eradicated worldwide. In the UK, diphtheria, polio and scarlet fever are relatively rare, and measles and whooping cough much diminished.

Nevertheless, there is no room for complacency. Tuberculosis, thought to have been almost eliminated, has shown a recent increase. The steady control of air pollution following the Clean Air Act, 1958, has become more difficult with the increase in traffic in cities and with other more complex pollutants. There is a significant increase in childhood asthma. Even more disturbing has been the increase in the number of reported cases of food poisoning – 77,557 in 1996. Indeed, the greatest public health scares of the last few years have all centred on food, its production and its preparation for consumption. Notable have been the revelations that most mass-produced poultry and eggs may be contaminated with salmonella and bacteria, while beef may cause *E. coli* poisoning or be the source of CJD (Creutzfeldt–Jacob disease) via cattle infected with BSE (bovine spongiform encephalopathy).

Overall life expectancy has increased during the last 50 years (Table 9.1), partly due to primary care services' efforts to prevent and treat ill-health. Primary health care is now much better organized, with the majority of GPs working in group practices supported by teams of other health professionals and by social workers. Most practices have attached nurses trained in community care, health visitors and midwives. They have direct access to physiotherapy, chiropody, language and hearing therapy, occupational therapy. It is not uncommon to have a counselling service.

But preventing illness is not the only responsibility. The other work relates to the care and treatment of those who are ill. Only 12% of patients attending their GP will end up in a hospital out-patients, clinic and only 2% in a hospital bed. Following the changes brought in by the 1990 Act and the new 1990 GP contract, NHS trusts and GPs alike have incentives to introduce a wider range of patient services in primary care, for instance minor surgery and consultant clinics at the surgery as well as

Table 9.1

Life expectancy (England and Wales)

	1951	1995
Men	65.8	74.4
Women	70.8	79.6

sessions from complementary therapies such as acupuncture and hypnotherapy. In addition to GP surgeries and health centres, there may be other clinics run in suitable community facilities such as church or school halls but this is becoming rarer as GP premises are improved. The majority are looked after by the primary care team, headed by a general practitioner.

See Chapter 12 for details of professional services in primary care

The emphasis on the desirability of looking after patients in their own homes arises not only because of the high cost of hospitalization but because removing the patient, particularly the very old and very young, from home may create serious social and psychological difficulties. Young children can become badly distressed unless their parents are able to accompany them to the hospital and remain with them. Some elderly people admitted to hospital become observably more confused and dependent there. Attempts have been made to look after severely ill patients at home through 'Hospital at Home' schemes[29] but this is probably less cost effective than hospitalization; making the most economic use of professional time is difficult in such circumstances.

9.4.1   Family planning services

Family planning services are obtainable either from the GP at the surgery or from clinics run in other premises by NHS trusts or by contracted agencies such as the Family Planning Association or the Brook Advisory Centres for young people. These independent agencies also provide abortion facilities for those women having difficulty because of the consultant's opposition or because the NHS is unable to provide an adequate service. Male and female sterilization does not require hospital admission. Some health authorities fund Well Woman clinics. These provide a screening service, including smear tests to check whether cancer is present in the cervix, routine breast screening and advice about regular personal health checks. A similar service for men is usually only available in the private sector.

9.5   PREVENTION OF ILL HEALTH

The maintenance of health was a fundamental principle of the 1946 NHS Act. Conflicts of interest account in part for successive governments' weakness in tackling prevention. They do not wish to offend those commercial concerns who contribute to the country's wealth or to forego the tax revenues from the sale of admittedly harmful products. The role of the Health Education Authority reflects this dilemma.

It took 20 years for the Health Education Council to be established (1968) as a government-funded body. Until 1973 its medical research division conducted studies on such issues as the incidence of gonorrhoea, participation in measles immunization programmes and the causes of accidents at home. In 1987 it was renamed the Health Education Authority and given special health authority status, bringing it more closely under DoH control. It has been accused of being unduly

Figure 9.1

Main causes of death

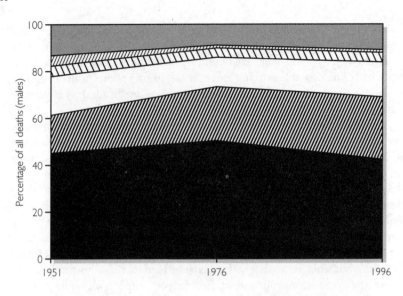

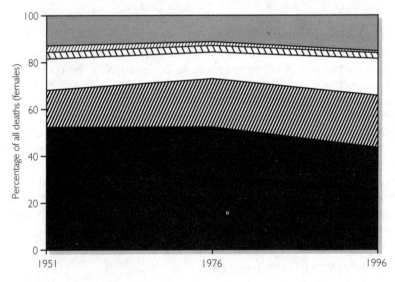

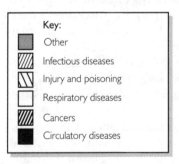

Source: compiled using data from the Office for National Statistics

compliant to the government's wish not to make enemies in the business world. Nevertheless it developed several national campaigns, such as 'Look After Your Heart', which helped to raise the public's consciousness of avoidable ill health. It was still criticized for failing to be effective, and in the early 1990s its future was uncertain. By 1998 it was still in existence as a special health authority.

How is effectiveness to be judged in this area? *Prevention and Health: Everybody's Business*[30] gave examples of successes, many of which resulted from public health measures initiated in the nineteenth century. In the twentieth century, immunization programmes and new drugs have helped to bring about further reductions in the incidence of disease. Disconcertingly, as one problem has been tackled another has arisen: young children survive to become part of an increasingly elderly population which makes new and greater demands on services; and, over time, the general pattern of illness and disease changes.

Governments have been unwilling to face the short-term unpopularity that some health-promoting measures may incur. For example, the protracted campaign to introduce legislation making the wearing of car seat belts compulsory could have been significantly shortened if support from health ministers had been unequivocal. Clear evidence from other countries was disputed by many MPs who preferred to discuss the issue as a question of infringement of personal liberty. The substantial reduction in serious and costly accidents since the law has been implemented shows the price of that extended discussion. Similar equivocation concerning banning tobacco advertising should also be costed in terms of avoidable illness and premature deaths.

A more targeted approach was forced on the government by the emergence of AIDS. There was a massive media campaign and earmarked funds. The success of this approach is easier to assess, but the expected explosion of the disease has not happened (Table 9.2) and health authorities have been able to reduce the facilities made available for patients with this disease. Improved drug regimens have also helped.

On the whole, it is left to pressure groups to remind the community of the risks associated with various lifestyles and the measures they can take to protect themselves. As in other industrialized nations, notably the USA, promoting good health has become more acceptable. Interest in physical fitness programmes, better diet, reducing smoking and excessive

Road deaths declined from 6352 in 1979 to 3599 in 1998

Smoking is estimated to cost the NHS between £1.54 and £1.7 billion each year and causes about 92,000 deaths (DoH briefing, November 1997)

	1985	1995
AIDS diagnosed cases	236	1524
HIV positive	2528	2225
Exposure category (%)		
Homosexual	67	57
Heterosexual	2	32
Injecting drug use	4	6
Contaminated blood	24	1

Source: government statistics

Table 9.2

AIDS in the UK

consumption of alcohol is growing. Health authorities were encouraged to set up health education departments in 1974[31]. 'Health promotion' and 'positive health' initiatives in the style of commercial advertising campaigns are needed to overcome the fatalistic attitude of the public. Young women have been seemingly impervious to the risks of smoking and young men to the increased cancer risk associated with unprotected sunbathing.

Prevention and Health, although a useful review, ended lamely by encouraging further discussion on ways in which people might help themselves to become fitter. It suggested that authorities should take action 'with whatever resources can be made available'. Over the years the problem has remained the same: the rhetoric of health promotion has often failed to engage with the population in general. Even within the NHS many see health promotion as an 'extra', which can be curtailed in times of financial difficulty. Governments also react in this way, which explains why the important messages of the Black report were ignored by the government in 1980. Cost implications were allowed to become obstacles to implementation.

Rather more positive government advice was contained in *Care in Action* (1981)[32], which specifically set out the components of a local strategy for health authorities to pursue. The issues to be addressed by this strategy included a policy on smoking, the development of genetic counselling and family planning, improvement in school health services, the extension of immunization, a programme for reducing heart disease, better health education in schools (particularly covering smoking and alcohol use), nutrition and preparation for parenthood, the reduction of accidents on the road and in the home, a renewed attempt to fluoridate water supplies, and further encouragement to maximize the contribution from voluntary, community and commercial organizations to improve health care. *The Health of the Nation*[33] (1992) stated the Conservative government's commitment to health promotion and disease prevention although, again, this did not extend to banning tobacco advertising. Labour's *Our Healthier Nation*[34] (1998) reiterated much the same messages that had been around for over 20 years.

Apart from support (stopping well short of legislation) for fluoridation, successive governments have neglected prevention of dental ill-health. The British Dental Association, in a submission to the Secretary of State in 1983[35], pointed out that the escalation of dental charges amounted to dental practitioners becoming 'tax collectors for the NHS'. This was acting as a deterrent to effective dental care, particularly among those most at risk. As a result, it was increasingly difficult to fulfil the DHSS Dental Strategy Review Group's aim of 'providing the opportunity for everyone to retain healthy functional dentition for life, by preventing what is preventable and by containing the remaining disease or deformity by the efficient use and distribution of treatment resources' (1981). The new dentists' contract attempted to move dental practice towards a preventive approach (rather than 'drill and fill') through financial incentives. One result was significant withdrawal of dentists

Fluoride added to the public water system reduces dental decay significantly; however, some see it as a pollutant

from NHS work (although this was also attributed to poor rates of remuneration).

Internationally, the World Health Organization (WHO) tries to encourage governments to do more. In 1985 it published *Health for All 2000*[36], an initiative to reduce the level of sickness world-wide by the complete elimination of some diseases. The WHO is also concerned to reduce inequalities and to reorientate health services towards primary care. It launched the *Healthy Cities Project*[37] in 1984. Compared with others, the UK has no excuse to be complacent as long as it continues to rate badly for heart disease and in relation to low standards of environmental health, to give but two examples.

Not all health risks can be dealt with by health promotion initiatives. Altering personal behaviour to reduce avoidable disease is notoriously difficult. The Comptroller and Auditor General calculated, in 1989, that the 180,000 deaths per annum from heart disease (27% of the total) cost the UK £500 million. Heart disease is heavily influenced by smoking and bad diet. The campaign to reduce smoking has been relatively successful; less than a third of the population now smokes. Improving diet has proved to be the more difficult aspect, although other Western countries have shown impressive reductions in heart disease where governments have been determined to change eating patterns away from highly saturated fat products. In the UK, the official approach to alcohol consumption has also been ambivalent even though the health cost to the nation of alcohol-related illness is large. A Royal College of Physicians report in 1987[38] reckoned that over 20% of all hospital admissions were alcohol-related.

9.6   HEALTH AND SAFETY AT WORK

A separate but linked aspect of health promotion exists in the occupational health services. Until recently there were enormous gaps in checks on the provision of safe and healthy working environments. Responsibility rested outside the NHS, shared between several government departments which organized inspectorates (alkali, clean air, explosives, factories, mines and quarries and nuclear installations). These were not uniformly effective, and the legislation did not require employers to inform their employees of the risks entailed in working under exposure to various dusts, fumes and chemical substances, nor to inform those who were not their employees of the risks entailed in entering such working environments. Occupational health services were set up independently by a number of firms and industries, but it was estimated that only 65% of factories with 100 or fewer employees had the service of a full-time or part-time doctor. Occupational health services were not included in the remit of the NHS in 1948, and many feel that this has led to their neglect and a poor understanding of their relevance to patterns of health and illness.

Originally an appointed factory doctor service was run by the Ministry of Labour, but it was only in 1973 that the Employment

See Chapters 6 and 12 for further details of dental services

Medical Advisory Service came into being. This was designed to work through the Department of Employment to provide advice to ministers, employers, trades unions and other interested parties on occupational health and hygiene, and medical aspects of training and rehabilitation. Only about 120 doctors were involved in this service all over the country, the Department of Employment taking the view that engineers, chemists and other specialists, rather than doctors, had the expertise to assess and change the working environment. In 1972 the Robens Committee published its report, *Safety and Health at Work*[39], and, 3 years later, its full proposals were embodied in the Health and Safety at Work Act, 1974, which unified responsibility for co-ordinating services with the Health and Safety Commission – an independent body with representatives from employer and employee organizations and the local authorities. The Commission took over the work of the Employment Medical Advisory Service and the former inspectorates, and operates through the Health and Safety Executive, which employs inspectors, engineers and doctors to enforce the application of the Act's provisions. Under these, all employers, employees and self-employed people (except domestic workers in private employment) are protected in the work setting, and risks to the health and safety of the general public arising from work environments must be prevented. This includes control of noise, emission of fumes, handling toxic materials and the risks of specific working environments.

The Act operates through a series of codes of practice and requires employers to maintain safe plant and equipment, safe systems of work and premises, to arrange for adequate training, instruction and super-vision, to provide facilities and arrangements for employees' welfare at work, to lay down a health and safety policy in writing and to inform employees about it. The legislation also covers all staff and practitioners in the NHS for the first time, and the Department of Health issues guidance from time to time relating to the particular hazards of work in the NHS.

Obviously, occupational health services vary: the requirements of heavy manufacturing industries will differ from those of non-mechanized service enterprises. Some firms have provided services far beyond the legal requirements, and have delegated responsibilities to special fire and safety officers and appointed medical advisers. In October 1978, regula-tions came into force enabling safety representatives and committees to be appointed by employees. These have the power to make regular inspections and reports on conditions in the workplace, to take the advice of health and safety inspectors and make representations to the management. The health and safety legislation can improve conditions over time, and create greater awareness of avoidable hazards.

The NHS used to be largely exempt from health and safety legislation by virtue of Crown immunity. This asssumed it was impractical, in legal terms, for the Crown, the legislature, to prosecute a state-run organi-zation for non-compliance: the Crown could not prosecute itself. The National Health Service (Amendment) Act, 1986, started the process of removing this exemption. First came the right of the Health and Safety Executive's inspectors, working closely with local authority environmental health officers, to check on food hygiene in hospital kitchens. By 1991, health authorities and trusts could no longer claim exemption from the recommendations of fire inspectors; this has proved expensive as they are obliged to improve fire escapes in old hospitals. Another important piece of legislation affecting hospitals is the Control of Substances Hazardous to Health Regulations[40], which impose a duty on all employers to protect their staff from exposure to contamination of various kinds. The full cost of removing Crown immunity for the health service is likely to be considerable, but it brings the NHS up to the standards required of other employers and service providers.

9.7 ACUTE HOSPITAL SERVICES

Although it is the stated objective of the NHS to promote health, the fact remains that most of its resources are devoted to the care and treatment of those who are sick and who are treated in hospital. The definition 'acute services' covers all urgent or serious episodes of ill health, and generally excludes routine services for children and the elderly (although children and old people may become acutely ill), women having babies, the mentally ill, the physically handicapped and those with learning disabilities. There are about 108,000 beds available for acute care. Acute services alone absorb some 49% of the total health budget.

How is acute care provided? In cases that are not emergencies, the GP refers the patient to a hospital consultant for advice about symptoms or for treatment that requires the consultant's special skills. The consultant has undertaken extensive training in his or her own speciality and has expert knowledge, access to sophisticated equipment and facilities and, in the case of the surgeon, particular technical skills. For those patients involved in accidents or sudden collapse, referral from a GP is not necessary and they can be taken directly to the accident and emergency department of the district general hospital or to the casualty department of the local GP hospital. Non-emergency, but not necessarily non-urgent, patients are referred by a GP to a specific consultant or group of consultants working in the appropriate speciality. The patient is given an appointment in the out-patient department, which is usually held at the district general hospital. In some districts, it may be at the GP hospital or health centre. The consultant, or another doctor in their medical team, examines the patient and makes a diagnosis, with the help of various tests and procedures such as blood, urine or tissue analysis, X-ray and other methods of body and organ scanning. This may require several hospital visits as an out-patient and sometimes in-patient treatment will then be prescribed. Treatment may involve invasive procedures such as surgery or radiotherapy or may be based on drugs. Supportive treatments from physiotherapists or occupational therapists are also available.

Table 9.3

Hospital attendances 1996/97
(England)

In-patients	8,381,000
Accident and emergency – new attendances	12,439,000
Out patients – first attendances	11,298,000

Source: *Government expenditure plans 1998/99* (Cm 3912)

Once the patient's condition has improved sufficiently, the consultant will discharge him or her back to the general practitioner. Florence Nightingale defined discharge from hospital as 'dead', 'well' or 'relieved', and the outcome must still be one of these. Although the percentage of the population admitted to hospital has remained constant at 9%, the distribution has changed markedly since 1982 (Table 9.4).

This change in case mix has a significant effect on workload. During the same period length of stay for acute patients decreased from 8.9 days to just over 5 (see also Section 9.7.2).

Table 9.4

Age groups admitted to hospital
(% of UK population)

	1982	1994
Under 5	13	8
Over 75	13	18

Source: Office of Health Economics (1997)
Compendium of Health Statistics. OHE, London

9.7.1 Cost effectiveness

See further discussion of effectiveness and audit in Chapter 10

The cost effectiveness of acute care is a controversial topic. Patients are submitted to an increasing array of sophisticated treatments at great expense to the NHS and yet the outcome may well be inconclusive. Nevertheless, patients' support for what doctors want is demonstrated by the enthusiasm for raising money for high-technology medical equipment. New procedures may well be less troublesome for the patient and may greatly improve accuracy of diagnosis and treatment. For instance, patients found air encephalograms (in which air was introduced into the cavities of the brain to demonstrate the presence or otherwise of a tumour) acutely uncomfortable, leaving them with a headache for several days. This has been replaced by computed tomography (CT) and magnetic resonance imaging (MRI), which give the doctor more information and subject the patient to no more discomfort than he or she would have from a routine X-ray.

The introduction of fibre-optics has enabled surgeons to perform keyhole surgery – operations on organs inside the body without having to open the patient's abdomen.

One of the most notable successes of the last 25 years has been joint replacement, particularly the hip. This has been achieved by the anaesthetist and orthopaedic surgeon working together with the instrument and prosthesis maker. With improved control over drugs and gases, the anaesthetist can now anaesthetize patients of any age without undue risk.

Orthopaedic surgeons have perfected the technique of joint replacement with the result that many elderly people, previously disabled and immobilized by degenerating joints, can continue to be active and independent.

New drugs have also had remarkable effects, but, at the same time, there have been a few controversial failures. There is also disturbing evidence of drug-induced illness due to side effects or the prescribing of unsuitable combinations of drugs. Nevertheless, compared with pre-NHS days, acutely ill or injured patients now usually have every chance of receiving a high standard of care and treatment wherever they are in the UK.

9.7.2   Targets

The 1976 Priorities document was the first realistic attempt to set targets for acute care in terms other than the number of beds in a hospital. It argued that there should be slower growth of resources for this service so that more could be done for the less advantaged services. The document endorsed the idea that the district general hospital should provide for the usual range of medical and surgical patients, as well as having a maternity unit, a psychiatric unit, a geriatric unit and children's department. Most DGHs have full-scale accident and emergency departments, and some also have ear, nose and throat and eye units. A few centres have more specialized departments, such as radiotherapy and neurosurgery. The Priorities document drew attention to important trends, many of which are still in progress. A key one is inpatients' length of stay. It has been reduced quite remarkably (Table 9.5). This is due to changes in medical practice, such as the earlier mobilization of surgical patients, new surgical techniques such as laser treatment for certain ophthalmic problems, which allow patients to be seen as day cases, and possibly also to general improvements in the home environment.

Key reference: DHSS (1976) *Priorities for Health and Personal Social Services in England. A consultative document.* HMSO, London.

Second, medical technology has continued to develop too fast for the NHS to be able to cope sensibly. The Priorities document said that the pressure to adopt new techniques and equipment had to be controlled, otherwise it would push up costs per case, even though patients might have to stay in hospital for fewer days. In the 1990s there was a growing recognition that medical practice needed to be scrutinized more openly and that evidence of effectiveness had to be taken into account. This has

1957	21
1976	10
1998	5

Table 9.5

Length of stay in hospital (average days, England)

not slowed the development of medical technology, the cost of which has been largely hidden. Probably much of the money released by the reduction of long-stay beds has been absorbed by the acute services.

The Priorities document listed the main areas of concern as reducing waiting-times; continuing with efforts to reduce the unequal distribution of services; facilitating medical advances; improving services for the elderly and for rehabilitation. How far have these aims been pursued?

9.7.3   Waiting lists

Success stimulates its own demand, and the NHS has failed lamentably to keep pace with that demand. So national waiting lists for surgical operations in 1998 stood at over 1 million despite the exhortations of successive government ministers. There is considerable controversy about the significance of long waiting lists in themselves[41]. Waiting lists represent the quantity of demand that it would ideally be reasonable to meet, whereas waiting times are ultimately within management's control. Many feel that waiting time should be seen as the more significant indicator. In any case, despite the waiting lists, urgency as determined by the severity of the condition still ultimately decides how soon most patients are admitted to hospital care.

There have been periods when the NHS's response has been fatalistic but successive governments have been determined to improve the situation. No other country experiences the same difficulties as the UK in regard to waiting lists. Whether lasting reform can be achieved, given the same levels of demand, without significant increases in funding is doubted by many. Nevertheless, this defeatism was rejected in 1990, when the Chief Executive of the NHSME suggested that if managers failed to reduce waiting lists, then their performance-related pay would suffer. In 1998 the Secretary of State for Health, Frank Dobson, reiterated this threat.

9.7.4   Inequalities

The unequal distribution of acute services was arguably exacerbated by the internal market, because competition provoked opportunism. This meant that the services being offered were not necessarily the most needed. The 1997 Labour government vowed (once again) to make the NHS a more equitable service.

See Chapter 14

9.8   MOTHERS AND BABIES

More pregnant women than ever before are now likely to have a satisfactory outcome to their pregnancy. The perinatal mortality rate has steadily declined and now rests at 8.7 per 1000 births (1996 figures) – Box 9.2.

However, this is still not as good a figure as that achieved by other Western countries, notably Sweden. Care of the pregnant woman is one of the areas most able to benefit from efforts made by professional health staff. Examination early in pregnancy by the GP and consultant obstetrician, regular supervision by the midwife and attendance at

Stillbirth	Baby delivered dead after 24 or more weeks' gestation.	
Perinatal mortality	Baby dying in the first week of life plus still births.	
Neonatal mortality	Baby dying in the first 4 weeks of life.	
Infant mortality	Baby dying in the first year of life.	

Box 9.2

Births and infant deaths

antenatal clinics, together with routine scanning and, in cases of risk, amniocentesis (testing the amniotic fluid surrounding the fetus for genetic abnormalities such as Down's syndrome and spina bifida) have all improved the chances of a successful birth and a healthy baby. The reduction in the number of unsatisfactory births (those with a suspect physical prognosis or just unwanted births) has been brought about by regularization of abortion facilities following the 1967 Abortion Act. Women are now able to obtain abortions fairly easily and it is estimated that up to one-fifth of all pregnancies are now terminated within the first few months. Therapeutic terminations of pregnancy are allowable at any point of gestation but are medically more risky as the pregnancy develops. The overall number of abortions notified in 1996 was 168,000.

Between 1971 and 1996, the UK's birth rate fell from 901,600 to 733,400. However, more babies survive than ever before: over the same period infant mortality fell from 17.9 per 1000 births to 6.1. The Priorities document emphasized the need for further improvement in special care facilities for newborn babies. Twenty years later there is a network of intensive care units based in the larger district general hospitals. This may mean that parents have to travel some distance to be with their child but the concentration of skills in one place assures sophisticated treatment. These units are run by a team of specialist paediatricians, anaesthetists and nurses with special training. The survival rate of premature and low birthweight and handicapped babies has increased, and this in turn has increased the survival rates of vulnerable individuals who may need further care later in life.

Some would argue that not all the changes are good for the mother. There has been continuing criticism that enforcing hospital deliveries causes a less than satisfactory experience for the mother. This was recognized in the 1993 *Changing Childbirth*[42] report. It followed a detailed report by the Social Services Select Committee[43], which had argued for more choice for mothers without sacrificing the safety of herself or her baby. There was a danger of over-medicalizing childbirth. For those with predicted normal births, it was reasonable to leave the midwife in charge provided she had emergency support if needed. In only one area around Bath, the Select Committee noted, had there been a determined attempt to provide mothers with an alternative to a central facility. There, some 33% of births take place in seven local units. Elsewhere a few midwife-led maternity units have been set up, usually in units formerly led by obstetricians. Overall only 2% of births take place at home although this figure is rising each year in response to mothers' demands. The move to hospitalization originally followed the recommendations of the 1959 Cranbrook report[44], at a time when only 60% of births were in hospital and maternal and perinatal mortality were causing concern. In 1970 the Peel report[45] stressed the need for an integrated approach to maternity care, which at that time was more difficult, given the tripartite divisions between the health services.

9.9 CHILDREN

One strong indication of health service effectiveness is the health of children. To oversimplify: a healthy child means a healthy adult. Child care starts by making sure that a baby's health is supervised from birth and that he or she is developing satisfactorily. Routine examinations detect hearing, speech or sight abnormalities, and the child can then be referred for suitable specialist treatment. Once at school, the child is examined by the school doctor at least twice during his or her school career, and has more regular supervision from nurses attached to the schools. Continuous scrutiny by teachers also helps identify health or developmental problems. They can also ask for the help of other health professionals, in particular those concerned with speech and language difficulties and clinical psychologists. Health problems among adolescents, arising from sexual activity or addiction to smoking, drugs or solvent abuse, make especially difficult demands, particularly as parents are not necessarily aware of some of the problems or feel themselves defeated by them. Some children suffer sudden illness and accidents. Over 44% of home accidents happen to children under 15; children are involved in 13% of road accidents.

The accident statistics must be treated with caution. Home accidents represent hospital-treated non-fatal accidents calculated from a sample of 20 hospitals. The road accident figure is calculated from police-reported road accidents

The hospital regime for acutely ill or injured children has changed for the better in the last 40 years. Much of this has resulted from pressure applied by the parents themselves and Action for Sick Children (previously the National Association for the Welfare of Children in Hospitals). Official reports, including the 1959 Platt report on the *Welfare of Children in Hospital*[46] and the Court report (1976) entitled *Fit for the Future*[47], have also been influential. In turn, such reports were influenced by the work of enlightened paediatricians such as McCarthy and Jolly, who did much to make the child's stay in hospital less of an ordeal. Most hospitals now have some facilities for parents wishing to stay with their children in hospital.

McCarthy first developed a mother and child unit at Amersham General in the 1950s

Surgical treatment of children is less common: routine tonsil and adenoid operations are no longer done and, as a result of more widespread dissemination of evidence of the relatively poor medical and cost effectiveness of grommet treatment for persistent glue ear, this operation is also declining. Self-contained children's departments have largely superseded previous arrangements, whereby children needing surgery were usually treated in the adult part of the hospital. With the increasing uptake of immunization, long-term in-patient care for children is now unusual, and the demand for specialist children's hospitals has decreased. Attention is therefore switching to sick children in the community with some paediatricians specializing in this area. In 1996 the DoH issued the document *Child health in the community: a guide to good practice*[48].

The Priorities document and *The Way Forward*[49] emphasized the need for better secure accommodation to ensure that adolescents were not remanded in prison. It now appears that residential services for adolescents and younger children were often run inappropriately. Evidence of the scandalous abuse of children continues to surface. This, together with revelations of the extent of sexual abuse of children, those in care and those living at home, caused great public concern in the 1990s. Health authorities are required to review their procedures for dealing with children who are suspected of having suffered sexual and other physical abuse. Diagnosis of child abuse is controversial and requires special training for clinicians. Statutory protection for children is provided by the Children Act, 1989.

In 1997 there were 32,400 children on child protection registers

9.10 PEOPLE WITH LEARNING DISABILITIES

Some babies are born with a learning disability or subsequently develop this impairment, despite improved care of mothers and babies during pregnancy and birth. Learning disabilities are not identifiable diseases; they result from malfunction during pregnancy, injury at birth or subsequently by accident, infection, drugs or a developing degenerative condition. The care of such people has to take account of this variety of causes. Classification is fraught with problems of definition. It has been customary to rely on intelligence quotient (IQ): those who score under 50 are reckoned to have severe disability and those between 50 and 70 mild disability. The IQ measure is controversial and not necessarily a good indicator of the needs of a person with a learning disability. Accordingly, this has led to attempts to define people in terms of their level of dependency on others, but this too has proved to be inexact. There are three or four severely disabled people per 1000 in the 15–19 age group. It is repeatedly found that highly dependent people with learning disability who were institutionalized can make radical progress in a different environment, becoming much more capable than the most optimistic professional staff would have predicted.

Interestingly, the name of the condition has troubled every generation and reflects the changing attitude of society to the problem. From the 'idiots' of the late nineteenth century, the descriptive and legal terms have included 'deficiency', 'subnormality' 'mental handicap', and now 'people with learning disabilities' or 'learning difficulties'. In other countries the preferred term is 'mental retardation'. The changes of label reflected changed attitudes. In the last 25 years there has been significantly more discussion on how best to look after people with learning disabilities. Most now live in the community. This may be in ordinary housing or in larger homes. A few still languish in hospital but this is usually because they have other problems; in particular, gross behavioural disorders.

A person with a learning disability is usually identified early by the health visitor or family doctor, and a programme of support for the family can then be arranged. The Children Act confirms the right of the disabled child to be treated like any other child. Attempts to integrate disabled children in ordinary schools have sometimes proved difficult. Disabled children are entitled to education up to the age of 19, although not all education authorities discharge their obligations in this respect. After 19, opportunity centres and sheltered workshops may give people with learning disabilities a place to go during the day.

The status of this speciality has gradually risen among professional health services staff, and managers no longer see it as a low-prestige area of work. The change was first stimulated by the recurring scandals arising from lack of appropriate care, starting with the Ely Hospital affair of 1969[50] and Pauline Morris's study *Put Away*[51] the same year. The most significant policy document was *Better Services for the Mentally Handicapped* (1971)[52], which was in effect a charter for people with learning disabilities. The long-term aim is to provide a more satis-factory environment for them. The traditional segregation from society is deplored; health, social services and educational authorities are encouraged to work together to provide an integrated, readily accessible service. Every effort should be made to support the families of such people. The 1976 Priorities document endorsed these aims and proposed considerable growth in the number of local authority training centres and residential homes. Staffing ratios in hospitals were to be increased to help improve the standards.

In 1975, the National Development Group was set up to lead the way to these better standards. Its regular reports were important in maintaining government commitment. Despite this, the group was disbanded in 1980, after the government published a review of the slow progress since the *Better Services* document. One reason was the conflict between professionals about the best way of providing care. Some staff were convinced that the increasing emphasis on community care was wrong, both for the community, who may feel threatened by people with learning disabilities in their midst, and for the people themselves, who may be discriminated against and might lose access to those facilities provided as a matter of course in specialist hospitals. The Jay report[53], published in 1979, fanned the flames of disagreement by suggesting that training nurses in mental handicap was inappropriate and that a less clinically based training would be better. In the event, faced with this professional controversy and because the financial implications were considerable, the government did not support the Jay recommendations.

Discharging of people from long-stay hospital beds has accelerated. In 1985 there were 42,000 designated hospital beds but in 1996 only 13,000. By the year 2000 nearly all mental handicap hospitals will have closed and former patients will have been relocated into the community. The majority of these people have no overriding medical condition that requires hospital services; *Caring for People* stressed the importance of individual assessments leading to more appropriate placements. Learning disability is now no longer a health care issue unless gross behavioural disorder or other physical or mental illness requires active treatment. Despite this, people's interests have to be safeguarded and the National Development Team, once part of the government's official advisory service, is now largely self-financed and works to protect people with learning disability by providing advice to those working with them.

9.11 THE PHYSICALLY DISABLED

Another numerically small group of people requiring considerable support is the physically disabled. This broad label covers people with a variety of conditions. Disablement may be due to injury, particularly the results of a road accident, infectious or degenerative disease, sudden medical emergencies such as a stroke or congenital abnormalities. The requirements of a disabled person will naturally vary according to his or her problem. At the most severe level the disabled person will need complete medical and nursing care in a hospital. All too often this care is provided in unsuitable accommodation: an acute ward where the arrangements are geared to a high turnover is not suitable for someone having to live there for a long period. Worse still for a younger disabled person is a ward of elderly patients, some of whom may be confused. Unfortunately, many health professionals tend to underestimate the potential for improvement in profoundly disabled people, particularly those with head injuries, those with multiple sclerosis and stroke victims. Without an early and co-ordinated attempt to estimate the rehabilitative potential or the appropriate scope for alleviation, the patient will not only fail to improve but may well develop further problems and deteriorate.

Following the passing of the Chronically Sick and Disabled Persons Act, 1970[54], health authorities started to develop special units for younger disabled people. Implementation of the policy was slow and in due course overtaken by the belief that every effort should be made to support people in their own homes. Where this is not possible charitable organizations, such as the Cheshire Homes, are more likely than hospitals to provide long-term care.

Disabled people who can continue living outside hospital may be usefully supported by cash benefits and visits from NHS staff. The state-funded Attendance Allowance subsidizes the cost of someone giving long-term physical assistance. Social services and health authorities are empowered to lend or give the disabled person an extensive array of physical aids to daily living. House adaptations can also be provided free of charge. Nevertheless, the disabled person may still find getting around away from home difficult; public buildings have not yet been adapted as thoroughly as the 1970 Act laid down. Work can be difficult to find for disabled people, particularly in a time of high unemployment. Sheltered working conditions are relatively limited and often provide very tedious work for the physically handicapped person of normal intelligence.

Physically handicapped people, unlike those with learning disability, are well able to speak for themselves, and pressure groups such as the Disablement Income Group and the Disabled Drivers' Association continue to put pressure on governments and social services and health authorities. Voluntary bodies also provide considerable support, both in the provision of residential accommodation and in advocacy for disabled people's needs.

9.12 MENTALLY ILL PEOPLE

It could be said that the physically disabled do better than the mentally ill because their condition does not attract the same amount of stigma. Mental disorder, unlike learning disability, is an illness and still frightens many people; primitive reactions to madness underlie their responses.

Large mental illness hospitals isolated from the community have now all but disappeared. The number of beds available – 39,000 in 1996 – was less than half those in use ten years previously, which in turn was half those available in the 1950s. The 1962 Plan envisaged the gradual closure of these hospitals, most of which were built following the asylum legislation of the second half of the nineteenth century. However, care in the community for mentally ill people has not been a great success; in 1998 the Secretary of State announced a review of the policy because it is increasingly felt that some people are a danger both to themselves and to others if they live without continuous supervision.

Questions remain unresolved. Do patients fare better left at home supported by visiting specialist staff, or do they recover more quickly if admitted to a hospital away from the environment that may have contributed to their illness? If the latter, should this be a small local unit close to their own community or is it better to use a larger hospital which, because of its size, can provide a wider range of therapeutic regimes? What are the most appropriate regimes of treatment and care?

Despite these questions, day care continues to develop, and can be particularly valuable in the support of those chronically ill people whose symptoms are an irritant to their families rather than a cause of profound family disruption. Day care is also more useful in looking after the elderly mentally ill. Whether senile dementia, now often referred to as Alzheimer's disease, is really a classifiable condition or merely a generalization for a range of behavioural problems found in old people is not clear. Admitting a patient to hospital because of episodes of confusion often increases their disorientation but, although support in their own homes surrounded by their own family and possessions is more humane, the strain on families should not be underestimated.

As with learning disability, the problem of definition is considerable. Alongside those radical views which hold that it is not individuals who are ill but society[55], opinions still differ about the nature of mental illness. Traditionally, patients are categorized into two main groups: the psychotic and the neurotic. Neurotic is used as a technical term. Those suffering from psychosis seem to others to have a poor perception of reality; they may be convinced that they are right and everyone else is wrong, and their delusions may be consequently bizarre. The person with neurosis characteristically has a view of reality which most other people would share, but has problems coping and is subject to anxiety and distress that can be sufficiently disabling to require professional support, in or out of hospital. Psychosis is found in all populations and cultures and does not appear to be related to class. Neurosis, however, is more specifically correlated with social conditions and class.

Treatment for the mentally ill varies even for the same conditions. Some psychiatrists, psychologists and nurses feel that the encouragement of self-help through group therapy is both humane and effective[56], while others rely more on helping the patient to cope by using drugs and in some cases, electro-convulsive therapy (ECT). Psychotherapy demands a long and time-consuming interaction with the patient. It is not widely provided within the NHS because of a shortage of resources as well as doubts in some professional quarters about its efficacy. The treatment of mentally ill people depends on satisfactory team working. The doctor, the clinical psychologist, the nurse, the social worker, the occupational therapist and others need to agree a treatment plan to obtain the best results.

The concept of the therapeutic community was first developed in Dingleton Hospital, Scotland in the 1970s

For many patients, their illness will be a recurring event. In order to take the stigma out of these episodes of ill health, the DoH's policy has been to encourage the development of community support, thus avoiding hospital admission. Earlier in the 1970s it was believed that stigma might be reduced if admission was to a mental illness unit in a district general hospital. There is declining support for this view.

Despite the uncertainty about effective therapies there have been some considerable improvements. In the mid-1950s there were over 150,000 people in mental illness hospitals. The consequent over-crowding meant that standards were very low and wards with over 60 patients were commonplace. The 1959 Mental Health Act did a great deal to reduce the numbers compulsorily admitted to hospital, and this, together with developments in drug therapy, started a gradual reduction in hospital numbers. The 1962 Plan predicted the closure of a substantial number of the older isolated mental illness hospitals to be replaced by smaller units attached to DGHs. In 1975 a white paper, entitled *Better Services for the Mentally Ill*[57], set out the government's long-term policies: more facilities to be provided within the community to keep the mentally ill out of hospital and, consequently, day hospitals, sheltered work and adequate home support all to be expanded. If people became ill enough for hospital, they should be admitted wherever possible to either the local DGH or, if old and mentally infirm, to the local community hospital: staffing ratios were to be improved, particularly medical, nursing and social work staff. Where older hospitals remained, renewed attempts should be made to improve standards.

The 1976 Priorities document supported these aspirations, but in 1979 the Royal Commission found that the policies were ambiguous, particularly regarding the closure of old mental illness hospitals. It said that, realistically, any government would have to accept that most mental illness hospitals would remain open for the rest of the century at least. Policy, therefore, should centre on providing a balanced service within which these hospitals could play a part. Financial stringency at the beginning of the 1980s forced many health authorities to review their strategies for the mentally ill.

The internal organization of the psychiatric services has worried successive governments. The Nodder report (1980)[58] supported the consensus team approach, but criticized the lack of direction shown by many of these teams. It advocated a more structured approach, with annual objectives and routine monitoring of achievement. The discussions leading to the 1982 reorganization ignored most of these recommendations, but, in some cases, unit management teams set up after 1982 operated along the lines suggested by Nodder.

Poor results may arise because objectives are poorly formulated or, in the case of secure units, because of implementation failures. The 1976 Priorities document proposed a secure unit for each region and capital monies were allocated immediately. Most of these were never built, either because of staff opposition or because of failure to agree on the type of patient who should be accommodated there. But pressure has continued to grow on how to deal with mentally ill people who have committed crime. The so-called 'special hospitals' were previously the sole responsibility of the Home Office. By degrees they have become the responsibility of the DoH. But their history has been troubled by clashes between the Prison Officers' Association and the more therapeutically inclined nursing staff. Health authorities are put under considerable pressure by the courts to look after people who are considered to be unsuitable for prison. They in turn have few facilities and, if they cannot arrange an admission to one of the special hospitals, they will buy care in an expensive private institution. The situation remains unsatisfactory.

Mental illness continues to be a priority for the government. New problems are developing, particularly those arising from drug and substance abuse. It is not always clear what regime is appropriate or which professional approach most suitable. Psychiatrists have shown an unwillingness to deal with challenging behaviour; psychologists and appropriately trained nurses may have more success with violent people. In addition the number of elderly people with mental disorders will continue to rise.

9.13 ELDERLY PEOPLE

The largest single category of patients is the elderly: at any one time, over half the beds in the NHS are occupied by people aged over 65, many of whom are admitted for acute conditions. Those under the care of geriatrician and other designated staff absorb some 11% of total health expenditure (1996). The proportion of elderly people in the population (currently around 18%) is expected to increase over the next decade. The rise in the number of the very old (those over 75) is predicted to be much higher. These statistics reflect steady improvements in child health since the beginning of the century rather than the increasing life expectancy in the elderly themselves. Broadly speaking, the longer you live, the longer you live. However, the physical quality of life diminishes and those over 75 are ten times more likely to see their general practitioner during a year than the rest of the adult population. Old age brings many symptoms, some, such as deafness, blindness and arthritis, due to physical degeneration, some because of mental incapacity. Ironically the mental confusion can be increased by the intervention of professional staff, so that an elderly person admitted to a geriatric assessment unit may appear more disorientated than before admission.

Opinion is divided as to how much treatment, as opposed to care, should be given to the very old. Geriatricians, anxious to attain the status accorded to their general physician colleagues, may be tempted to submit their patients to a battery of pointless clinical investigations. On the other hand, before geriatricians were appointed, the passiveness of care and lack of treatment given in many hospitals for the elderly was reminiscent of workhouse conditions. A balance has to be found between active intervention and letting life take its course.

Specialist care of old people is a phenomenon of the post-war era. Geriatricians attempt to see the patient as a whole person, concentrating on their environment as well as their health. Problems often arise after the discharge of an elderly person because insufficient account is taken of their home circumstances. Most elderly people in hospital are not in the care of the geriatrician, but have been referred to other specialists. Nevertheless, most district general hospitals now have specialist geriatric assessment units. Some have a policy that all medical admissions over the age of 75 are allocated to the geriatrician's team.

The proportion of old people in hospital or residential accommodation is still small. Most remain at home, requiring increasing support from health and social services. However incapacitated they may be, many elderly people wish to remain at home and may endure considerable physical and financial hardship to do so. Professional staff in the NHS know that more could be done and the elderly have become an increasingly important priority group. At times of financial stringency, it is often these support services which are cut first. The diffuseness of the problems makes coherent planning difficult. The need for specific plans for the elderly was recognized in the 1962 Plan, which said that every DGH should have an active geriatric unit where elderly patients could be assessed, even those who would subsequently need long-term care.

In 1978, the government brought out a consultative document called *A Happier Old Age*[59], which stressed the need to keep elderly people in the community for as long as possible, giving them support through home helps, district nurses, day centres and meals on wheels. It said that voluntary bodies should be encouraged to help in these tasks. The Royal Commission, a year later, supported this general view, but noted that geriatrics should remain part of the mainstream of medicine if a fully integrated service was to be provided. More active research into the problems of the elderly was encouraged.

As part of the encouragement of partnership between the public and private sectors, the 1982 Conservative government increased social security benefits to encourage elderly people to remain in such homes, rather than be admitted to NHS beds. The 1981 white paper *Growing Older*[60] did little more than support the general direction that policies had been taking for over a decade. Put simply, these policies supported the maintenance of elderly people in the community as long as possible. When illness necessitates hospital admission, this should be to an acute assessment unit, which had been shown to reduce the overall length of stay. Longer-term hospital care should be contemplated only for the most dependent. By the end of the 1980s most long-term care was being provided in the independent sector.

Caring for People[61] (1989) stated that there were over 6 million people with some sort of disability. Others have put the figure even higher. Many disabled people are elderly and have multifaceted problems. The process of individual assessment is therefore crucial to deciding what best to do in matching the needs and wishes of the elderly person to the available resources. Despite some criticism, the *Health of the Nation*[62] white paper was widely welcomed for focusing attention on the outcomes of care. There is evidence that health authorities have yet to appreciate the significance of the growing numbers of elderly. Governments have been criticized repeatedly for not allocating sufficient resources to keep up with the increase in demands from the elderly.

The biggest revolution over the last 10 years has been the substantial removal of long-stay beds from the NHS. This had never been an explicit policy although the Conservative government gave considerable support to the development of the independent sector. In some respects smaller nursing homes provide a more acceptable alternative, especially if they are conveniently placed near other members of the family. But the development of nursing homes has been haphazard. Their standards also vary enormously and their regulation puts great demands on health authorities, which some are unable to meet. In addition those patients with means are expected to pay for most of their health care, which would be free to the rest of the population. This unsatisfactory situation was acknowledged and a Royal Commission set up in December 1997 produced their extensive report *With Respect to Old Age* 15 months later[63]. Among their recommendations were the proposals that health and social services budgets for the elderly should be pooled; that patients requiring state aid should be allowed to keep £60,000 of personal assets rather than the previous limit of £16,000; and that in any case all personal care in nursing and residential homes should be free with the patient making contributions for domestic costs if they had sufficient assets to do so. Crucially, the Royal Commission rejected the idea that there was a 'demographic timebomb', and accordingly maintained that 'the costs of care were affordable'. They did not accept that private insurance to top up state support was sensible, particularly as many private insurers were averse to taking on the risks of illness in old age. The government received many of these recommendations guardedly.

CONCLUSION

This chapter has surveyed the main plans and policies for patients developed by the NHS. It is evident that many of these have been little more than statements of good intent. Only the 1976 Priorities document made a real attempt to match policies with resources, and this was quickly stifled by the worsening general economic climate of the next two decades. Since then attention has tended to focus on alternatives to direct provision by the NHS, in the hope that this will raise standards and redistribute the financial burden of care.

REFERENCES

1. The National Health Service Act, 1946. HMSO, London.
2. Ministry of Health (1956) *Report of the Committee into the cost of the National Health Service* (Guillebaud report). HMSO, London (Cmnd 9663).
3. Ministry of Health (1962) *A Hospital Plan for England and Wales* p. iii, para. 1. HMSO, London (Cmnd 1604).
4. DHSS and Welsh Office. Central Health Services Council (1969) *The Functions of the District General Hospital* (Bonham-Carter report). HMSO, London.
5. DHSS (1980) *The Future Pattern of Hospital Provision in England. A consultative document.* HMSO, London.
6. Ministry of Health (1945 and 1946) *Hospital Survey.* HMSO, London.
7. Ministry of Health (1963) *Health and Welfare – the Development of Community Care.* HMSO, London.
8. DHSS (1976) *Priorities for Health and Personal Social Services in England. (Consultative document).* HMSO, London.
9. DHSS (1977) *The Way Forward.* HMSO, London.
10. DHSS (1976) *Sharing Resources for Health in England. A report of the Resource Allocation Working Party (RAWP).* HMSO, London.
11. DHSS (1976) *Joint Care Planning: Health and Local Authorities.* Circular HC(76)18/LAC(76)6. HMSO, London.
12. DHSS (1977) *Joint Care Planning: Health and Local Authorities.* Circular HC(77)17/LAC(77)10. HMSO, London.
13. DHSS (1976) *Prevention and Health: Everybody's Business. A consultative document.* HMSO, London.
14. DHSS (1981) *Care in Action – A Handbook of Policies and Priorities for the Health and Personal Social Services in England.* HMSO, London.
15. DHSS (1981) *Care in the Community.* HMSO, London (see also HC(83)6/LAC(83)5 on *Care in the Community and Joint Finance*).
16. DHSS (1980) *Report of the working party on Inequalities* (Black report). HMSO, London.
17. DHSS (October 1983) *The NHS Management Inquiry* (Griffiths report). DHSS, London.
18. DoH (1992) *Health of the Nation.* HMSO, London (Cm 1986).
19. DHSS (1975) *A Guide to Planning in the NHS.* HMSO, London.
20. DHSS (1976) *NHS Planning System.* HMSO, London.

21. DHSS *Steering Group on Health Services Information* (Körner committee). Various reports from 1982 onwards.

22. DoH (1989) *Caring for People: Community Care in the Next Decade and Beyond*. HMSO, London (Cm 849).

23. DoH (1998) *The new NHS: modern – dependable*. HMSO, London.

24. DHSS (1982) *Planning in Partnership*. HMSO, London.

25. Audit Commission (1986) *Making a Reality of Community Care*. Audit Commission, London.

26. DoH (1988) *Community Care: Agenda for Action* (second Griffiths report). HMSO, London.

27. op. cit. *Caring for People*.

28. Bosanquet, N. and Gray, A. (1989) *Will you still love me?: New opportunities for Elderly People in the 1990s and beyond*. Research Paper No. 2. NAHAT, Birmingham.

29. Clarke, F. (1984) *Hospital at Home: the alternative to general hospital admission*. Macmillan, Basingstoke.

30. op. cit. *Prevention and Health*.

31. DHSS (1974) *Health education* HC HRC(74)27. DHSS, London.

32. op. cit. *Care in Action*.

33. op. cit. *Health of the Nation*.

34. DoH (1998) *Our Healthier Nation*. The Stationery Office, London.

35. British Dental Association (1983) *NHS Dental Treatment: What it costs and how the cost has risen*. British Dental Association, London.

36. World Health Organization (1985) *Health for All 2000*. WHO, Copenhagen.

37. World Health Organization and Liverpool University UK (1985) *Healthy Cities Project*. WHO, Copenhagen.

38. Royal College of Physicians (1987) *A great and growing evil*. RCP, London.

39. *Safe and Healthy at Work* (Robens report). HMSO, London (Cmnd 5034).

40. Statutory Instrument *Control of Substances Hazardous to Health Regulations 1988*, S.I. 1657 (came into force 1 October 1989).

41. Yates, J. (1987) *Why are we waiting?* Oxford University Press, Oxford.

42. DoH Expert Maternity Group (1993) *Changing Childbirth* (Cumberlege report). HMSO, London.

43. House of Commons Social Services Committee (1980) *Report on Perinatal and Neonatal Mortality* (Short report). HMSO, London (Cmnd 8084).

44. Ministry of Health (1959) *Report of the Maternity Services Committee* (Cranbrook report). HMSO, London.

45. DHSS, Central Health Services Council (1970) *Domiciliary Midwifery and Maternity Bed Needs* (Peel report). HMSO, London.

46. Ministry of Health, Central Health Services Council (1959) *The Welfare of Children in Hospital* (Platt report). HMSO, London.

47. DHSS Committee on Child Health Services (1976) *Fit for the Future* (Court report). HMSO, London (Cmnd 6684).

48. DoH (1996) *Child health in the community: a guide to good practice*. The Stationery Office, London.

49. op. cit. *The Way Forward*.

50. DHSS (1969) *Report of the Committee of Enquiry in to Allegations of Ill treatment of Patients and Other Irregularities at Ely Hospital Cardiff* (Howe report). HMSO, London (Cmnd 3795).

51. Morris, P. (1969) *Put Away*. Routledge and Kegan Paul, London.

52. DHSS Welsh Office (1971) *Better Services for the Mentally Handicapped*. HMSO, London (Cmnd 4683).

53. DHSS (1971) *Committee of Enquiry into Mental Handicap Nursing and Care* (Jay report). HMSO, London (Cmnd 7468).
54. See also Ministry of Health Circular HM(70)52, *Chronically Sick and Disabled Persons Act, 1970.*
55. Szasz, T. (1976) *The Myth of Mental Illness.* Harper and Row, New York; and Illich, I. (1977) *The Limits to Medicine.* Penguin Books, Harmondsworth, UK.
56. Jones, M. (1982) *The Process of Change* Routledge and Kegan Paul, London.
57. DHSS (1975) *Better Services for the Mentally Ill.* HMSO, London (Cmnd 6233).
58. DHSS (1980) *Organisational and Management Problems of Mental Illness Hospitals* (Nodder report). HMSO, London.
59. DHSS (1978) *A Happier Old Age.* HMSO, London.
60. DHSS (1981) *Growing Older.* HMSO, London (Cmnd 8173).
61. op. cit. *Caring for People.*
62. op. cit. *Health of the Nation.*
63. Royal Commission on Long Term Care (1999) *With Respect to Old Age.* The Stationery Office, London (Cm 4192-1).

10

EFFECTIVENESS, PERFORMANCE, QUALITY AND OUTCOMES

In any one year there are millions of consultations between doctors and patients, in surgeries and clinics, millions of operations, dental treatments, prescriptions for medicines.

Box 10.1

NHS activity (UK, millions) 1996

GP consultations	325
Out-patient department attendances	45
Hospital day cases	3
In-patient admissions	11
Surgical operations in hospital	6
Prescription items dispensed by chemists	550
Courses of dental treatment	31

Source: Office of Health Economics (1997) *Compendium of Health Statistics*. OHE, London

The statistics provide an indication of the volume of work the NHS carries out. However, they also raise questions. Were all those prescriptions absolutely necessary? Were all the operations carried out appropriate to every patient's condition? Are all GPs providing the same level of service to each person they see? In short, how does the NHS ensure that the service it provides is not only effective in clinical terms but is also cost effective and of high quality? This chapter examines attempts by the NHS to grapple with these fundamental issues.

10.1 EVIDENCE-BASED MEDICINE

Good medical practice has always involved examining and testing the clinical effectiveness of health care treatments and interventions. At a minimum, interventions need to do no harm, but clearly, to justify their use, treatments need to improve health. This may seem self-evident, yet a significant proportion of the treatments and services provided by the NHS (and, indeed, all health care services around the world) do not have a sound evidence-base as to their clinical effectiveness. So what exactly constitutes sound evidence?

Establishing the clinical worth of a treatment requires a scientific approach to the generation of experimental evidence, and the randomized control trial (RCT) is generally recognized as the methodological 'gold standard'. Testing the health impact of a treatment, drug or surgical procedure is surprisingly difficult. One of the key problems is isolating the effect of the medical intervention from the many other factors which influence people's health. Age, sex, wealth, upbringing, social class and genetic inheritance are all factors which, to differing degrees, have an impact not only on health status but also on the propensity to benefit from treatment. RCTs aim to neutralize the effects of such health determinants by randomly allocating individuals in an experimental study to two groups; a control and trial group – the latter receiving the treatment to be tested and the former receiving either nothing or a placebo. In this way any effects of the treatment on individuals' health can be, in theory, attributed to the treatment. One of the first RCTs carried out was a Medical Research Council (MRC) trial of streptomycin and reported by Bradford Hill in 1951. Since then, estimates of the proportion of treatments tested using an RCT vary, from as low as 10–20% up to 50–70%.

Integrating the results of evidence from RCTs (and other types of investigations) into daily medical practice is the key aim of evidence-based medicine[1]. There can be problems in translating the results of trials into action at an individual patient level because they are not usually constructed to reflect actual services, and often use extensive rules for excluding various patients (see Section 10.2). Nevertheless, ignoring the best available evidence inevitably means that medical practice becomes outdated.

There is a long history of the delayed uptake of the results of clinical findings (examples taken mainly from Haines and Jones[3])

Lemon juice to prevent scurvy was shown to be effective by James Lancaster in 1601. James Lind repeated Lancaster's experiment's nearly 150 years later, and the British navy eventually adopted the prophylactic at the start of the nineteenth century.

More recently, despite evidence of the beneficial effects of **steroids on the production of fetal lung surfactant**, many women in premature labour were not given this treatment.

A 1991 study[4] indicated that there was inadequate use of **prophylactic anticoagulants** in patients undergoing orthopaedic surgery.

Thrombolytic treatment for myocardial infarction was shown to be clinically effective more than a decade before it became widely advocated.

Dilation and curettage (D&C) has been shown to be 'therapeutically useless and diagnostically inaccurate'[5]. But in 1992/3, it was still the fourth most commonly performed surgical procedure in the NHS.

Box 10.2

Examples of delays in changing medical practice[2]

Despite increasing indications of lack of evidence either to support the provision of many treatments or to explain many examples of variations in medical practice or to justify delays in changing outmoded treatments (see Box 10.2), it is only in the last 5–10 years that the NHS has

Figure 10.1

Stages in the process of evidence-
based medicine

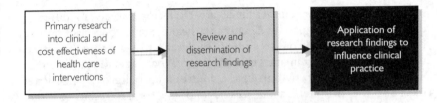

started to devote resources in a systematic way to generating the necessary primary research, and in particular to implement an NHS-wide approach to evidence-based medicine as indicated in Figure 10.1.

The appointment of Professor Sir Michael Peckham to the new post of Director of Research and Development in 1991 signalled a commitment by the Department of Health to evidence-based medicine. At that time ministers agreed to establish a research and development (R&D) strategy for the NHS. Two documents, *Research for Health*[6] and *NHS R&D Strategy: Guidance for Regions*, were published in 1991. These set out the first policy statements of the NHS R&D strategy. Early work on the strategy focused on ensuring that regions and other NHS bodies established appropriate systems and structures to manage their contributions to the R&D strategy, and built links to the many academic and charitable organizations concerned with health service research, including the major research councils (such as the MRC).

Apart from funding primary research, the R&D strategy has spawned a range of initiatives aimed at improving the scientific basis for health care. These included tackling the dissemination of research, for example through guidelines on best practice. In addition, regions were encouraged to generate, collate and disseminate guidance for trusts and purchasers on clinical effectiveness. Two important centres were also established – the UK Cochrane Centre and the NHS Centre for Reviews and Dissemination. The former (named after the epidemiologist Archie Cochrane; an ardent proponent of the RCT) is part of an international network of organizations dedicated to the systematic collection and review of currently available evidence from RCTs and other types of studies, which make results available to medical practitioners and others. The latter provides a similar reviewing service and also produces the *Effective Health Care Bulletins*[7], which collate information from many trials on specific disease problems.

Funding for research, development and dissemination is derived from a national levy, which, in 1998/9 amounted to £426 million (just over 1% of the total NHS budget). Around 80% of the levy is allocated back to NHS trusts and primary care providers to allow them to initiate or host research themselves. The remainder funds the national R&D programme, including sums allocated by regions.

Effective Health Care Bulletins have included: screening for osteoporosis to prevent fractures; stroke rehabilitation; the management of subfertility; the treatment of persistent glue ear in children; the management of menorrhagia; management of cataract; total hip replacement and compression therapy for venous leg ulcers

10.2 HEALTH OUTCOMES

A key aspect of evidence-based medicine at the level of individual treatments and care, and at a whole health care system level, is the *outcome* of a health care intervention. While the NHS has been very good at collecting, collating and disseminating information on the *inputs* to health care (finance, staffing, etc.) and *process* (operations performed, throughput, etc.), traditionally it has been poor at measuring and monitoring the outcomes of the care it provides. There are a number of reasons why this has been the case.

First, routine monitoring of the outcomes of interventions provided by the NHS would be unnecessary if all interventions were thought to be effective. Apart from the mounting evidence that not all interventions are in fact effective, even if all the treatments and services provided by the NHS had been subject to the evaluative scrutiny of RCTs, their implementation in *practice* is likely to lead to differences in outcome for at least three reasons. Variations in service organization, the skill of health care professionals and differences between study populations and those offered treatment in practice can mean that RCT results rarely replicate the effects achieved in the real world.

Second, measuring the outcome of health care interventions means measuring performance of individual clinicians, and as such can raise difficult issues concerning professional autonomy and accountability.

Third is the technical problem of defining what an outcome actually is, attributing it to a specific health care intervention and hence identifying what needs to be measured in practice.

Despite these difficulties, the importance of assessing outcomes has long been recognized. It is needed at a variety of levels within the NHS: patients, treatments, health authorities, and for the system as a whole. In the early 1990s, the Department of Health funded work to address the problem of defining outcome in health care. The Chief Medical Officer's Annual Report for 1991 (p. 81)[8] noted three definitions (Box 10.3).

Outcome	An end result which is attributable to intervention, or lack of intervention. The end result may manifest itself as a change in status, which may be absolute, or relative to expectation, e.g. deterioration in health when the expectation is no change.
Health outcome	An end result expressed in terms of health which is attributable to any intervention, i.e. not only a health services intervention. Health includes broader aspects such as function, social handicap, well-being and health-related quality of life, and relates to patients', public and professional values and expectations.
Outcome of health service	Any end result (health or otherwise) which is attributable to a health services intervention.

Box 10.3

Outcome definitions

In 1991 the DoH also commissioned the Faculty of Public Health Medicine to produce suggestions for hard measures of outcome. A consultation document, *Population Health Outcome Indicators for the NHS*[9], was published in 1993, but integration of the suggested measures into routine monitoring of outcomes has been slow. The DoH also set up a joint policy group/management executive unit – the Central Health Outcomes Unit – in order to work on the development and application of health outcomes assessment. The establishment of the UK Clearing House on Health Outcomes in Leeds in 1991 (funded by the Department of Health and the health departments in Northern Ireland, Wales and Scotland) aimed to provide a centrally coordinated source for clinicians and researchers on health outcomes. The new national performance framework (see Section 10.3) advocated by *The new NHS*[10] included health outcomes among its six dimensions of performance for the NHS.

Apart from the need to grapple with the measurement of outcomes of health service interventions, it is also necessary to measure the health of the population directly in order to inform policy and needs assessments by purchasers and to direct and monitor initiatives such as the *Health of the Nation*[11]. To this end, the DoH commissioned *Health Survey for England* in 1991[12]. The survey (of around 3000 people) focused on data related to cardiovascular disease and its associated risk factors. Subsequent surveys were expanded, and collected data on a wider range of health factors, including general measures of health status.

10.3 PERFORMANCE

Since the 1980s, the Department of Health has developed a package of statistical measures – performance indicators, or health service indicators (HSIs) – which draw together a whole range of financial and other performance measures for the NHS. These have provided a useful source of performance comparisons. The introduction of the internal market and the requirement for providers to publish prices for the procedures GP fundholders were allowed to buy added a dimension to financial performance comparisons. The requirement to publish prices for extra-contractual referral (ECR) procedures also provided a source of information for purchasers to use in order to compare the performance of providers. The accuracy of these prices was doubtful given current accounting systems, however. The financial performance of trusts has, since 1991, been monitored largely via three key financial duties: meeting a required financial return; achieving break-even on income and expenditure; and remaining within their external financing limits (EFLs). Of the 430 trusts in England in 1996, only one-third managed to achieve all three duties and just under one-half managed to break even on their income and expenditure[13].

The new NHS argued the case for the need to abolish the internal market. But it also recognized the need to address the problem of inconsistent and variable financial information available to purchasers and trusts to judge their performance. With evidence that the cost of similar operations in different parts of the country varied by as much as four times, the white paper outlined proposals for a *national schedule of reference costs* and a *national reference cost index*[14], which would provide benchmarked targets for trusts to aim for (see Section 10.4).

The new NHS also addressed performance across a number of fronts. Six areas were identified to constitute elements of a national performance framework:

- health improvement;
- fair access;
- effective delivery of appropriate health care;
- efficiency;
- patient and carer expectations of the NHS;
- health outcomes of care.

A consultation paper, *The National Framework for Assessing Performance*[15], was published in January 1998, setting out the government's strategy for measuring and monitoring performance across these six dimensions. Table 10.1 shows, for each of them, examples of aspects of performance suggested by the framework.

The performance measures to emerge from the national performance framework consultation are designed for internal use within the NHS. However, there is the question of whether, and if so, how, the general public should be involved in assessing the performance of the NHS. For example, in the wake of a number of highly public failures in cancer screening and in particular the deaths of a number of children undergoing cardiac surgery at the Bristol Royal Infirmary, the Secretary of State, Frank Dobson, announced the publication, in October 1998, of a package of clinical indicators covering various aspects of hospital care; in particular, death and complication rates following operations[16]. These indicators were made publicly available.

One of the difficulties (and not just for the public) with such indicators is how to interpret them. Ranking hospitals on the basis of crude death rates following surgery, for example, provides only a partial picture of performance. Those hospitals that take particularly difficult or complex cases are likely to have higher death rates than those that have simpler more straightforward cases. To isolate the impact of a *hospital's* performance on outcome, it is necessary to adjust the crude rates for such factors as severity, comorbidity (other ill health which the person may have in addition to their main illness) and age. Statistical techniques exist to deal with these issues, but they can also confuse the search for straightforward comparisons of performance.

10.4 VALUE FOR MONEY

An ongoing aim of the Department of Health is to use the resources at its disposal as efficiently as possible. Maximizing the value the NHS

Table 10.1

Aspects of performance in six areas of care

Areas	Aspects of performance
I Health improvement	The overall health of the population, reflecting social and environmental factors and individual behaviour as well as care provided by the NHS and other agencies
II Fair access	The fairness of provision of services in relation to need on various dimensions: • geographical • socio-economic • demographic (e.g. ethnicity, sex) • care groups (e.g. people with learning disabilities)
III Effective delivery of appropriate health care	The extent to which services are: • clinically effective (interventions or care packages are evidence-based) • appropriate to need • timely • in line with agreed standards • provided according to best practice service organization • delivered by appropriately trained and educated staff
IV Efficiency	The extent to which the NHS provides efficient services, including: • cost per unit of care/outcome • productivity of the capital estate • labour productivity
V Patient/carer expectations of the NHS	The patient/carer perceptions on the delivery of services, including: • responsiveness to individual needs and preferences • the skill, care and continuity of service provision • patient involvement, good information and choice • waiting times and accessibility • the physical environment; the organization and courtesy of administrative arrangements
VI Health outcomes of care	NHS success in using its resources to: • reduce levels of risk factors • reduce levels of disease, impairment and complications of treatment • improve quality of life for patients and carers • reduce premature deaths

obtains for every pound it spends and minimizing wasteful uses of resources is not merely a question of saving money or in some way economizing; spending scarce resources on inappropriate or ineffective services means that less is available to be spent on appropriate and effective services. The 'cost' of wasting resources is thus the lost (health) benefits that could have been obtained from spending them more wisely.

Conventional economic wisdom suggests that there are likely to be inefficiencies in a large, complex and resource-hungry organization such as the NHS. In addition, as a public organization, reliance on the personal initiative or 'public-spiritedness' of those responsible for committing resources is unlikely to squeeze out all such inefficiencies.

10.4.1 Cost improvement programmes

One incentive for actively encouraging the more efficient use of scarce resources is the 'cost improvement programme' (CIP) introduced in

1984. Districts were expected to release money from their main budgets by running services with greater efficiency, not by cutting services. The target was usually set at about 1% of districts' total budget by the DoH. Initially such efficiencies were readily identifiable, for example more careful spending on ancillary services. But it became progressively harder to find candidates for improvement and therefore to reach the target without reductions in service levels[17].

Having exhausted 'easy' savings, it was then necessary to look at the core of the expenditure, patient care itself. In the past doctors were given a relatively free hand to treat their patients as they wished, without giving much consideration to the financial consequences. This changed as attempts were made to raise the awareness of costs generally in the NHS. It was first called 'clinical budgeting' then redubbed 'resource management'. It aimed to help those who make decisions about patient care to do so with an idea of the actual costs of their decisions. It is a system for looking ahead at intended decisions; it required doctors to conduct regular reviews of expenditure against the speciality budgets they create. Incentives can be built in, to permit one speciality's savings to be returned to it for its own development schemes.

What should these budgets include? Should nurses be counted in or are they part of the hospital's overall responsibility? If nursing costs fall on a speciality budget, the doctors might wish to reduce the number or seniority of the hospital's nurses in order to make savings. But this might be unacceptable to the hospital's chief nurse if it would reduce nursing standards or hinder his or her authority to deploy nurses throughout the hospital. The only sanction a doctor who overspends experiences is pressure from his peers.

A version of CIPs remained part of the DoH's managerial efficiency toolkit even after the internal market was introduced. Each year districts were set an efficiency target – measured by the 'purchaser efficiency index' – which they were expected to build in to their contractual arrangements with their providers. Targets were usually set at around 2–3% each year. Unlike CIPs these were not just concerned with realizing cash (and to an extent non-cash) savings for redeployment, but with improvements in 'technical efficiency', or achieving more activity for every pound spent. The index was similar to an overall measure of technical efficiency known as the cost-weighted activity index. Figure 10.2 shows how the English NHS increased its technical efficiency between 1981/2 and 1995/6. The figure shows that, while spending on the NHS has increased in real terms, the number of patients the NHS has treated has increased even more, hence the cost-weighted activity index has increased (since 1981/2, by nearly 40%). However, the efficiency index has been heavily criticized[18]. Although the DoH attempted to modify it to meet these criticisms, *The new NHS* proposed its abolition.

The DoH's national framework for assessing performance (see Table 10.1) has attempted to find alternatives to the efficiency index which do not encourage potentially perverse incentives. The *national schedule of*

The purchaser efficiency index was a relatively crude measure of technical efficiency, and was calculated by dividing the change from one year to the next of a weighted sum of activity (in-patients, day cases, out-patients, etc.) by the annual change in real spending to produce this activity. The index was widely criticized within the NHS for failing to capture the full range of service provision and quality of service, and also for encouraging perverse incentives

Figure 10.2

Cost-weighted activity index: a measure of technical efficiency (English hospital and community health services)

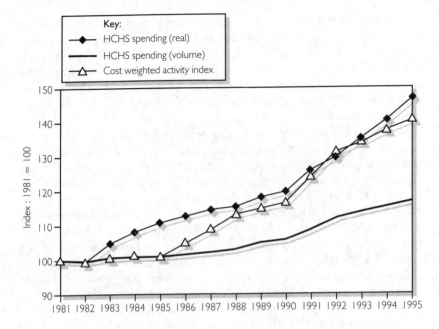

Source: statistics compiled from DoH (1995, 1997) *Government expenditure plans 1996/97 and 1998/99*, (Cm 3212 and 3912). HMSO, London

reference costs and the related *cost index* are part of the performance framework's drive to encourage the efficient use of resources. In addition, measures such as average length of stay, the cost per 'unit of care' (e.g. cost per case detected by screening), generic prescribing rate, day case rate and labour productivity indices will be used to provide broad comparators across purchasing organizations and to set targets for achievement. Although this avoids the problems created by highly aggregated measures of efficiency such as the efficiency index, the problem of interpreting the resultant *collection* of performance indicators re-emerges. Moreover, as the national performance framework makes clear:

> *[While] it is reasonable to suppose that differences between health authorities may in part be driven by differences in performance ... there may also be other factors beyond the control of health authorities, which lead to variations and confound comparisons between one health authority and another. (p. 17)*

10.5 ACCOUNTABILITY

The Secretary of State for Health is politically accountable to Parliament and the party in power is accountable to the electorate through general elections. The people responsible for running a public service are held accountable by the community at large in various ways. First, the Permanent Secretary and the NHS Chief Executive are formally designated as accounting officers and have to report to Parliament for the proper expenditure of public money. They are required to appear before the Public Accounts Committee to answer points brought up by the Comptroller and Auditor General. They may also have to answer criticisms publicized by the Audit Commission, which took on the responsibility for NHS audit in 1990. The abolition of the regions and the lack of non-executive directors in the new regional offices could be seen as strengthening central control and tightening the accountability chain (with regional directors accountable to the Chief Executive). Another instrument of review is the Health Committee, a select committee of the House of Commons made up of MPs from government and opposition parties.

See also Chapter 3

The monitoring of the NHS has grown more rigorous, as has that of central government. Following the 1982 reorganization a system of ministerial reviews was set up. Initially each regional chairman was summoned to meet one of the ministers annually. From 1989 this was changed to become a more detailed investigation by the NHSME Chief Executive of the regional general manager, assessing the performance of the region over the last 12 months, comparing it with the objectives that had been agreed, and at the same time examining the plans and the resources likely to be available for the coming year. This review was confirmed formally in a letter to the regional general manager, which effectively became a contract for regional performance. As well as these links between the centre and the regions, increasingly other meetings were encouraged such as the so-called 'bilaterals' where, for example, a regional director of finance met with his or her counterpart on the NHSE. The abolition of the regions and the direct accountability of the regional directors to the Chief Executive has changed this system of corporate contract review at the regional level.

Successive governments have sought new ways of making the NHS more accountable, and this has brought about its own tensions. At times the NHS has been asked to make inappropriate changes inspired by short-term expedients. But often governments have witnessed the thwarting of their plans for change by the capacity of the NHS to maintain the status quo. Some governments are more prescriptive than others: the 1974–9 Labour government issued a detailed policy document *Priorities for Health and Personal Social Services in England* in 1976[19], whereas the Conservative document *Care in Action* (1981)[20] was far less detailed, allowing health authorities to make their own judgements about priorities. By the late 1980s more detailed schemes were being introduced, targeted on such specific problems as breast and cervical screening programmes, waiting lists and active measures to combat the spread of AIDS.

Health authorities are monitored to check that they have implemented the policies, and it has been found, not for the first time, that co-operation in implementing policies can be bought: the NHS is much more likely to accept a change if the directive is accompanied by earmarked funds. The publication of *The Health of the Nation* in 1992 (and its updated and refocussed version, *Our Healthier Nation*[21], in 1997) has further encouraged the NHS to be concerned with promoting health as well as treating sickness.

All health authorities are accountable for the proper spending of public money. The Permanent Secretary and the Chief Executive at the DoH are the designated accounting officers who must answer any expenditure questions put to them by the Public Accounts Committee. Health authorities' accounts are externally audited to satisfy the government that public funds have been properly used, and each health authority has its own audit staff. The 1990 NHS and Community Care Act transferred responsibility for the government's audit, previously undertaken by the DoH's own audit staff, to the Audit Commission which must report to the Secretary of State any unlawful expenditure or financial loss. But their remit is much wider than this, and they undertake various surveys to assess value for money. The National Audit Office, responsible to the government for scrutinizing all public authorities, also conducts reviews of services from a financial perspective. For example, a study into the use of operating theatres[22] demonstrated poor use of this expensive facility.

At the time of each reorganization the government has claimed it is delegating more authority down the line. But in 1993 this principle was called into doubt by major scandals in the West Midland and Wessex regions, where computer procurement had been mismanaged to the extent that many millions of pounds were squandered. Similar scandals in the private sector had led to the setting up of the Cadbury Committee on corporate governance[23]. A DoH Task Force on this topic culminated in the publication of an Executive Letter on *Codes of Conduct and Accountability (EL(94)90)*[24]. Other guidance was also aimed at improving board performance[25]. Greater delegation also requires more rigorous accountability.

Health authorities now have less of a role in direct purchasing of health care for their populations, but they have an important role in holding their local PCGs to account – both financially and in terms of an agreed health care strategy (the health improvement programme). The creation of PCGs, and drawing GPs into the NHS management and decision-making process creates particular tensions with regard to accountability. While PCGs, health authorities, trusts and local authorities all work to an agreed health improvement programme, GPs – the leading professional group within PCGs – are not employees of the NHS, but independent contractors. However, PCGs are in charge of the bulk of the resources the NHS spends on health care. Given the large sums of public money that PCGs control, how is accountability for spending (and implementing national policy directives) ensured? The key is the health authorities, with whom PGCs now have to draw up an 'accountability agreement', which will then be monitored by the authority. In addition, PCG chairs are directly accountable to health authority chief executives, who have the power to approve their appointment. In turn, health authority chief executives are held financially accountable to the DoH for their local PCGs.

National monitoring of the NHS takes place in other ways. The Health Advisory Service (HAS) was set up by Richard Crossman in 1969 following the report on mismanagement and cruelty to mentally handicapped patients at Ely Hospital in Wales[26]. Originally the HAS operated through four teams but this has been altered so that reviews of service for people with learning disabilities are now undertaken by the Development Team for the Mentally Handicapped (see Chapter 9), leaving the HAS to look at services for the elderly, the mentally ill and, more recently, services for abusers of drugs and other substances. HAS reports were initially confidential but are now published. Health authorities are expected to take the recommendations very seriously and to prepare regular reports on their implementation. The membership of HAS teams is drawn from the NHS itself and this factor makes it less easy to disregard their reports.

Another body set up under the 1990 NHS and Community Care Act is the Clinical Standards Advisory Group, whose job is to advise ministers and to make investigations into matters of clinical care. It is not yet clear whether this group will promote specific national clinical standards and to what degree it may be used by ministers to put pressure on the medical profession. At an individual level, the Health Service Commissioner can act on behalf of those who have not been satisfied with a health authority's investigation of their complaint, providing it is not of a purely clinical nature.

10.6 QUALITY

The subject of quality in health care is problematic. What do we actually mean by a 'quality' service? Ultimately, of course, the quality of a service is reflected in the outcome of treatment. In this sense quality really means (medical) effectiveness and appropriateness (that is, a patient receives not only a treatment that works but also one from which they benefit). Quality standards, controls and assurance are important instruments for achieving improvements in health status. They do not have any inherent value. Methods for improving quality, and hence the outcomes, of services range from hospital and doctor accreditation to organizational and managerial 'quality' marks guaranteeing that a particular process, shown to deliver good outcomes, is always used.

What does the public think of the health services? Are they confident that the expenditure and the organization of health care provides appropriate benefits? Table 10.2 shows the considerable differences in the public's attitudes in ten developed countries. By monitoring the quality of the services provided and in particular the work of doctors themselves, it is possible to see where there is specific scope for reform.

Another element of the national performance framework is the National Institute for Clinical Excellence (NICE), a new special health authority charged with promoting high quality health care and promoting guidance on clinically and cost-effective health care. The consultation document *A First Class Service*[27] set out the government's

Table 10.2

Public attitudes to health care services

	Minor changes needed (%)	Fundamental changes needed (%)	Completely rebuild system (%)
Canada	56	38	5
Netherlands	47	46	5
West Germany	41	35	13
France	41	42	10
Australia	34	43	17
Sweden	32	58	6
Japan	29	47	6
United Kingdom	27	52	17
Italy	12	46	40
United States	10	60	29

Source: adapted from Harvard-Harris-ITF, 1990 Ten-Nation Survey. In, Blendon, R. et al., Data Watch: Satisfaction with health systems in ten countries. *Health Affairs,* **10**(2), 185–92

CEPOD was launched in 1988 and has published the results of three national surveys (completed on a voluntary basis by clinicians) concerned with the quality of the delivery of anaesthesia and surgery and the perioperative care of patients

BS 5750 on Quality Systems is a 'kitemark' of the independent British Standards Institute, awarded to businesses and organizations to indicate that they follow a predetermined set of standards and processes. It does not necessarily give an indication of the quality of the eventual outcome of the process

See discussion in Section 9.7.2

approach to the issue of quality in the NHS and indicated that the NICE would have a central role in promoting quality, with the Commission for Health Improvement (CHI) acting as a monitor of trusts' and purchasers' moves towards the care standards laid down in the national service frameworks.

Although purchasers have stipulated strong commitments to the provision of high-quality services in their contracts with providers, there is little evidence that purchasers or providers have found reliable ways to measure and monitor quality. Recent initiatives such as the *Patient's Charter*[28], the Confidential Enquiry into Perioperative Deaths (CEPOD) and the limited use of the quality standards BS 5750 or ISO 9000 by providers are a step forward with regard to quality. Waiting times targets are unlikely to be an adequate reflection of service quality.

10.7 CLINICAL GOVERNANCE

It used to be accepted that clinicians would automatically provide the best care they could and that patients could therefore have complete faith in their doctor's judgement. Over the last 10 years there has been increased emphasis on the need for clinicians to be held to account for their decisions. The much publicised failure of two Bristol cardiac surgeons to attain reasonable success rates in their heart operations on children gave the government the opportunity to insist on much more stringent and visible procedures for reviewing clinical performance.

The notion of systematically analysing the quality of care patients receive from individual clinicians seems sensible, but it did not get significant government backing until the 1989 white paper *Working for Patients*[29]. This required all doctors to undertake audits of their professional work. *Working Paper 6*[30] defined audit as '...the systematic, critical analysis of medical care, including the procedures used for diagnosis and treatment, the use of resources, and the resulting outcome and quality of life for the patient.' The key aim of medical and clinical audit is to establish reflective practice as an integral part of the process of care and treatment. Accreditation, on the other hand, is a prospective process which aims to make sure that services can be supplied to a proper standard initially. The process allows a provider to demonstrate that it has the capability to provide services to stated standards. These standards may be about the quality or the quantity of inputs (for instance, staff), or they may concern the process (the manner of working of those staff), or they can be a statement of the expected outcomes or outputs (what those staff did). Although the process of accreditation can be mechanical, at its best it provides an opportunity for a provider and a purchaser to develop a constructive relationship. It is essentially less judgmental than audit and less punitive than contract monitoring.

In the UK accreditation has been developed relatively slowly. In the USA, in comparison, the Joint Commission on the Accreditation of Hospitals has long been in business. Currently in the UK the most widely used system has been developed by the King's Fund, which has a division devoted to Health Services Accreditation. There are also schemes such as Investors in People and ISO 9000 and its successors, which aim to provide national and international benchmarks of good practice in industry generally but which can be usefully applied to the NHS.

Key reference: Scrivens, E. (1995) *Accreditation – Protecting the Professional or the Consumer?* Open University Press, Buckingham.

In the UK explicit monitoring of patient experience had been in the hands of bodies such as the Health Advisory Service and the National Development Team. But these bodies were mostly concerned with the longer-stay patient; it was left to the Royal Colleges to institute their own systems for setting standards for more acute care and these were not generally open to public scrutiny. The scrutiny of general practice was almost entirely reserved to the review of prescribing practice, and then largely in financial terms.

It is admittedly difficult to organize coherent and systematic clinical performance reviews[31]. Valuable work had been undertaken nationally through CEPOD and the long-standing enquiries into perinatal and maternal mortality. It was now necessary to incorporate similar systems of scrutiny into all aspects of clinical care.

The opportunity came with Labour's *The new NHS*, which committed the NHS (para. 3.5) to a new system of clinical governance aimed at continuous improvement. The detail was spelt out both in *A First Class Service* in June 1998 and in the guidance, 3 months later, on the setting up of Primary Care Groups[32]. Clinical governance, for the setting up of which chief executives were held accountable, was described on p. 33 as follows:

Clinical governance can be defined as a framework through which NHS organisations are accountable for continuously improving the quality of their services and safeguarding standards of care by creating an environment in which excellence in clinical care will flourish.

Implementing clinical governance is not without its difficulties. It is not always easy to agree on a clinical standard; what is good practice to some may not be to others. For instance in obstetrics there are widely divergent views on the best place for delivery. Some maintain all births should be in well equipped central departments while others maintain that low-risk births – at least a third of all births – are best undertaken in a less clinical setting. Secondly, statistics which are used as indices of practice are not always reliable and are subject to misinterpretation. Thirdly clinicians are undoubtedly accountable but to whom – their patient, their profession, the management or the government? Fine if all concur but where they do not, to whom is the doctor most accountable? Finally, if a clinician is found to be working to too low a standard what reasonably can be done given that sanctions sometimes punish the patient as much as the doctor?

Clinical governance is undoubtedly time-consuming and if undertaken insensitively can ruin the delicate relationship between managers and doctors. Other clinical professions also need to be involved in reviewing not only their own practice but also the nature of their co-operation with each other; there are instances where the patient suffers because of inadequate communication among clinicians or confusing treatment regimens.

The general Medical Council issued two pamphlets in July 1998, *Good Medical Practice* and *Maintaining Good Medical Practice*

Conclusion

Reorganizations may come and go, but many of the fundamental issues discussed in this chapter remain. The emergence of the concept of evidence-based medicine over the last 5 years has re-emphasized the need to appraise critically the scientific basis of medical practice. It draws together performance-related themes in clinical research, economics and management. The NHS has been at the forefront internationally in recognizing the investment required for research and development if health services are to keep abreast of developments in medical technology. The importance of an evidential underpinning to medical care is increasingly being recognized at organizational, managerial and policy levels. Such questions of new (and existing) health care interventions as 'Does it work?', and the supplementary economic question 'Is it worth it?' are increasingly being asked in the context of the NHS's organizational changes.

References

1. Sackett, D. L., Richardson, W. S., Rosenberg, W. and Haynes, R. B. (1997) *Evidence-based Medicine: How to teach and practice EBM.* Churchill Livingstone, London.

2. These examples are taken from: Appleby, J., Walshe, K. and Ham, C. (1995) *Acting on the Evidence*. Research Paper No. 17. NAHAT, Birmingham.

3. Haines, A. and Jones, R. (1994) Implementing the findings of research. *British Medical Journal* 308: 1488–92.

4. Laverick, M. D., Croal, S. A. and Mollan, R. A. B. (1991) Orthopaedic surgeons and thromboprophylaxis. *British Medical Journal* 303: 549–50.

5. Lewis, B. V. (1993) Diagnostic dilation and curettage in young women should be replaced by outpatient endometrial biopsy. *British Medical Journal* 306: 225–6.

6. *Research for Health: A Research and Development Strategy for the NHS*, 1991. HMSO, London.

7. Universities of Leeds and York, DoH (1992–) *Effective Health Care Bulletins* (published by NHS Centre for Reviews and Dissemination from 1994).

8. DoH (1992) *On the State of the Public Health 1991. The Annual Report of the Chief Medical Officer of the Department of Health*. HMSO, London.

9. DoH (1993) *Population Health Outcome Indicators for the NHS*. A Consultation Document. HMSO, London.

10. DoH (1997) *The new NHS*. The Stationery Office, London (Cm 3087).

11. DoH (1992) *The Health of the Nation*. HMSO, London (Cm 1986).

12. OPCS (1993) *Health Survey for England 1991*. HMSO, London.

13. DoH (1998) *Departmental Report: The Government's Expenditure PlansL 1998/99*. The Stationery Office, London (Cm 3912).

14. DoH (1998) Press release, June 14th 1998.

15. NHSE (1998) *The new NHS: Modern and Dependable: A National Framework for Assessing Performance*. Consultation Document. NHS Executive, Leeds.

16. DoH (1998) Press release, June 9th 1998.

17. King's Fund Institute (1989) *Efficiency in the NHS*. Occasional paper No. 2. King's Fund, London.

18. See for example Editorial (1993) Efficient Purchasing. *British Medical Journal* 307: 4–5.

19. DHSS (1976) *Priorities for Health and Personal Social Services in England*. A Consultative Document. HMSO, London.

20. DHSS (1981) *Care in Action – A Handbook of Policies and Priorities for the Health and Social Services in England*. HMSO, London.

21. DoH (1998) *Our Healthier Nation*. The Stationery Office, London.

22. National Audit Office (November, 1987) *Use of Operating Theatres in the NHS*. HMSO, London.

23. *The Financial Aspects of Corporate Governance* (Cadbury report), December 1992. Gee & Co., London.

24. DoH (1994) *Code of Conduct and Code of Accountability* (EL(94)90). Department of Health, London.

25. Wall, A. (1993) *Healthy NHS Boards*. NAHAT, Birmingham.

26. DHSS (1969) *Report of the Committee of Inquiry into Allegations of Ill-treatment and other Irregularities at the Ely Hospital, Cardiff*. HMSO, London (Cmnd 3975).

27. DoH (1998) *A First Class Service: A Consultation Document on Quality in the NHS*. NHS Executive, London.

28. DoH (1991) *The Patient's Charter*. HMSO, London.

29. DoH (1989) *Working for Patients*. HMSO, London (Cm 555).

30. DoH (1989) *Medical Audit Working Paper No. 6, Working for Patients*. HMSO, London.

31. See, for example, Kerrison, S. *et al*. (1994) Monitoring Medical Audit. In: *Evaluating the NHS Reforms* (ed. Robinson, R. and Le Grand, J.). King's Fund, London.
32. DoH (1998) *The New NHS – Developing Primary Care Groups* HSC 1998/139. NHS Executive, Leeds.

STAFFING – DOCTORS AND NURSES

11

It is said that nearly one million people work in the NHS: clinicians, therapists, managerial and support staff. The boundaries of their work are constantly changing, as are their conditions of employment. The next two chapters give a brief history of each group, their present working arrangements, their pay and likely developments.

In very approximate rounded figures, the staff in the main categories are shown in Table 11.1.

	No.	%
Nurses, midwives, health visitors, auxiliaries and assistants	352	44
Administration and estates	167	21
Scientific, therapeutic and technical	99	12
Medical and dental	85	11
Support services	70	9
Ambulance	15	2
Other	3	1
Total	**791**	**100**

Table 11.1

NHS staff (1996, England, approx., whole-time equivalents thousands)

Source: Office of Health Economics (1997) *Compendium of Health Statistics*. OHE, London

The number of people employed (as opposed to whole-time equivalents) rose from just over 400,000 in 1951 to 940,600 in 1996, an increase of 235%. The only group which has declined is support staff, due to efficiency initiatives and contracting out.

11.1 DOCTORS

The development of medicine as a scientifically based understanding of health and disease has depended on the pace of discoveries in the natural sciences. The last 100 years have seen the most rapid changes, although important landmarks date earlier than that. This part of the chapter is concerned with the professional organization of doctors, their education and training, their distribution, their working arrangements in the NHS and their remuneration.

11.1.1 What do doctors do?

Broadly speaking, doctors are in three groups; those working primarily in hospitals, those in general practice, and public health doctors in community medicine, a much smaller group than the other two (see Table 11.2).

All doctors undergo the same training leading to qualification after 5

Table 11.2		1986	1996
Doctors (numbers; whole-time equivalent thousands)			
Hospital			
	Consultants	12.7	17.6
	Other career grades	0.7	3.0
	Registrar	8.5	10.2
	Other junior grades	12.4	16.9
	Other (clinical assistants, etc.)	2.1	2.0
	Total	**36.4**	**49.7**
GPs			
	Principals	24.5	26.9
	Assistants	0.3	0.7
	Trainees	1.7	1.3
	Total	**26.5**	**28.9**
Public health doctors			
	Consultants at region	–	–
	Directors of public health at HA	0.14	0.10
	Other senior staff	3.05	2.21
	Trainees	0.28	0.30
	Total	**3.47**	**2.61**

Source: DoH

years followed by a pre-registration year working in a hospital in general medicine and general surgery. Once registered by the General Medical Council, they can select the branch of medicine they wish to pursue (see Section 11.1.3). In hospital medicine, certain choices tend to be much more popular than others. It is not unusual for a registrar to have to change career direction because progress in his or her first choice is blocked or limited. Equally, some specialities are so short of applicants that attaining a consultant post can be rapid, after obtaining the required postgraduate qualifications and working in recognized junior jobs. Competition is considerable in such specialities as nephrology, cardiology, infectious diseases, general surgery, obstetrics and gynaecology, ophthalmology, neurosurgery or paediatric surgery, but less so in geriatrics, venereology, chemical pathology and anaesthetics.

The normal time-scale for a newly qualified hospital doctor's promotion is 1 year as a house officer, 2–3 years as a senior house officer, and no more than 7 years as a specialist registrar. Care is taken by the medical profession to ensure that the number of specialist registrars nationally does not exceed the likely number of consultant vacancies but occasionally this does not work out and specialist senior registrars may have to make a late change in their career aspirations.

The clinical work is organized around a basic unit called a 'firm', composed of one or two consultants and a varying number of more junior grades. Patients referred to hospital by a GP for in-patient or out-patient treatment become the responsibility of a specific consultant, who has to make decisions about their diagnosis, treatment, referral and discharge. The consultant is helped by junior doctors and by a variety of nursing and paramedical staff, and delegates some of the work to them while retaining full personal responsibility. In practice, the specialist registrars have some autonomy, although they are responsible to their consultant, and they supervise the work of the house officers. The discretion given to each grade of junior doctor varies considerably from firm to firm, and depends on the nature of the clinical work, the number of staff involved and the personality of the doctor. Teaching of junior medical staff, medical students and other hospital staff may also play a part in the work of the firm.

For general practitioners the path is simpler. A three-year post-qualifying vocational course is obligatory and includes experience in such relevant hospital specialities as general medicine, paediatrics and obstetrics, together with a period as a supervised trainee in a general practice and an elective period of the trainee's choice. At the end of this, the new GP seeks his or her own appointment in a practice. The competition is unequal across the country, with inner-city areas the much less popular choice.

Public health medicine, traditionally considered the least prestigious choice, has recently started to attract more interest from those wanting to take a wider perspective on health. Their specialization starts at registrar level. The most senior appointments are as directors of public health in health authorities.

There are still far more male doctors than female doctors, although over 50% of medical school graduates are women. Attempts have been made through the Women Doctors Retainer Scheme, introduced in 1972[1], to enable previously unemployed women doctors to undertake part-time work to keep in touch with their profession. The retraining scheme[2], inaugurated in 1969, made special arrangements for women to work part-time at registrar level. Inevitably, women do better in shortage specialities and community medicine, and in those specialities where there are permanent sub-consultant-grade posts, known as associate specialist or staff grades.

Doctors, particularly junior hospital doctors, have habitually worked long hours. The problem is partly a consequence of attempting to provide continuity of care, although the quality of that care is undermined by tiredness and errors if they have had to spend too many hours on duty. A report published in 1990[3] found that for a sample of over 400 doctors, the house officers spent an average of more than 90 hours per week on duty, including the time actually spent with patients and at the hospital on call for emergencies. Following this there has been a determined attempt to reduce the hours and all NHS trusts are now required to make arrangements to reduce junior doctors working hours to the standard 40 hours per week. Where this is not possible extra duty payments are made. Maintaining the optimum number of doctors on duty is not easily achieved. Because all junior doctors are regarded as trainees, periods of study absence have to be allowed. This may oblige general practices and hospitals to employ locums for short-term cover. Governments have discouraged the use of locums on the grounds of expense and because, as temporary staff, they tend to offer a less informed service. Many GPs have now set up agencies to provide 24-hour cover over relatively wide areas.

Despite long hours, lengthy training, the need for continuing study and the competition for promotion, medicine remains a popular profession. It commands social prestige, considerable respect, reasonable remuneration and its members exercise extensive power in the NHS at all levels. Within their ranks each main group has its own distinctive culture.

11.1.2 Professional organizations

Before 1700 the medical profession was firmly divided into three groups: physicians, surgeons and apothecaries, of whom physicians had the highest status. The Royal College of Physicians of London was founded in 1518; members were graduates of Oxford and Cambridge Universities who had received religious and classical education and, subsequently, often studied medical subjects in European universities. Surgeons, on the other hand, were not scholars but craftsmen organized in a guild that was associated with the barbers, and they were licensed to perform the small range of procedures that could be carried out on unanaesthetized patients. The third group, apothecaries, were tradesmen who, from 1617 were licensed by the Society of Apothecaries to sell drugs prescribed by physicians. Until 1700, treatment was essentially carried out in patients' homes. However, the position changed between 1700 and about 1850, partly because that period saw the rise of the great voluntary hospitals which provided the setting for developments in surgery; in comparison, the techniques and abilities of physicians hardly advanced. The prestige of surgeons rose and, in 1745, the Company of Surgeons was founded, cementing their independence from the barbers and enabling educational standards to improve; by 1800 the Company had become the Royal College of Surgeons of England.

Apothecaries also advanced, and by 1703 they were entitled to see patients and prescribe medicines themselves. The result was that they became the 'general practitioners' for the middle classes and the poor. The Apothecaries Act of 1815 gave the Society of Apothecaries the right to license those who had served a 5-year apprenticeship and passed examinations, and some physicians took this qualification as well. As the voluntary hospitals were closed to these practitioners and only employed the services of those recognized by the Royal Colleges, the distinction between consultants and general practitioners became established. The Society of Apothecaries pioneered improvements in the standard of education and in raising the status of practitioners far more than the universities or Royal Colleges did. From 1842 to 1844, 16 practitioners were licensed by the universities of Oxford and Cambridge, 37 by the Royal College of Physicians and 953 by the Society of Apothecaries.

Despite this success, unqualified practitioners flourished (the 1841 census showed over 30,000 doctors, while the first Medical Directory, published in 1845, listed only 11,000 qualified practitioners), and demand arose for a single licensing authority and a single professional qualification permitting practice in any branch of the profession. The strongest pressure for such a licence came from the Provincial Medical and Surgical Association. This body was founded in Worcester in 1832, and drew so much support that, by 1855, it had changed its name to the British Medical Association. The campaign resulted in the passing of the Medical Act, in 1858, which created the General Council of Medical Education and Registration[4]. It is now called the General Medical Council (GMC) and has 50 members representing the Royal Colleges, the universities, the Crown and the profession at large. Its duty is to maintain a register of practitioners, licensed by recognized authorities, and to supervise the educational standards of training institutions. In practice, the GMC relies on medical schools to maintain standards in undergraduate training, and on the Royal Colleges for postgraduate and specialist training. Hospitals are constantly reminded of the power of the Royal Colleges to remove training approval from hospital posts, and this threatened sanction has done much to improve standards of training and also to promote such facilities as medical libraries.

Following the Merrison report in 1975[5], the GMC constitution was changed, and greater attention has since been paid to registration matters, particularly of overseas doctors, who make a significant contribution to the NHS. The GMC is also concerned with disciplinary matters and has the power to remove a doctor from the Medical Register, totally or for a limited period, in cases of serious professional misconduct or for such criminal convictions which would make it undesirable for that person to continue in practice.

Other medical corporations have been established, including the Royal College of Obstetricians and Gynaecologists (1929), the Royal College of General Practitioners (1952), the Royal College of Pathologists (1962) and the Royal College of Psychiatrists (1971).

The Royal Colleges and other medical corporations are not trades unions for doctors, but bodies mainly concerned with post-registration training and development, and, until comparatively recently, they represented only the élite specialities of the profession. The British Medical Association (BMA) emerged as the spokesman for the 'underdog' general practitioners. It threatened Lloyd George's government with destruction of the National Health Insurance Scheme through GPs' refusal to co-operate just as the scheme was about to be implemented. The opposition was dropped in 1912 when the government agreed to the demand for a higher rate of remuneration for GPs. Before that time, the out-patient departments and dispensaries of the voluntary hospitals provided treatment, subsidized by the charitable organizations, and thus represented an alternative source of treatment for people, instead of going to a general practitioner who contracted to work for a friendly society, if private treatment could not be afforded.

The 1911 Act had the effect of greatly increasing the numbers of people entitled to medical benefit through membership of the approved societies, and hence safeguarded the level of GPs' incomes under the National Health Insurance Scheme. Rivalry between GPs and hospital doctors was considerable, and the BMA set out the terms of their relationship in a code of ethics which made the GP responsible for his patients while the specialists could be consulted for opinion and advice on diagnosis and treatment. This enabled GPs to maintain lists of patients without the fear that, if any of them were referred to a hospital doctor, they would be taken over. To the present day, hospital doctors do not have a list of registered patients for whom they assume continuing responsibility, whereas GPs do.

Other bodies have emerged to protect doctors' interests, including the Hospital Consultants and Specialists Association and the Medical Practitioners Union, but the BMA is still regarded as the foremost and legitimate voice for all doctors, whether or not they are members. Its role in the setting up of the NHS in the 1940s has been described in Chapter 2, and, since that time, its internal organization has been modified, such that it mirrors the structure of the NHS. Hospital doctors are represented in the BMA by its Central Committee for Hospital Medical Services, while GPs are separately represented by its General Medical Services Committee. The constituents of these two committees are, respectively, the Regional Committee for Hospital Medical Staffs and the Regional Committee for Local Medical Committees, on which doctors working in the NHS are represented. The BMA's leadership has not always been regarded by individual doctors as being in touch with their interests; on a number of occasions the BMA has been publicly unable to present a convincing view of the profession's position. One factor which may contribute to this impression is that there are three separate bodies (or sets of bodies) acting for the profession – the medical corporations for professional representation, the GMC for discipline and self-regulation, and the BMA for pay negotiations.

11.1.3 Medical education

The training of doctors involves a large element of practical experience, and, in the past, students were apprenticed to physicians, surgeons and apothecaries, the university part of their training representing a relatively small element. The balance has now altered, although this tradition has had a substantial influence on the style of undergraduate curricula, and postgraduate education is still mainly in the hands of the professional organizations rather than the universities. By 1858 there were 11 medical schools in London and at least 10 in the provinces apart from the universities of Oxford and Cambridge. By 1914, all except four of the present provincial university medical schools were open.

Before the First World War, the teaching of clinical subjects was provided by physicians and surgeons who, although in private practice, gave their services to the hospitals where students were apprenticed as clerks and dressers for short periods. Pre-clinical subjects were taught by doctors engaged in clinical work who often did not specialize in these subjects. The Haldane report[6], published in 1918, strongly criticized these features and recommended there should be full-time clinical teachers of university status, and that units of medicine and surgery, under clinicians with professorial status, should organize and provide the clinical teaching. It was not until the 1920s, however, that things began to change, and this was partly due to the establishment of the University Grants Committee (now the Higher Education Funding Council for England and its equivalents elsewhere in the UK), which was given responsibility for financing the universities.

The medical schools were becoming steadily more dependent on the universities for funds. Research and specialization extended as a result but, by 1944, the idea of full-time specialist units had not really been implemented, and there were only seven full-time chairs in medicine, four in surgery and two in obstetrics. In that year, the Interdepartmental Committee on Medical Schools published its report (the Goodenough report)[7]. It reaffirmed the main points of the Haldane report and proposed full-time professorial units in obstetrics and gynaecology as well as in medicine and surgery. It suggested that pre-medical studies should be started by potential medical students at secondary school and continued at medical school, and that, after qualification, one year of pre-registration hospital work under supervision should provide the necessary practical experience before a newly qualified doctor could work alone.

The pattern of undergraduate education was further investigated by a Royal Commission chaired by Lord Todd, from 1965 to 1968[8]. At that time, students with high passes in biology, chemistry and physics 'A' level examinations were admitted to medical schools for five terms of preclinical instruction in anatomy, physiology and biochemistry. After examination, the students then studied for three more years, partly in the hospital wards and partly in formal lectures. The subjects included medicine, surgery and sometimes psychiatry. They took examinations in these subjects, too, before obtaining their qualifying degree (MB, BS or MB, ChB or MB, BChir), and then had to spend one further year in approved training posts as house officers before being registered. There was no compulsory further education, although a junior doctor wanting to advance his or her career in certain specialities would have to take further instruction and examination, leading to Membership of the Royal College of Physicians (MRCP) or Fellowship of the Royal College of Surgeons (FRCS), for example.

Equivalent qualifications were also issued by the Conjoint Board of the Royal Colleges of Physicians and Surgeons (MRCS,LRCP) and by the Society of Apothecaries (LMSSA)

The Todd Report was a comprehensive document that questioned the assumptions on which medical education had been based and made several radical recommendations about its future organization. It suggested that the undergraduate curriculum should be broad and flexible, to include sociological subjects and to cover the whole concept of human biology in the preclinical stage, possibly leading to a medical science degree after three years. Four broad modules covering (1) medicine and surgery, (2) psychiatry, (3) obstetrics, gynaecology and paediatrics and (4) community medicine and general practice should constitute the clinical stage, but the qualifying doctor should not be expected to be fully trained. Subsequently, the programme for postgraduate training should be systematically planned to give wide-ranging experience in carefully approved posts, for both hospital special-ists and general practitioners, through the development of postgraduate training centres in the district general hospitals. The report also suggested that the number of places in medical schools should be doubled by 1990, that the twelve London schools be merged into six expanded schools and the postgraduate schools consolidated with them, closer links being forged all over the country between the medical schools and multi-faculty universities.

Following the Todd recommendations, three new provincial medical schools – Southampton (Wessex Medical School), Nottingham and Leicester – were set up. The suggestion regarding medical school numbers has been challenged following concern that there might be too many doctors to allow satisfactory career progression. By 1983, the BMA argued that medical school intake should be held at the 1979 level and even that assumed a considerable increase in the number of GPs consequent on a reduction of list sizes to an average of 1700. This target is yet to be achieved (see Table 11.3).

Postgraduate education is of equal importance and here too there have been changes. Central councils for postgraduate medical education exist for England and Wales, Scotland and Northern Ireland, with responsibility for monitoring standards and advising the regional postgraduate committees. Joint higher training committees have been set up for a number of specialities, to define the scope of special education within the specialities, to establish criteria for posts and inspect them, to recommend patterns of appointments and to provide accreditation. There is, similarly, a Postgraduate Training Committee for General Practice. In 1976, the National Health Service (Vocational Training) Act was passed, creating a legal framework for the future regulation of training for doctors wishing to become general practitioners.

The training of postgraduate doctors has been criticized educationally for the lack of proper supervision and practically because working hours were too long to allow appropriate study time. Accordingly, in December 1993 the DoH Chief Medical Officer Sir Kenneth Calman issued a report, *Hospital Doctors: training for the future*[9], recommending a more streamlined approach by replacing the previous senior and registrar grades with a new specialist registrar grade which should not be held for more than seven years and should have a certificate of completion. This is now replacing the former grades of registrar.

11.1.4 The distribution of hospital doctors

Career progression in hospitals is still difficult to manage. As the DHSS *Medical Manpower*[10] paper pointed out in 1978, hospital medical staffing structure is an 'uneasy pyramidal shape', which was then maintained largely by the employment of overseas doctors and by using junior doctors as 'pairs of hands' rather than trainees. The time spent as a registrar has decreased and theoretically all specialist registrars should become consultants. A few may not achieve this status for a variety of reasons, and become associate specialists instead, whose duties are more limited. Some departments such as casualty departments in smaller general hospitals may rely on such doctors.

The organization of hospital doctors in the NHS was first set out by the Spens Committee on the remuneration of consultants and specialists in 1948[11]. There have been a number of modifications since that time: first, as a result of the recommendations of the Joint Working Party on Medical Staffing Structure in the Hospital Service (the Platt report)[12] in 1961, then the Todd Report suggested an increase in training posts between the registrar and consultant grades. This was rejected by the Royal Commission in 1979[13], which proposed three grades after registration: assistant physician (or surgeon), a grade with a tenure of about four years, and physician, which could be either a final post or act as a training post for the consultant grade. This proposal was not accepted and neither was the suggestion in the King's Fund study *The Organisation of Hospital Clinical Work*[14], a year later, that there should be two grades of consultant – which, it claimed, would encourage mobility and allow consultants to change and develop their interests within their speciality. At present they may hold the same contract for 30 years, although, with the transfer of their contracts from regions to NHS trusts after the 1990 Act, tenure is not quite so secure.

Ensuring a steady flow of suitably trained doctors has always been difficult. In 1981, the House of Commons Social Services Committee (the Short report)[15] endeavoured to deal with the problems which had been troubling the NHS for some years. It recommended increasing the number of consultants and improving the training of hospital doctors aspiring to be consultants. These proposals were not received well by consultants, although they were welcomed by the junior staff. In subsequent discussions, it became clear that a reduction in juniors' working hours in smaller specialities would mean the consultants themselves being first on-call on some occasions, which they found unacceptable.

Previous reports on medical organization had been criticized initially, only to be implemented later on, and the DHSS issued a circular early in 1982, HC(82)4[16], which accompanied the government's response to the Short report and welcomed and supported most of the report's recommendations. In particular, regions were asked to prevent further expansion of senior house officer posts and to draw up plans aimed at achieving, by 1988, a ratio of 1:1 of consultants to training-grade posts and to evaluate the cost of this.

The call to increase consultant numbers was echoed in the report *Achieving a Balance*[17] issued by the Department of Health, the Joint Consultants' Committee of the BMA and the regional chairmen in July 1987. The implementation of these proposals was assisted by the Joint Planning Advisory Committee (JPAC), which had been set up in 1985 to advise the DoH and Welsh Office on the number of posts in the medical and dental training grades needed to meet expected demand in service specialities and research.

Overseas doctors tend to have an unpredictable effect on staffing plans. The GMC's introduction of more stringent language and accreditation procedures has reduced their numbers, as a significant proportion fail these tests. Some overseas countries such as India are now less willing to support UK training for their doctors.

11.1.5 General practitioners

The split between general practitioners and hospital doctors that emerged in the eighteenth and nineteenth centuries still exists, and general practice, although it has consistently attracted about 50% of qualifying doctors in the lifetime of the NHS, remains the somewhat less prestigious choice. Both the Royal College of General Practitioners and the General Medical Services Committee (GMSC) of the BMA have worked hard to improve the standing of general practice, and there is a growing recognition of the fact that general practice, as the key element of primary medical care, is the area where more planning of services and scrutiny of the outcome of treatment is able to alter the balance in the whole pattern of health care. Following the National Health Service and Community Care Act 1990 the power of GPs increased relative to their consultant colleagues because, through purchasing, they had some control over what consultants do. Nevertheless, claims that general practice is in crisis periodically recur.

Between 1949 and 1978 the number of GPs increased by 36%, compared with an increase of hospital doctors of well over 100%. The continuing increase in GP numbers has allowed the average list size to decrease, so that in 1996 there were 32,960 principals with an average list size of 1821. It is the aim of the BMA to reduce the list size to 1700. Within these figures there are variations as to size of practices (see Table 11.3) and list sizes per GP (see Table 11.4).

In order to secure an even distribution of GPs throughout the

Table 11.3

GP practices (1996, England and Wales)

No. of doctors	No. of practices	% of total
1	2863	30
2	1876	15
3	1423	15
4	1257	13
5	933	10
6	645	6
7+	535	5

Source: *Royal College of General Practitioners Information Sheet, September 1997*

Table 11.4

GPs' average list size (1996, UK)

England	1885
Wales	1724
Scotland	1495
N.Ireland	1731
Average	1821

Source: *Royal College of General Practitioners Information Sheet, September 1997*

country, the National Health Service Act, 1946, established a nine-member independent body called the Medical Practices Committee (MPC), responsible for controlling the number of GPs operating in any one area. They did this by introducing four categories; designated areas, with an average list of over 2500; open areas, between 2101 and 2500; intermediate areas, between 1701 and 2100; restricted areas, 1700 or less. HAs are responsible for reporting vacancies to the MPC and making recommendations regarding the filling of posts, which will take into account population changes and other developments. HAs fill the vacancies once they have been authorized by the MPC. In a restricted area, the MPC cannot recommend approval, whereas financial inducements are offered to those wishing to practise in designated areas. The 1990 contract (discussed further below) encouraged GPs to undertake more primary care; some also continue with hospital work as clinical assistants or hospital practitioners, paid directly by the NHS trust concerned.

11.1.6 Community medicine/public health

Although major improvements in public health had been brought about in the nineteenth century by doctors whose standing was then high, over 100 years later this speciality is held in relatively low esteem by the rest of the medical profession. The majority of infectious diseases have been brought under control, and legislation has long since improved the environment to the point where clean air and water can be assumed. However, significant and repeated outbreaks of food poisoning, of diseases caused by new types of environmental hazards and newly identified viruses, have increased awareness that maintaining the public's health cannot be taken for granted; measures are still needed to protect the population.

The speciality of community medicine was meant to have been given impetus by the 1974 reorganization. Instead it became increasingly demoralized and understaffed. The reasons for this decay started when former medical officers of health, autonomous public health specialists employed by the local authorities, found themselves transferred to district or area management teams, where their often powerfully individualistic style of working was deemed inappropriate. Their role became ambiguous thereafter: were they to manage medical work, and if so, whose? Or were they primarily responsible for overseeing the care of the health of the community at large? Despite the Hunter report[18], which had called for the amalgamation of these doctors' managerial and clinical responsibilities, and the 1979 Royal Commission's opinion that community physicians should contribute to planning, health education, epidemiology and environmental health, their role and status diminished. In January 1986, Sir Donald Acheson, Chief Medical Officer to the DoH, was asked to make a special study of the state of public health, and he reported 2 years later. In *Public Health in England*[19], he proposed that each district should have an appropriately trained Director of Public Health, together with at least one other consultant and a specialist in infection control, probably trained in microbiology. Acheson's report completed what some regarded as the emasculation of their speciality by making each new Director of Public Health (DPH) managerially accountable to the District General Manager.

Slowly, however, particularly following the 1990 Act and the emphasis placed on epidemiologically based needs assessments to inform the contracting process and on evidence-based medicine (see Chapter 10), attitudes are changing. The now obligatory annual report from the Director of Public Health is proving a useful instrument for raising the consciousness of health authorities, the professions and the public to the broad challenges facing health care.

11.1.7 Doctors and management

The participation of hospital doctors in management and their contribution to the efficiency of the hospital service was a major theme of the 1974 reorganization, and stemmed from the fact that doctors were in a position to direct the use of costly resources with varying, but often considerable, degrees of autonomy. After discussions between the Minister of Health and the profession in 1965, the Joint Working Party on the Organization of Medical Work in Hospitals was set up to discuss the progress of the NHS, and particularly to review the hospital service. It produced three reports (1967, 1972, 1974[20]), known as the Cogwheel reports because of the design printed on their covers. The first report recommended the creation of divisions of broadly linked specialities, with representatives from among consultants and junior medical staff who would constantly appraise the services and methods of provision within the division.

Such divisions were likely to be set up on a faculty or speciality basis, such as surgery, medicine, obstetrics, pathology, etc. Representatives of each division were to come together in each hospital as a medical executive committee, which would co-ordinate the work and views of the division and provide a link with nursing and administration. The sort of problems they might consider could include bed management and the organization of out-patient and in-patient resources. Most hospital groups gradually implemented this scheme, and, by 1972, the second report was able to identify the essential elements of an effective Cogwheel system and to report that, in large acute hospitals particularly, the system had been helpful in dealing with improved communications, reductions of in-patient waiting lists and the progressive control of medical expenditure. The third report suggested that Cogwheel should continue to deal with issues where the agreement and action of hospital doctors was the main need, while problems requiring strong collaboration between all the professional groups, both within the hospitals and in community services, should be the province of the district management teams and their health care planning teams. It would still be appropriate for Cogwheel systems to concentrate on efficiency issues, and it would be helpful for hospital doctors to see their clinical freedom in the context of team work and the necessity of sharing resources.

Cogwheel has been the basis for subsequent initiatives to involve doctors in managerial issues. It was not until HC(82)1[21] that clear directions were given on how clinical members were to be appointed to the DMT following the 1982 reorganization; the consultant should be elected by the consultant body and the GP by all GPs in a district. Following the 1982 reorganization, unit management teams were also set up, usually as a triumvirate of doctor, nurse and administrator, although some had additioal hospital doctors and GPs. The role of these teams was not altogether easy to determine, nor was their corporate relationship to the DMT. The 1983 Griffiths report proposals[22] recommended modification to this type of team decision-making. Ironically, it was hospital doctors' criticisms of consensus management which probably did most to encourage the Secretary of State to commission the Griffiths report in the first place. The resulting proposal, that there should be a general manager at district and unit level, led the BMA to say that such a post should be held by a doctor, even though many doctors were doubtful that filling the role would be practicable, given their relative or total lack of management training and their prime commitment to patient treatment, which would allow little time for the managerial role. In the event, 19% of unit general managers' jobs in 1986 were held by doctors.

In the late 1980s, formal involvement of doctors in management was brought into focus again by the decision to appoint clinical directors. Under this system, which superseded the Cogwheel structures, one doctor heads a team of clinical colleagues, usually a single speciality, and is held responsible for the appropriate working of that speciality. Doctors need to be involved closely in the decisions about health care, but cannot spend too much time away from their patients. A study by the Institute of Health Services Management in 1990[23] found that various approaches were being adopted for the appointment of clinical directors because the simple model, with one doctor in charge of all the other clinical staff of the team, had been seen as unacceptable. It would have challenged a doctor's clinical autonomy as well as the professional integrity of nurses and other workers. Whatever the local arrangements, the appointment of clinical directors does seem to be helping clinical staff to become more aware of the costs of care and the importance of setting priorities within cash limits[24]. These posts are now essential, with the introduction of clinical governance and the increasing importance of doctors being seen to be accountable for their clinical decisions.

See Chapter 10 for fuller discussion

11.1.8 Doctors' pay and conditions

Doctors' pay has often posed governments difficulties. Doctors' negotiators are no less dedicated than those of other workers and industrial action is not unknown. When the NHS began, systems for employing the services of doctors had to be carefully worked out and negotiated between the government and the profession. Two committees, under the chairmanship of Sir Will Spens, reported in 1948 on the remuneration of general practitioners[25], consultants and specialists. They recommended pay scales for consultants and junior hospital doctors, arrangements for part-time contracts for consultants and a system of distinction awards which would provide for a significant minority the opportunity to earn incomes comparable with the highest that can be earned in other professions. For GPs, the Spens committee recommended a graded scale of incomes, leading to an average net income for doctors at age 40 to 50, which would be paid out of a central pool. The income would be made up of a capitation fee for each patient on a GP's list, including a fixed allowance for practice expenses, plus payments for certain individual items of service. The figures for all doctors were quoted at 1939 money values, leaving to the government the decision about which increases would establish and protect the status of these incomes relative to each other and to other professional incomes, in the context of rising inflation.

The adjustments fixed by the government were not acceptable to the BMA in respect of GPs' incomes, and, after negotiations had broken down, the matter was referred to adjudication in 1953. Mr Justice Danckwerts awarded the GPs a substantial increase and said that the size of the central pool should be related to the total number of GPs and not to the population covered by the NHS, in order that required increases in the numbers of GPs would not be discouraged. The result was that some of the increased incomes were paid directly into a special fund from which GPs could draw if they spent money on improving or building new surgery premises.

The BMA again made a claim for increases in 1956, but this time on behalf of hospital doctors as well as GPs. The health ministers did not agree to it and the matter was referred to a Royal Commission under Sir Harry Pilkington, which sat from 1957 to 1960[26]. It recommended new levels of remuneration, but also that a standing review body of 'eminent persons of experience in various fields of national life' should keep medical and dental remuneration under review, making recommendations which were, on the whole, to be accepted without alteration, directly to the Prime Minister. The effect of setting up this review body in 1963 was to end the practice, initiated by Spens, of calculating doctors' pay increases in relation to the rate of inflation. However, at the same time, it left the pay settlements in the hands of a body, separate from the Ministry, that could be advised but not instructed by the government. The Whitley Council system for collective bargaining and determination of the pay was intended for all staff but the Royal Commission was persuaded to recommend the end of direct negotiations between representatives of the health departments and the profession on Whitley Councils through the creation of a permanent independent review body.

The Review Body
The Review Body on Doctors' and Dentists' Remuneration was duly set up, consisting of six members and the Chairman, Lord Kindersley. Its terms of reference were 'to advise the Prime Minister on the remuneration of doctors and dentists taking any part in the National Health Service'. Twelve reports were issued between 1963 and 1970,

and these concerned the basic rates of pay for different grades of doctors and dentists as well as particular aspects of remuneration, including distinction awards. The Review Body constructed its recommendations after receiving evidence from doctors' and dentists' representatives, from the Ministry/DHSS, and factual information about changes in the cost of living, the movement of earnings in other professions and the state of recruitment in the profession.

However, GPs were not satisfied with the awards made to them by the Review Body, and, in 1965, a crisis developed with the BMA asking GPs throughout the country to sign undated resignation forms which would be used or not, depending on the outcome of negotiations with the Minister. In March 1965, Kenneth Robinson (the Minister of Health since October 1964) largely accepted the GPs' suggestion for a completely new contract, as outlined in the BMA's publication *A Charter for the Family Doctor Service*[27]. This set out a radically revised scheme of payments, including a 5-day working week, 6 weeks' paid annual holiday, payments for out-of-hours services, an independent corporation to make long-term loans to GPs for building or improving surgery premises, ending the pool system, direct reimbursement for practice expenses, ancillary help, and several other items.

The gap between the incomes of GPs and hospital consultants was narrowed. A notable achievement of the whole dispute was, however, to encourage group practice from purpose-built or modified premises, through the setting up of the General Practice Finance Corporation, and the reimbursement of a greater proportion of practice expenses, which encouraged employment of ancillary staff. It also reduced the burden of signing National Insurance certificates, to which GPs had strongly objected.

In March 1970, the Twelfth Report of the Review Body[28] recommended a general increase of 30% for doctors and dentists to be introduced over 2 years, because their pay had been falling behind increases for other professions. The government accepted this for the training grades of doctors and dentists, but agreed to only half the awards for career grades in hospital and general practice work, referring the balance to the National Board for Prices and Incomes. Lord Kindersley and the members of the Review Body resigned on the day after this announcement in June, and the BMA advised its members not to co-operate with the NHS administration. These sanctions were lifted after the general election in 1970, in return for assurances from the new Conservative government that the reference to the National Board for Prices and Incomes would be withdrawn. In November, the government set up three new review bodies to handle the pay negotiations for groups in the public sector where the negotiating machinery had been unsatisfactory: doctors and dentists in the NHS; the chairmen and board members of the nationalized industries; and the armed forces. These review bodies had interlocking membership and their secretariat was provided from the Office of Manpower Economics. The new terms of reference for the Doctors' and Dentists' Review Body (chaired by Lord

In fact 17,800 forms were eventually returned

Halsbury) laid down that their recommendations would not be referred to another body (this had been the reason for Lord Kindersley's resignation) and would not be rejected or modified unless it was unavoidable.

Lord Halsbury resigned as Chairman of the Review Body after the Fourth Report[29], published in July 1974, had been rejected by the profession who expressed their lack of confidence in him. The Review Body continued its work without a chairman, and published a supplement to the Fourth Report at the end of the year. This was accepted by the government and the profession. Annual reports have been issued since then. Tension regarding Review Body recommendations has remained a feature of governments' relationship with doctors. The funding of pay awards over the last 10 or 12 years has not matched the actual awards, however. Although governments have made up most of the difference between the pay award and funds already allocated to the NHS, from the 1980s onwards it increasingly left a deliberate funding gap, which had to be filled by DHAs (and later NHS trusts) by funding the money through efficiency savings. In 1992, the Chancellor of the Exchequer, Norman Lamont, introduced a 1.5% pay ceiling for the public sector, in an attempt to curb government spending in the face of a huge deficit between tax revenues and expenditure. The ceiling affected the Review Body pay recommendations which were effectively ignored by the government. In 1994, the government stated its requirement to keep the rise in the public sector pay bill as close to zero as possible. Again, the Review Body's pay recommendations were ignored. Although NHS trusts had the power to negotiate pay and conditions for their clinical staff, few were prepared to step outside national conditions.

The 1990 GPs' contract

A major change in GPs' pay was embodied in the new contract, implemented on 1 April 1990. The negotiations leading to this were protracted and, at times, bitter. The profession's own leaders in the BMA found the terms they had agreed with the Secretary of State were rejected by the majority of their membership. By August 1989 a revised contract was agreed and sent out to all GPs and, although it too was unpopular, the Secretary of State decided to impose it anyway. A vigorous campaign of opposition, involving patients, did not change his mind.

The new contract (see Figure 11.1) gave greater emphasis to the core of the GPs' remuneration, the capitation fee. Better financial incentives were introduced to encourage more health promotion than before, and attaining targets for immunization and cervical smears is rewarded with cash. Since the implementation of the contract there does appear to have been a corresponding increase in activity in targeted areas but there has been little evaluation of possible detrimental effects of the new target payments on other areas of GPs' work not attracting special payments. To help the GPs there has been a marked increase in practice support staff (Table 11.5).

Main components	% of income*
Capitation	63
Standard capitation fees	
Deprivation payments	
Registration fees	
Child health surveillance	
Target payments	
Cervical cytology	
Childhood immunizations	
Pre-school boosters	
Allowances	17
Practice allowances	
Seniority awards	
Postgraduate education allowances	
Rural practice payments	
Trainee supervision grant	
Out-of-hours allowances	
Items of service fees	16
Night visits	
Temporary residents	
Contraceptive services	
Emergency treatment	
Maternity	
Vaccinations and immunizations	
Sessional	4
Health promotion payments	
Minor surgery	
Teaching medical students	

*The percentages are based on a practice with four partners
Source: adapted from Ellis, N. (1997) *The General Practitioners Handbook.* Radcliffe Medical Press: Abingdon

Figure 11.1

General practitioners' income

In 1997 HAs were permitted to employ GPs on a salary. Although many GPs view salaried status with horror, preferring to keep their semi-independent contractual relationship with HAs, others, unwilling to take on the business commitments that come with joining a practice, have been happy to become salaried. It has also been useful to HAs in filling positions in areas with insufficient doctors.

GPs must be available to their patients for 26 hours per week, and they can no longer give up full responsibility to a deputy or locum. A new allowance was introduced for GPs who train medical students and

	1986	1996
Practice managers	0	6.5
Secretarial/reception	21.9	35.3
Nurses (attached staff from DHA/Trusts not usually included)	2.5	9.8
Others	5.0	7.6
Total	**29.4**	**59.3**

Source: *Health and Personal Social Services Statistics, 1997.* HMSO, London

Table 11.5

Practice staff (thousands whole-time equivalents, England)

who, themselves, take part in regular postgraduate activities. The overall intention was to reward doctors who provide a high quality of service, though many GPs expressed the worry that the contract would merely increase administrative procedures. There seems little doubt, however, that the new contract and the fundholding scheme has put more managerial and administrative pressure on GPs. *The new NHS* groups all GPs into Primary Care Groups run by doctors and nurses. After initial enthusiasm, doubt set in about how this would work and the managerial pressure it would put on doctors[30]. At the same time there was renewed anxiety that that there will be insufficient GPs in the future.

11.1.9 Hospital doctors

Relations between hospital doctors and the government were not so troublesome until about 1972 when dissatisfactions with the form of consultants' contracts arose. The consultants' view, expressed mainly through the BMA, was that they had been required to take on several new responsibilities without adequate pay adjustments. At that time, their contracts specified the minimum number of hours to be worked, depending on whether the doctor had opted to work full-time for the NHS or part-time, in order to take on private work also. Discussions between the consultants and the DoH continued inconclusively, and after the 1974 general election replaced the Conservatives with a Labour government, the new Secretary of State for Social Services, Barbara Castle, took up the consultants' problem. She proposed to make full-time NHS work financially more attractive than part-time work. In addition, she proposed to recast the distinction awards system (see below) entirely by creating two new pay supplements: a medical progress supplement (to award valuable innovations in medical research or academic study, like the old awards) and a service supplement (to reward overburdened consultants in unpopular regions or unfashionable specialities, which the old awards neglected). Negotiations on these proposals were stormy, and took place in the context of the Review Body's deliberations on a claim from the consultants for a large interim backdated increase. At the beginning of 1975, the BMA called on consultants to 'work to contract' (i.e. to do no more than the minimum they were required to do) to demonstrate their opposition to the government's proposals, and their rejection of the Review Body's decision not to grant them an interim award. The disruption caused by the consultants' action was quite widespread; it ceased late in 1975.

At about the same time, however, junior hospital doctors commenced 'work to contract', in support of their claims for a new contract to recognize the long hours and heavy responsibilities they had to shoulder. Again, the negotiations were acrimonious, but a settlement was reached later in 1975 when the Review Body priced two new types of supplement that junior doctors could receive if they worked extra hours over a newly defined basic working week of 40 hours. The cost of this settlement turned out to be more expensive than the Review Body had calculated, because of the way the health authorities awarded the new supplements. In addition, hospital work levels were significantly reduced as a result of the consultants and junior doctors 'working to contract', and this showed up as increased waiting times for out-patient appointments and in-patient admissions.

The junior doctors' new contract took effect from February 1976. Subsequent discussions focused on the reduction in junior doctors' working hours and revised training arrangements. In 1994 the DoH issued the circular *The new deal: plan for action*[31] which obliged HAs and trusts to work together to reduce working hours and to provide more satisfactory shift arrangements to allow for reasonable time off and time for study.

Negotiating pay for doctors and some of the other professional groups runs no more smoothly now than it did 20 years ago. The Review Body was set up to avoid recurrent disputes and to arrive at settlements which would be fair to the profession and to the taxpayer who foots the bill. In the event, the effect of greater militancy among members of the medical profession, and government attempts to control the rate of pay increases, has put great strains on the ability of both sides to negotiate acceptable pay and terms of work under the NHS. Intrinsic problems persist. When first set up, the Review Body seemed to be more sensitive and more influential than the Whitley Council, but it has also been politically more vulnerable to governments who can negotiate on the assumption that doctors will not be able to invoke support from other groups of NHS staff or their trade unions. The professional representatives of the Review Body are not always in accord, and junior medical staff have had serious disagreements with their parent body, the BMA. Another lever in the negotiations is relativities. Doctors have been able to demonstrate from time to time that they have done less well over time than other professional groups.

Other aspects of hospital doctors' pay have also given rise to dispute. The system of distinction awards makes extra annual payments to some 34% of consultants (Table 11.6). In 1998 the Secretary of State announced a review of merit awards in the wake of a case in Bristol where a consultant surgeon who had been struck off for bad clinical practice even though he was in receipt of a significant merit award. The system of allocating these awards is conducted by doctors themselves through regional committees, managers being involved only in nominations to the lowest of the four levels of award. The awards have national status and are funded centrally. The cost in 1994/95 was around £109 million.

	% basic salary	value of award
A+	95	£54,910
A	80	£40,460
B	60	£23,120
	No % award but 5 discretionary points	£2300–11,560

Source: British Medical Association

Table 11.6

Merit and Distinction Awards (1998)

The changed managerial climate of the late 1980s brought a more rigorous approach to doctors' employment through the requirement that each consultant's work plan should be agreed with the local management to ensure that they matched service needs. This was endorsed in one of the papers[32] accompanying *Working for Patients*, and led some consultants to fear that they could be expected to work more under non-medical direction than they considered compatible with their professional status. Management's view was that greater efficiency required a clear contract with the consultants, specifying what is to be done, and when. Increasing emphasis on evidence-based medicine and on comparing consultants' workloads is eroding some of the autonomy that consultant doctors thought was their professional privilege. It remains to be seen whether this will influence consultants' motivation.

Another initiative aimed at improving the quality of service was the white paper's emphasis on the importance of medical audit. The Confidential Enquiry into Perioperative Deaths (CEPOD)[33] examined, in three regions, all deaths within 30 days of surgical operation; this survey was later extended to the whole country. Every district is required to have clinical audit committees managed by the doctors themselves. The outcomes, reported anonymously, can be made available to local management. In due course, participating in medical audit could be made a contractual obligation. The medical profession's opposition to the 1989 white paper was vociferous, but as had happened before, once the reforms were under way, doctors in hospitals and general practice decided it was simpler to accept change.

See Section 10.7

11.2 NURSING

The practice of nursing, which takes various forms, aims to promote health, prevent illness, restore health and alleviate suffering. Nurses are by far the most numerous NHS staff: in 1996 there were 352,300 (whole-time equivalents) nurses employed and, in an average acute services NHS trust, their salaries amount to well over 40% of the total budget, a level of expenditure, therefore, that has to be managed particularly effectively. After the 1974 reorganization, the nursing profession underwent several fundamental changes in practice and organization. This part of the chapter first provides a historical review of the origins of the various parts of nursing and then reviews recent events that have promoted nursing as an independent profession no longer subordinate to medicine.

11.2.1 History of nursing

Hospital nursing

Hospital nursing is rooted in the work of the nursing orders of the religious houses of the Middle Ages. Men and women who became monks and nuns were called by a sense of vocation to alleviate the sufferings of sick people. The oldest hospitals, St Bartholomew's (1123) and St Thomas' (1215) were founded to reflect this concern. Even with the founding of voluntary hospitals in the eighteenth century nursing standards were often poor. Matters improved in the nineteenth century when Elizabeth Fry founded an Institute of Nursing at Guy's Hospital where women were trained under the influence of Quaker teaching.

Florence Nightingale (1820–1910), traditionally the founder of modern nursing, rejecting her upper class background, went to the Crimea in 1854 and redeemed the apparently hopeless situation of the army hospitals in that war. Returning with a secure reputation, she devoted the rest of her long life to public works and in particular to establishing nursing as a respectable profession. The Nightingale Training School at St Thomas' was the forerunner of many others. The ward sister became the keystone of nursing care, carrying out the wishes of the doctors and training her own staff. At the top of the hierarchy was the matron, in charge of nursing and housekeeping. Matrons shed these other responsibilities only in the 1950s. Nurse training in poor-law infirmaries, fever hospitals and lunatic asylums took longer to set up, and there was no recognized training for nursing mentally ill patients until 1891 when the Royal Medico-Psychological Society started to issue certificates.

Nursing needed statutory recognition to become a secure profession. The matter was resolved in 1919 with the passing of the Nursing Registration Acts, which established the General Nursing Council (GNC). The GNC maintained a register of nurses trained in approved institutions who had passed examinations after 3 years of study and supervised practice. The Nurses Act 1943 recognized the scope for employing more practical nurses and accordingly approved a 2-year training to enrolment. The 1949 Nurses Act incorporated male nurses into the main register (they had had their own register since 1919) but not until the Sex Discrimination Act, 1975, were men allowed to train as midwives. Currently some 10% of nurses are men. The GNC was superseded by the United Kingdom Council for Nursing, Midwifery and Health Visiting in 1983 (under review in 1999). Progress on the professional status of nursing came with 1966 Salmon report and the fundamental changes to training of the early 1990s (see below).

Community nursing

Community nurses – that is, district nurses, health visitors and midwives – unlike their hospital counterparts had always worked independently. The history of district nursing is closely associated with philanthropists such as William Rathbone in Liverpool and the Queen's Institute of District Nursing, set up with money given at Queen Victoria's silver and golden jubilees at the end of the nineteenth century. The Queen's Institute accepted nurses who were already registered and gave them further training to equip them to work in the community. Under the NHS Act, 1946, local authorities became responsible for organizing home nursing and, at first, tended to use Queen's Institute nurses on an agency basis until they began recruiting and training their own staff.

The title 'health visitor' probably first came into use in 1862 when a voluntary body, the Ladies' Sanitary Reform Association of Manchester and Salford, paid staff to visit people in those towns, concentrating on cleanliness, healing the sick and advising mothers on the care of their children. In 1875, the Royal Sanitary Institute (now the Royal Society of Health) was founded to promote the health of the people and began to set examinations for sanitary inspectors. In 1892, Florence Nightingale started a course at Buckinghamshire Technical College where 'health missionaries' were trained to meet the needs of 'home health-bringing', and the women thus trained were employed by the local council to visit people in need. The Royal Sanitary Institute set examinations for health visitors and school nurses from 1906, and, in 1908, the London County Council decreed that all health visitors should hold an accredited certificate approved by the Local Government Board.

The scope for improvements in health at that time is demonstrated by the infant mortality rate (deaths in the first year of life), which was 163 per 1000 live births at the turn of the century and 6.1 in 1996. Acts passed in 1907 and 1915 requiring births to be registered provided the means of identifying the problem, and from then health visitors have continued to concentrate on infant and maternal welfare. The Jamieson report (1956)[34] endorsed this emphasis.

In recent years health visitors, traditionally the most highly trained nurses, have had difficulty in defining their role given the overlaps with district nursing, health promotion and social work. Their professional association changed its name to Community Practitioners and Health Visitors Association in January 1997 in an endeavour to encapsulate their broader role and recognize those of its 17,000 members who worked in community roles, such as school and practice nurses, but who were not trained health visitors.

District nurses' work has become more demanding with earlier discharges from hospital and the general development of community care. An Audit Commission report[35] noted that district nurses treated 2.75 million patients a year at an estimated cost of £660 million. Given the ageing workforce, the report urged trusts and health authorities to review what district nurses were doing, with a view to a more rational allocation of work and to ensuring that skills were maintained.

Midwives
Midwives have been recognized from earliest times. Only in the late nineteenth century did richer families prefer a doctor to deliver their babies, principally because the majority of midwives were said to be untrained, often ignorant and of 'very low character', epitomized in Dickens' character Mrs Gamp. Their standards started improving again with the foundation of the Midwives Institute in 1881 by a group of women who wished to strengthen the status of the midwife. The 1902 Midwives Act established the Central Midwives Board to keep a roll of approved midwives and to ensure adequate training programmes and standards of good practice. The Ministry of Health, created in 1919, then took over supervision of the Board.

Midwifery was practised in hospitals, in independent nursing homes and at home. There was a need to regulate arrangements and in 1948 local health authorities were given the statutory duty to provide a domiciliary midwifery service and to supervise standards of practice. Hospital management committees had to provide sufficient facilities for a mother to have her baby in hospital if she so wished. Following the recommendations of the Cranbrook report (1959)[36] and the Peel report (1970)[37], hospital confinement has become the norm. This change has greatly affected the nature of the work midwives do, now that hospital obstetric services rely so much on medical expertise and sophisticated technical procedures for antenatal tests and monitoring. Those working only in hospital or only in the community may lose some of their skills, unless they are part of an integrated system which allows them experience in both settings. The 1993 report *Changing Childbirth*[38] is a boost to their professionalism.

See Section 9.8

11.2.2 Principal reforms

In 1963, shortages of trained nurses and the apparent decline in the status of nursing prompted the government to set up a review of the profession under the chairmanship of Brian Salmon. Its report, published three years later[39], noted that the title 'matron' was applied equally to nursing heads of hospitals whether they had 10 beds or 1000, and that the distinction between their duties and functions had become increasingly unclear. It was said that job titles were themselves anachronistic now that men held 'sister' and 'matron' posts. The report, therefore, recommended a much clearer hierarchy to recognize that in nursing, as in other professions, there were intrinsic differences between top, middle and first-line management. Policy was the responsibility of the top manager, the chief nursing officer; programming policies was what middle managers, principal and senior nursing officers were there to do; and the practical delivery of nursing remained with the first-line nurse, nursing officer, charge nurse or sister, and staff nurse.

- Nursing should share equal status with medicine and management.
- Nursing should be organized to differentiate between:
  - policy-makers – top management;
  - those who programme policy–middle management;
  - those who control its execution–first-line management.
- A new 5-level grading structure should reflect this.
- Non-nursing duties should be removed from nursing supervision.
- Nurses should receive managerial training appropriate to their grade.
- The scope and function of nursing committees should be reviewed.

Box 11.1

Salmon report 1966

The recommendations were accepted and it was agreed that 16 pilot schemes should be set up and evaluated. There was impatience to move faster, so the evaluation exercise was never seriously undertaken. This proved unfortunate. Doctors and administrators were always rather scornful of the idea of nurses as managers, caricaturing the new ranks as 'clipboard-carrying nurses' who would be at a loss if faced with a patient. Nurses themselves did not always implement the new structures wisely, and, by too slavishly following the Salmon report's blueprint for several managerial levels, they created unnecessarily complicated local hierarchies. But the report did establish the professional head of nursing as an equal with his or her administrative and medical colleagues. This was later upheld through full-status membership of the management teams at district, area and region, following the 1974 reorganization.

There were also changes in the organization of community nursing. The 1968 report from the National Board for Prices and Incomes[40], as well as urging implementation of the Salmon structures to improve the pay prospects of more senior hospital nurses, noted that the fragmentation of community nursing services should be counteracted by designating similar senior posts. Following this, the DHSS set up a working party, under the chairmanship of E.L. Mayston, to consider how far the Salmon management concepts were applicable to community nursing. Its report was published in 1969[41] and commended by the Secretary of State to local authorities employing community nurses.

The Mayston report noted that health visitors were concerned with the health of families as a whole, health education, the early detection of abnormalities in children and school health. It recognized that district nurses provided skilled care in people's homes under the clinical direction of GPs, and recommended that they be attached to GP practices more securely in order to facilitate integrated care.

Box 11.2

The Mayston report 1969

- Every local health authority should have a chief nursing officer.
- The senior nursing structure should be immediately reviewed.
- There should be three levels of nursing management.
- Management training should be given to senior community nurses.

Local health authorities restructured their nursing hierarchy accordingly, appointing a director of nursing services accountable to the medical officer of health for all nursing and midwifery services in the community. Because the 1974 reorganization then amalgamated the management of community and hospital services, the two nursing structures had to be brought together in each district under the District Nursing Officer. Some specialization remained, unlike in the social work services, where reorganization based on the Seebohm report[42] had introduced the concept of the 'generic' social worker to respond to all types of client needs.

Within districts community nursing was usually allocated to its own nursing division headed by a divisional nursing officer. In some AHAs, community nursing remained in the control of the areas rather than the districts because, for instance, the organization of child health services benefited from a coterminous boundary with the local county education authority.

There were also a few posts for nurses at area and regional level to participate in strategic planning. These opportunities away from practical nursing provided more ambitious nurses interested in management with a good career path similar to that of administrators and other senior specialists. It was the reductions in these very opportunities that caused much of the resentment when, 10 years later, general management was introduced. Nurses were potential candidates for the role of District General Manager but, in the event, few applied and even fewer were appointed. From holding the rank of a district management team member and the status of a chief officer accountable directly to the health authority, they became subordinates of the DGM. At unit level there was a similar effect, as the head nurse was made responsible to the unit general manager instead of the district nursing officer. The Royal College of Nursing campaigned vehemently through 1985, protesting at this loss of status, and stressing the indisputable fact that only nurses were with the patient 24 hours in the day. They argued that this gave them a position that had to be reflected in representation at the highest levels of decision-making. But the concept of general management did not allow this. Where nurses did become general managers they quickly learnt that they could not wear two hats: the generalist perspective had to be paramount, whatever the incumbent's professional background.

By 1990, nurses had accepted the new position, probably encouraged by their experience that, in most districts, nursing services were not valued any less, even with the slight loss in status. Indeed, in some cases, the middle managers and first-line nursing staff expressed preference for the new arrangements, welcoming the opportunities they now had to convince general managers of the importance of their role, and eliciting much support in the process. The period after 1984 was difficult for the displaced chief nursing officers, as they adapted to jobs with less managerial scope, such as quality assurance and planning.

Following the 1990 reforms, nurses again found themselves on decision-making boards. Their membership was obligatory within NHS trusts, optional at health authority level. But in the majority of trusts this did not mean that this nurse directly managed all the nurses, only that she/he was head of nursing practice. Opinion remains divided as to the wisdom of separating these functions.

Nursing is not just a task-orientated activity, with procedures carried out according to prescribed routines. According to *The Extended Clinical Role of The Nurse*[43], the nursing process, as it came to be called, should concentrate on the patient as a whole. This led to the idea of a 'primary' nurse, later called a 'named nurse', who was assigned to a small group of patients on the ward and was primarily responsible for their care. Traditionalists complained that this led to less efficiency on the wards, but it has undoubtedly encouraged nurses to be more knowledgeable about those they care for.

In the community, the increasing number of nurses attached to GP practices brought its own organizational problems, mainly because many GPs still had patients scattered around the locality and the overlap between neighbouring practices was considerable. This meant that nurses from several practices were working in the same area with a consequential waste of resources. The 1986 Cumberlege report *Neighbourhood Nursing – A Focus for Care*[44] recommended that the advantages of having nurses attached to practices could be retained, and that better deployment would result, if they were organized to serve communities of between 10,000 and 25,000 population. The report was disparaging about the practice nurses employed directly by GPs, saying they lacked the necessary skills and were professionally isolated. However, the 1990 GP contract ignored this criticism, giving emphasis to the continued employment of practice nurses and encouraging expansion (for instance into management) without always the requisite training proposed by *The new NHS*, which continues to emphasize the importance of community nurses in commissioning health care, through the involvement of nurses in primary care groups.

Further developments in practice seem set to continue, with nurses taking over some of the doctor's duties such as limited prescribing and patient assessments, and with nurse practitioners taking their own referrals. Overall, though, it seems that the profession had a brief taste of managerial influence in the 1970s, while mostly it still works under the ultimate supervision of doctors in hospital and community settings.

In an effort to rally morale, particularly of senior nurses, in 1989 the Chief Nursing Officer of the Department of Health published *A Strategy for Nursing*[45]. The document examined practice, staffing, education, leadership and management, and reviewed the changes taking place, or needed, to establish the profession as an equal partner with the others involved in looking after the patient.

11.2.3 Education and training

The General Nursing Council was set up in 1919 and survived, with various modifications, until 1 July 1983, when it was superseded by the United Kingdom Central Council for Nursing, Midwifery and Health Visiting (UKCC), which was established by the Nurses, Midwives and Health Visitors Act, 1979. The impetus for this change came from the report of the Committee on Nursing, known as the Briggs report, published in 1972[46]. As well as its more general concerns about nursing, it addressed the statutory framework controlling the professions of nursing and midwifery and their educational needs. The three branches of nursing had a different statutory history, and Briggs said that this needed remedying so that a more coherent approach to education and training could be developed.

The 1979 Act repealed the Nurses' Acts of 1957, 1964 and 1969, as well as amending a large number of clauses of other Acts concerning nursing. The new Act required the UKCC to establish and improve standards of training and professional conduct, to determine rules for registration and for maintaining a single professional register and to protect the public from unsafe practitioners. The UKCC was supplemented by national boards for each country in the UK. In particular, these boards have to provide, or arrange for others to provide, courses of training leading to registration, and they have an important role in fostering post-registration courses now usually developed by universities. Review of their working in 1998 led to a government proposal to repeal the present arrangements and set up a single UK Nursing, Midwifery and Health Visiting Council[47] which aims to strengthen regulatory powers and co-operation with kindred professions, given the changing boundaries of clinical responsibility.

The 1979 Act lowered the minimum age for entry to nursing training to 17 and imposed a common standard of entry qualifications for first-level nurses. The Briggs report discussed the concept of a 'common portal of entry' whereby, instead of registered and enrolled nurses having to pursue different training schemes, all those intending to nurse would undertake a common core course of study, specializing only thereafter. This worried those who felt that the entry requirement would be too low to select nurses capable of high academic achievement, or so high it would deter the good practical nurse. This point was ultimately addressed by the proposals of *Project 2000*, published in 1986[48].

Project 2000 marked a major change, aiming to exchange apprentice status for true student status. Students are now supernumerary to the ward workforce. The initial core course lasts for 18 months, after which the trainee proceeds to a specialist branch such as children or mental health. There is now concern that specialization takes place too early and that there is dearth of 'general' nurses in the middle grades. Nurses are now required to keep their professional practice up to date through post-registration education and practice (PREP); failure to do so will compromise their registration which has to be renewed every 2 years. Previously only midwives were subject to this reassessment process on a 5-year basis.

Implementation of *Project 2000* was hampered by its cost and the administrative difficulties. The report of Working Party 10[49], associated with the 1990 NHS reforms, gave control of nurse education to the regions, and schools of nursing were then transferred to universities who were themselves going through substantial expansion.

In order to provide substitute staff for the student nurses who previously undertook a significant part of basic nursing, the nursing auxiliary (general) or nursing assistant (mental illness) grades are filled by health care assistants, of whom 16,800 are formally designated. There are still many others who work in nursing without nursing qualifications. The trend to give these staff training is being pursued by the Qualifications and Curriculum Authority.

11.2.4 Nurses' pay

Nurses are a powerful group in the NHS because of their numbers. They have always been able to command the sympathy of the general public. Despite this, nurses' pay has not always compared well with rates in other countries. Although UK nurses are usually assumed to be underpaid, their position relative to other groups has varied. For most employees in the public sector, pay awards have seldom reflected the true costs of living; by degrees, the pay of NHS workers has fallen further behind the general level of settlements, which has provoked crises in relations with the government and repeated calls from the staff for recognition of the justice of their claims. Nurses had not traditionally been militant but this altered in the late 1960s with the Royal College of Nursing's 'Raise the Roof' campaign.

Discontent persisted until the government commissioned Lord Halsbury to examine nurses' pay. His first report, in 1974[50], gave substantial awards to most grades of nursing staff, and some increase in holiday allowances. The benefit was gradually eroded although a Review Body had been set up as an alternative to the Whitley Council to determine nurses' pay. A new approach, agreed in 1988[51], aimed to assess all the nursing responsibilities and allocate nursing grades according to agreed criteria. On the face of it this was a much fairer system than before, where some nurses had been undertaking more responsible work than others and yet had been receiving less pay. Unfortunately, this enquiry into clinical grading caused a storm of discontent. Many nurses disagreed with the assessments made by their managers, claiming that they took more responsibility than their manager said. In turn, the nurse managers would not agree to nurses claiming responsibilities that they regarded as superfluous or outside their competence. Doctors inflamed the situation by supporting the nurses' appeals against the managers, in pursuit of personal patronage and loyalty to the nursing staff with whom they worked.

Thousands of nurses lodged formal appeals and the hearings were only completed in 1994. What had begun as steps towards a rational and fair grading system ended by provoking more opposition among nurses to their employer than anything before. The experience was not all bad, however; at the end of the assessment exercise, management for the first time had a complete picture of what nurses were doing and to what standard of competence. There was now an explicit system for deciding the correct mix of skills for each type of clinical work.

Senior nursing staff, although dissatisfied over status, had held on to their advantageous pay rates and conditions of service throughout the 1980s. For example, the right to retire early with accelerated pension benefits continued, even after the original reason for such payments (living in and therefore being constantly on call) had long since ended. In 1991, a new pay scale for senior nurses was introduced to mirror that already in place for senior managers. The effect of this was to remove a long-standing difference between managers and nurse managers, which had caused the nurses considerable resentment. There are perennial crises in nursing and in 1997 the Minister for Health, Baroness Jay, announced a campaign to recruit more nurses for training and to encourage those already trained to stay in nursing. Despite this their next pay award was implemented in stages.

CONCLUSION

Doctors remain the lead professional group in the NHS, despite the development of trained NHS general managers, particularly in the 1980s and 1990s. Although managers of the largest NHS trusts have seen their pay rise appreciably, doctors seem able to remain the best paid group of health care staff overall. This is partly because their contracts have advantageous elements not available to others: for example many consultants can do private work in addition to their NHS contract[52]. Doctors have also managed their own profession in ways that have reinforced their autonomous position at the top of the health workers' pyramid. This is not unique to the medical profession or to the UK, of course. Whether doctors can maintain their pre-eminent status in the future is at least questionable, given that they are being held much more accountable, not only by the government but also by their patients. There are dangers: patients need to trust their doctors. Putting them under too much pressure may destroy this delicate but essential requirement and lead to the law courts. If the use of litigation became much more prevalent, it could threaten fundamentally the doctor–patient relationship.

Although doctors traditionally may be seen as the leading group in the health service, nurses in fact provide the vast majority of care to patients in hospital and in the community. For most hospital patients, contact with doctors is small and intermittent compared with the involvement with nurses. For those receiving care from health visitors, district nurses and other community-based nurses, the nurse is the main health professional. As with many kinds of personal service, the history of nursing has been one of greater professionalization through the creation of national representative and regulatory bodies, formalization of entry qualifications and increased training. Along with this professionalization has come greater responsibility. Tasks once seen as the domain of doctors are now routinely carried out by nurses and this trend is continuing. But there has been a counter-trend whereby some of the autonomy attached to nursing may decline as doctors lead clinical and managerial teams more explicitly. The new training has led to some anxiety that day-to-day nursing care is now in the hands of less capable staff and that some of the traditional standards attached to nursing may be lost.

REFERENCES

1. DHSS (1972) *Women Doctors' Retainer Scheme* Circular HM(72)42.
2. DHSS (1969) *Redeployment of Women Doctors* Circular HM(69)6.
3. Dowie, F. (1990) *Patterns of Hospital Medical Staffing. Junior Doctors' Hours, Interim report.* British Postgraduate Medical Federation, London.
4. Further Medical Acts, passed in 1956 and 1969, consolidated amendments to the membership and powers of the Council.

5. *Committee of Enquiry into the Regulation of the Medical Profession* (1975) Report of the Committee (Merrison report). HMSO, London (Cmnd 6018).

6. Ministry of Reconstruction (1918) *Report of the Machinery of Government Committee* (Haldane report). HMSO, London (Cd 9230).

7. Ministry of Health (1944) *Report of the Interdepartmental Committee on Medical Schools* (Goodenough report). HMSO, London.

8. *Royal Commission on Medical Education* (1968) Report of the Royal Commission (Todd report). HMSO, London (Cmnd 3569).

9. DoH (1993) *Hospital Doctors: training for the future. The report of the working party on specialist medical training* (Calman report). DoH, London.

10. DHSS (1978) *Medical Manpower – The Next Twenty Years.* HMSO, London.

11. Ministry of Health and Department of Health for Scotland (1948) *Report of the Interdepartmental Committee on the Remuneration of Consultants and Specialists* (Spens report). HMSO, London (Cmnd 7420).

12. Ministry of Health and Department of Health for Scotland (1961) *Medical Staffing Structure in the Hospital Service: Report of the Joint Working Party* (Platt report). HMSO, London.

13. Royal Commission on the National Health Service (1979) *Report of the Royal Commission.* HMSO, London (Cmnd 7615).

14. King's Fund (1979) *The Organisation of Hospital Clinical Work.* Project Paper No. 22 King's Fund, London.

15. House of Commons Social Services Committee Session 1980–81 Fourth report. *Medical Education with Special Reference to the Number of Doctors and the Career Structure in Hospitals* (Short report). House of Commons, London.

16. DHSS (1982) *Hospital Medical Staff: Career Structure and Training* Circular HC(82)4. HMSO, London.

17. DHSS, BMA Joint Consultants' Committee, RHA Chairmen (1987) *Hospital Medical Staffing: Achieving a Balance.* London.

18. DHSS (1972) *Report of the Working Party on Medical Administrators* (Hunter report). HMSO, London.

19. DoH (1988) *Public Health in England* (Acheson report). HMSO, London. (Cm 289).

20. Ministry of Health/DHSS (1967, 1972, 1974) *First, Second and Third reports of the Joint Working Party on the Organisation of Medical Work in Hospitals* (Cogwheel reports). HMSO, London.

21. DHSS (1982) *Health Service Development. Professional Advisory Machinery* Circular HC(82)1. DHSS, London.

22. DHSS (1983) *The NHS Management Inquiry* (Griffiths report). DHSS, London.

23. Dixon, M. *et al.* (1990) *Models of Clinical Management.* Institute of Health Services Management, London.

24. See for example, Audit Commission (1994) *Trusting the Future: Towards an Audit Agenda for NHS Providers.* HMSO, London.

25. op. cit. Spens report.

26. Royal Commission on Doctors' and Dentists' Remuneration (1960) Report of the Royal Commission (Pilkington report). HMSO, London (Cmnd 939).

27. BMA (1965) A Charter for the Family Doctor Service. *British Medical Journal* 189: 89.

28. Review Body on Doctors' and Dentists' Remuneration. (1970) *Twelfth Report* (Kindersley report). HMSO, London (Cmnd 4352).

29. Review Body on Doctors' and Dentists' Remuneration (1974) *Fourth Report* (Halsbury report). HMSO, London (Cmnd 5644).

30. Hunter, D. J. and Marks, L. (1998) *The development of primary care groups: policy into practice*. NHS Confederation, Birmingham.

31. DoH (1994) *The new deal; plan for action* Executive Letter EL(95)17. DoH, London.

32. DoH (1989) *Working for Patients: Working Paper 7* para. 2.5. HMSO, London.

33. *Confidential Enquiry into Perioperative Deaths*, 1987. Nuffield Provincial Hospitals Trust, London.

34. *Working Party in the Field of Work, Training and Recruitment of Health Visitors* (1956) Report of the Working Party (Jamieson report). HMSO, London.

35. Audit Commission (1999) *First Assessment: a review of district nursing services in England and Wales*. Audit Commission Publications, Abingdon, UK.

36. Ministry of Health (1959) *Report of the Maternity Services Committee* (Cranbrook report). HMSO, London.

37. DHSS, Central Health Services Council (1970) *Domiciliary Midwifery and Maternity Bed Needs* (Peel report). HMSO, London.

38. DoH, Expert Maternity Group (1993) *Changing Childbirth* (Cumberlege report). HMSO, London.

39. Ministry of Health and Scottish Home and Health Department (1966) *Report of the Committee on Senior Nursing Staff Structure* (Salmon report). HMSO, London.

40. National Board for Prices and Incomes (1968) *Pay of Nurses and Midwives in the NHS Report No. 60*. HMSO, London (Cmnd 3585).

41. DHSS, Scottish Home and Health Department, Welsh Office (1969) *Report of the Working Party on Management Structures in the local Authority Nursing Services* (Mayston report). HMSO, London.

42. Home Office (1968) *Report of the Committee on Local Authority and Allied Social Services* (Seebohm report). HMSO, London.

43. Royal College of Nursing (1979) *The Extended Clinical Role of the Nurse*. Royal College of Nursing, London.

44. DHSS (1986) *Neighbourhood Nursing – a Focus for Care* (Cumberlege report). HMSO, London.

45. DoH, Nursing Division (1989) *A Strategy for Nursing – a report of the Steering Committee* (Poole report). DoH. London.

46. DHSS (1972) *Report of the Committee on Nursing* (Briggs report). HMSO, London (Cmnd 5115).

47. DoH (1999) *Report on a review of the Nurses, Midwives and Health Visitors Act 1997 – the government's response*. DoH, London.

48. UKCC (1986) *Project 2000: A New Preparation for Practice*. UKCC, London.

49. DoH (1989) *Working for Patients. Working Paper 10: Education and Training*. HMSO, London.

50. DHSS (1974) *Report of the Committee of Enquiry into the Pay and Related Conditions of Service of Nurses and Midwives* (Halsbury report). HMSO, London.

51. DHSS (1988) *Clinical Nurse Grading Structure* Advance Letter NM1/88. DHSS, London.

52. Yates, J. (1995) *Private Eye, Heart and Hip*. Churchill Livingstone, London.

12

OTHER STAFF AND HUMAN RESOURCE ISSUES

In the public's mind, doctors and nurses are the most important people in the NHS, and indeed they are the most numerous, making up 55% of all NHS staff (see Table 11.1). Nevertheless, there are many other staff – therapeutic, scientific, domestic and managerial – without whom the NHS could not operate. This chapter gives a brief account of them and then reviews aspects of industrial relations, pay and training that affect all staff.

12.1 DENTISTS

In the seventeenth and eighteenth centuries there was no distinct profession of dentistry, but some barber-surgeons became known as 'operators for the teeth'. As scientific study of the teeth advanced, some practitioners were able to become very skilled specialists while others, who remained unskilled and unqualified, obtained their work through advertising. In 1878 the Dentists Act empowered the General Medical Council to examine and register suitably qualified dentists, but unqualified dentists continued to practise. The British Dental Association was founded in 1880 and dentistry became recognized as a profession. However, unregistered practitioners continued to flourish, and many of them were inadequately trained. It was not until 1921 that a new Dentists Act dealt with this by effectively closing the profession to anyone who was not trained at a school of dentistry recognized by the newly created Dental Board. The Act made the Dental Board responsible for keeping a register and for investigating cases of misconduct, but the GMC retained control over disciplinary action and the power to license practitioners.

A further Dentists Act, in 1957, established the General Dental Council as the single statutory licensing and registering body, taking on the functions of the Dental Board and the GMC (in relation to dentistry). It supervises the standard of dental examinations and teaching, and keeps the register of dentists who have obtained professional qualifications from one of the 14 approved schools of dentistry in the UK. (There are also two postgraduate schools.) Currently, around 700 students a year are admitted to study for either a degree (Bachelor of Dental Surgery, BDS) or a diploma (Licentiate in Dental Surgery, LDS). The training takes five years and, once trained, dentists pay an entry and retention fee to have their name on the register. Practitioners' names can be erased if they commit a felony or if they are found guilty of professional misconduct by the Council's disciplinary committee.

The Dentists Act 1983 revised the membership of the Council.

There are now 29 members, of whom 18 are registered dentists elected from among themselves, four are the chief dental officers of England, Wales, Scotland and Northern Ireland, six are lay people nominated by the Queen on the advice of the Privy Council and one is a dental auxiliary. The President is elected from this membership. In addition, three members of the General Medical Council can join discussions on dental education and examination issues. Those universities with dental schools can also send one member each (two for the University of London) who are additional to the 29 members and must themselves be dentists.

12.1.1 History of dental services

Before the NHS was founded, the general state of dental health was very poor. The School Medical Service, established in 1907, made provision for the dental care of mothers and children of pre-school age, but less than 2% of the eligible population made use of this and, although dental benefits were available under the National Health Insurance scheme to 13 million of the working population, only about 6% made claims. After 1948, the NHS provided dental services in each arm of the tripartite structure. Hospital dentists specialized in dental surgery or orthodontics (the straightening of children's teeth) and were graded in the same way as hospital medical staff. Some worked in dental departments of general hospitals and others worked within specialist dental hospitals. Local authorities were obliged by the 1944 Education Act to provide free dental inspection and treatment for all children in maintained schools, and they also cared for the dental health of expectant and nursing mothers.

In 1974, the reorganization changed only the administration of dental services; it did not alter this pattern of clinical work. Hospital dental surgeons (consultant oral surgeons and orthodontists) remained employees of the regions (or, in the case of teaching areas, the AHA(T)), and junior dental staff were employed by the districts. Local authority dental staff were transferred to the new areas which became responsible for community and school dental services throughout the area. General dental practitioners remained in contract with the family practitioner committees. The 1982 reorganization fragmented these arrangements by devolving the area responsibilities to each district, which appointed a district dental officer accountable to the DHA. Dental Advisory Committees ceased to be statutory in 1982, but most districts have one. These committees exist to give expert opinion on the provision of dental services; they are not concerned with the relations between the profession and its employers or with the internal organization of the profession.

Dental care is provided by general dental practitioners, to whom patients refer themselves for regular care; each episode of treatment is self-contained. The contract agreed in 1990 (see below) encourages patients and dentists to enter into a more continuous arrangement. There has been increasing concern that more deprived families are not seeking treatment. Dentists have been encouraged to maintain contact with these patients and the capitation payments were raised in 1998 by 25% for treating deprived children under the age of six. This followed an initiative from the DoH in 1997 *Investing in Dentistry*[1], which aims to tackle the unequal distribution of dentists and to encourage continuing professional education.

Children's teeth today generally have a much lower incidence of caries than in the past, but some groups such as elderly people and the handicapped, particularly those who live in residential care, need special attention from community dentists mainly employed by trusts. Specialist departments of dentistry in hospitals comprise the third branch of dental practice, where oral surgery, orthodontic and other restorative treatments are undertaken, the latter often with other surgeons specializing in plastic surgery or ear, nose and throat work.

12.1.2 Dentists' pay

As with doctors, dentists have one body to represent them professionally (the British Dental Association), one statutory body to regulate and control their practice (the General Dental Council) and separate bodies to negotiate their pay. Since 1960, their pay has been determined by the permanent Review Body which was established following the recommendations of the Royal Commission on Doctors' and Dentists' Remuneration[2]. Community dentists also became NHS employees from 1974, bringing their pay within the scope of the Review Body. Hospital and community dental staff receive a salary from their trust, but the system for general dental practitioners is more complicated.

Before 1948, general dental practitioners received most of their income from private practice, and a committee[3] was appointed to work out a scheme for the average weekly chairside hours being worked, and the health departments and the profession jointly worked out fees for different items of service that should provide this level of income. However, the initial demand for dentures and dental treatment was enormous, so dentists worked more hours and received higher incomes than had been anticipated. The government imposed limits on top earnings, and charges for dentures were introduced in 1951. Demand gradually declined, but because full information about dentists' total earnings (including private practice) and practice expenses was not available, the health departments and the BDA jointly discussed how to fix future levels of remuneration. The BDA demanded removal of the limit on top earnings, but the DoH was insistent, although new rates for items of service were offered, to raise the ceiling for top incomes. The BDA was not enthusiastic about this, but a survey of its members showed that a majority were not against this system of payment, so it was accepted.

The Royal Commission on Doctors' and Dentists' Remuneration made some specific recommendations about the pay of dentists, and it confirmed that general dental practitioners' pay should be based on fees for items of service. The Doctors' and Dentists' Review Body advised the government on the average net income that dentists should receive for working a specified number of chairside hours per year. The Dental Rates Study Group (a committee of representatives from the profession and the DoH under an independent chairman) assesses from time to time the level of dentists' practice expenses from information provided by the Inland Revenue, in order to determine average gross earnings, and hence draw up a scale of fees to produce average earnings of that level. The effect of this system was gradually to reduce the fee for a given treatment as more of those treatments were carried out faster or more efficiently. The system was called 'the treadmill' because it rewarded dentists for doing a greater number of those treatments. It tended to reward restorative work (fillings) rather than preventive treatment. The costs of general dental services to the NHS were therefore controlled to some extent by the degree of accuracy of the Dental Rates Study Group's calculations.

The Dental Practice Board in Eastbourne has to give prior approval for discretionary fees which can be claimed for treatments where a range of possible costs exists. Its records indicate the number and range of different courses of treatment that are given under the NHS, but no comparable figures exist for the extent of private treatment and for the number of people who do not go to a dentist at all.

As with other services of the NHS, many patients are exempt from dental charges: young people under 18 (19 if they are still in full-time education), mothers during pregnancy and for a year thereafter and anyone receiving income support or family credit under the social security system. Elderly people on low incomes may also be eligible, after a social security means test, to a certificate allowing them financial help. Dental charges for those who pay now amount to around 80% of the dentist's remuneration from the state.

12.1.3 The 1991 dentists' contract

Introduction of a new contract for dentists in 1991 caused some dissension, as did that of the family doctors. Although most dentists soon endorsed what they conceded was in the interests of themselves and their patients, many dentists have reduced their NHS work to concentrate on their private practice because payments under the new contract were felt to be too low. The main elements of the new contract shift the emphasis away from self-contained episodes of treatment towards continuing care, giving an incentive to undertake preventive rather than solely restorative work. Dentists thus receive a capitation fee for each patient they agree to care for over a 2-year period, renewable at any time by mutual agreement. Under this arrangement patients are entitled to emergency cover; this was formerly available only if the dentist voluntarily agreed to provide an emergency service. Dentists also receive capitation fees for children in their care, and about 20% of their monthly income is derived from capitation fees.

The system of obtaining approval from the Dental Practice Board before undertaking a particular treatment has been simplified.

Combining private and NHS treatment is now permitted, although not on the same tooth. Dental practices are, like GPs, required to provide their patients with an information leaflet that lists the individual dentists and their qualifications as well as other facilities provided, surgery hours and access for disabled people. The contract also requires dentists to keep up to date with developments in research and practice, and entitles them to improved maternity, sickness and early retirement benefits.

12.1.4 Dental staffing

There are about 18,500 dentists in practice in the UK (1997). On average, each dentist will deal with 2000 episodes of dental care per year. There are considerable regional variations in the incidence of dental disease, with the industrial north of England and Scotland having poorer dental health than the south. A corresponding variation in the distribution of dentists shows there are proportionally more dentists in areas with proportionally more people in the higher social classes. In order to strengthen the service, some dentists favour greater use of dental auxiliaries. These staff work with dentists, dealing with all the administrative duties as well as preparing instruments, mixing filling materials and processing X-rays. Dental hygienists are trained in schools of dentistry to be able to clean, scale and polish teeth, and they also play an important part in giving advice to patients about dental hygiene. In the school dental service, dental therapists are trained to carry out simple fillings, extract milk teeth and clean, scale and polish the teeth of school children; they also teach them about the importance of proper oral hygiene. Although the number of auxiliary staff is small (their remuneration is negotiated through Professional and Technical Whitley Council B), they can clearly take on the routine work under supervision and allow the dentist to apply his or her specialist skills and knowledge more widely. The General Dental Council controls their professional conduct through a subcommittee, the Dental Auxiliaries Committee.

Dental technicians are needed to make dentures, crowns, inlays and other appliances. They serve an apprenticeship in a dental laboratory, a hospital or a commercial firm, or they can undergo full-time training. Many general dental practitioners use the services of a commercial laboratory. In hospital departments, technicians also work in connection with the treatment of facial injuries.

12.2 OPHTHALMIC STAFF

The Worshipful Company of Spectacle Makers was given a Royal Charter in 1629, and opticians date their professional origins back to this time. However, it was not until the mid-nineteenth century that instruments for examining the eye and investigating refractive errors were invented, thus enabling the scientific diagnosis and treatment of sight disorders to develop. Qualified doctors specializing in the study of the eye took on the work of sight testing, as did the opticians who also sold spectacles. In 1895, the British Optical Association was founded, its aim being to achieve state registration for opticians, which would eliminate unqualified practitioners and establish professional status for the duly qualified. In 1923, a register of the Joint Council of Qualified Opticians was instituted, and the Council promoted a bill for state registration. But the BMA was against it, since it regarded doctors as being exclusively qualified to detect disease, and stated that all sight testing should be carried out under medical supervision. Most of the approved societies under the National Health Insurance scheme required the people they covered to go only to a practitioner on this register or to a doctor for sight testing.

In 1953, the Crook report[4] recommended that a General Optical Council should be established, to maintain a register of ophthalmic and dispensing opticians and to exercise governing and disciplinary powers over them. This was implemented by the Opticians Act, 1958. The General Optical Council gave opticians their independent professional status and restricted legal prescribing and dispensing of spectacles to them (or registered medical practitioners). The necessary qualifications for registration of ophthalmic opticians after 3 years' full-time study are granted by the Worshipful Company, the British Optical Association and the Institute of Ophthalmic Science. Dispensing opticians obtain qualifications for registration after 2 years of full-time study, 3 years' day release or a 4-year correspondence course, from the Association of Dispensing Opticians or with the Dispensing Certificate of the British Optical Association. Most dispensing opticians are members of the National Ophthalmic Treatment Board (NOTB) Association, and practise from medical eye centres that this body monitors.

See Section 6.6

Opticians' pay is negotiated through the Optical Whitley Council, although most of them dispense non-NHS lenses and frames as well. An optician does not have a list of patients like a GP, but is paid a separate fee for each item of service, under the terms of his contract with the health authority. Patients also pay charges for lenses and frames, which virtually cover the cost of them to the optician.

Until 1983 the ophthalmic service had been very stable for a variety of reasons. First, apart from the development of plastic, multifocal and contact lenses, there have been no major technical advances in the production of spectacle lenses. Secondly, over the age of 45, an increasingly large section of the population needs to wear spectacles. Thirdly, the manufacturing process for NHS lenses is basically unchanged, so that production cost increases have been lower than increases in manufacturing costs in general. This stability has helped the NHS considerably, because the constant and wide demand for spectacles can be met by opticians who can extend their incomes through non-NHS work. The NHS has been able to provide an adequate comprehensive service that was not fully integrated with the medical service, yet the existence of demand for private treatment had made it worthwhile for opticians to undertake NHS work as well.

The Health Services Act, 1984, removed the monopoly from opticians and allowed spectacles to be supplied by any retailer. This move was stimulated by the belief that the monopoly had kept the cost of non-NHS frames and lenses unduly high, particularly when compared to other countries. However, the proposal went much further and abolished the supply of NHS frames and lenses to all but children and certain people on low incomes. Although consumer representatives initially welcomed these reforms because of the opportunity to buy spectacles at a lower price, the ophthalmic profession was highly critical. They said it would mean that many people needing spectacles would obtain them without an eye test, thus endangering their sight and even their own and other people's safety.

12.2.1 Orthoptists

Orthoptists investigate squints and other defects of binocular vision. They work with medically qualified eye specialists and treat only patients referred to them by doctors. The majority of patients are children, and most orthoptists are women. The British Orthoptic Council was founded in 1930 and runs a full-time 2-year course leading to a diploma. The Board of Registration of Medical Auxiliaries registered orthoptists until 1966, when the Orthoptists Board of the Council for Professions Supplementary to Medicine (see Section 12.4) was set up to take this over.

12.3 PHARMACISTS

The pharmacists' profession can also trace its origins back three or four hundred years, but it developed from two distinct lines. The Society of Apothecaries was founded in 1617, and its members dispensed medicines on the order of physicians as well as prescribing and dispensing medicines direct to patients themselves. Chemists and druggists were retail shopkeepers who did not prescribe, but prepared and sold medicines in competition with the apothecaries. The Apothecaries Act of 1815 allowed apothecaries to charge for their professional advice to patients as well as for the medicines they dispensed, and this encouraged them to become more like general medical practitioners. The chemists and druggists progressively took over as the dispensers of physicians' prescriptions.

The Pharmaceutical Society of Great Britain was formed in 1841, and the Pharmacy Acts of 1852 and 1868 gave it the statutory duty to register pharmaceutical chemists who had obtained its diploma after training and examination, and to prevent those who were not pharmaceutical chemists or chemists or druggists from dispensing medicines or selling poisons. Under the National Health Insurance scheme only registered pharmacists could dispense medicines prescribed for insured people (except in remote areas where the doctors themselves could dispense their prescriptions).

Under the National Health Service, separate arrangements are made for dispensing medicines in the hospitals and the community. The Hospital Pharmaceutical Service employs registered pharmacists and technicians to prepare and dispense medicines to hospital in-patients and out-patients as prescribed by hospital doctors. The General Pharmaceutical Service involves retail pharmacists in dispensing medicines prescribed by general practitioners, under contract with the health authority). In 1974, AHAs appointed area pharmaceutical officers to supervise the hospital pharmaceutical services, even though each district probably had a district pharmacist. After 1982, most districts appointed a district pharmaceutical officer who transferred to health authorities after the 1990 Act.

Pharmacists undertake a 4-year degree course and then have a further year of pre-registration training accredited by the Royal Pharmaceutical Society. They can then choose whether to go into the hospital service, to become a retail chemist or to join industry in research or marketing. Pay negotiations for retail pharmacists are handled by the Pharmaceutical Whitley Council, and their central representative body is the Pharmaceutical Services Negotiating Committee. The National Pharmaceutical Union was founded in 1920 as a trade association for individual retail pharmacists. In recent years it has changed its brief to include the interests of employee pharmacists, and has also admitted company chemists to membership – this group now forms the majority of its members and it has changed its name to the National Pharmaceutical Association.

12.4 OTHER PROFESSIONAL STAFF

The work of the different professional staff in the health services is extremely varied, but overall it represents an identifiable and essential component in the whole programme of clinical care, without which medicine and nursing would be of limited effectiveness. Most of these practitioners undergo training that is as long and thorough as nurses' training. As medicine has become more sophisticated, specialization within the profession has increased, and with it has come the need for specialist supporting staff to provide the necessary backup services.

A number of landmarks should be mentioned before the individual professions are discussed. The first was in 1936, when the British Medical Association set up an independent Board of Registration of Medical Auxiliaries, incorporated under the Companies Act. Its object was to maintain and publish the National Register of Medical Auxiliary Services, listing those people who had satisfied the Board of their qualifications to practise. This arose because the doctors had become concerned that some of the techniques could involve risks if administered by untrained people. The result was that the professional organizations of dispensing opticians, dietitians, orthoptists, physiotherapists, speech therapists, chiropodists and radiographers became recognized by the Board, and their members were bound to work only under the direction of a doctor, while the doctors undertook to refer patients only to duly qualified practitioners. This arrangement could not stop unqualified practitioners from working, since registration was entirely voluntary. In this context, a committee was set up by the Minister of Health after the inception of the NHS, to consider 'the supply and demand, training and qualifications of certain medical auxiliaries employed in the NHS'. The result was the Cope report[5] and in 1954 regulations were introduced for the qualifications required for state registration of eight categories of staff by the NHS: chiropodists, dietitians, medical laboratory technicians, occupational therapists, physiotherapists, radiographers, remedial gymnasts and speech therapists.

In 1960, the Professions Supplementary to Medicine Act was passed. This established the Council for Professions Supplementary to Medicine (CPSM), and seven boards, one for each of the professions mentioned below (Table 12.1), excluding speech therapists. The boards were made legally responsible for the preparation and maintenance of registers, for prescribing qualifications required for state registration, and for approving entrance requirements, training syllabuses and training institutions.

Table 12.1

Training institutions for professions supplementary to medicine (1998)

Chiropody	14
Dietetics	9
Occupational therapy	31
Physiotherapy	32
Radiography	22
Speech and language therapy	16
Orthoptics	3

Source: Council for Professions Supplimentary to Medicine

They can remove practitioners from the register for professional misconduct and impose penalties for the improper use of the designation 'state registered'. In 1966 the provisions of the Act were extended to include orthoptists. The Board of Registration of Medical Auxiliaries continued to provide for voluntary registration of chiropodists, orthoptists, dispensing opticians, operating theatre technicians, technicians in venereology, audiology technicians and certified ambulance personnel. The CPSM is itself composed of one member from each of the boards, six nominees of the medical corporations and the GMC, four nominees of the Privy Council (including the Chairman) and four other nominees, a total of 21. The CPSM's future is under review.

These professions have gradually become more independent and now expect to be recognized as equal within clinical teams. After 1984, the heads of these paramedical departments became managerially accountable to the district general manager. The introduction of trusts following the 1990 reforms has fragmented many of these professions as the individual specialists within them become more geographically scattered. This has caused considerable concern that standards strengthened through professional unity would be harder to sustain.

There are other health care professions not under the supervision of CPSM. Nor are an increasing number of complementary therapies, which increasingly work alongside doctors and other therapists.

Physiotherapists	29,448
Medical laboratory scientific staff	20,917
Occupational therapists	19,427
Radiographers	19,179
Chiropodists	8,007
Dietitians	4,537
Osteopaths	2,500*
Orthoptists	1,267
Chiropractors	1,200+

Table 12.2

Other health care professional staff (UK, 1998)

*Estimate for the year 2000. +Estimate for the year 1999
Source: Council for Professions Supplementary to Medicine

12.4.1 Chiropodists

Chiropodists treat superficial ailments of the feet, and maintain the feet in good condition. In the eighteenth century chiropodists also cared for hands. They specialize in the treatment of existing deformities with appliances and special footwear, diagnosing and treating local infections, as well as preventive care, including the inspection of children's feet. Most chiropodists work in the community, holding clinics and making domiciliary visits. Many work privately. They work independently and do not require referral from a doctor, whereas those working in the hospitals work far more through referrals.

The Incorporated Society of Chiropodists was founded in 1912 to promote study and training and to improve services for poor people. The London Foot Hospital was founded in 1913, the first specialist hospital of its kind. A number of other professional organizations grew up and, in 1937, five of these were recognized by the Board of Registration of Medical Auxiliaries. They amalgamated to form the Society of Chiropodists in 1945, but there continued to be a range of bodies examining and registering chiropodists. The 1954 regulations laid down conditions for state registration and employment in the NHS, and the Chiropodists Board of the Council for Professions Supplementary to Medicine replaced these in 1963. In that year, it became the single body responsible for state registration, following a 3-year full-time course at an approved training centre. By 1990 several degree courses were available.

NHS treatments, including those done at patients' homes, are carried out by both NHS employed chiropodists and, where there is a shortage, private chiropodists who receive a fee from the NHS. The demand for chiropody outstrips supply, particularly for the priority groups – the elderly, the handicapped, expectant mothers, school children and some hospital patients. In 1996 there were 97,000 new NHS patients receiving on average a course of nine treatments. In 1977 the DHSS issued circular HC(77)9[6] which recommended various measures to the AHAs to enable them to make better use of their existing resources. Of particular importance was the suggestion that 'foot care assistants' could be employed to carry out simple treatments such as basic foot care and hygiene, for which the skills of the fully trained chiropodist were not necessary.

12.4.2 Dietitians

A dietitian applies knowledge of nutrients contained in food, the effect of preparation and cooking of them and their use by the body, to advise on suitable diets as part of the treatment of illness, as well as constructing diets for people with chronic disorders (e.g. diabetes, kidney disease). Most dietitians work in hospitals, following up patients through out-patient clinics. In addition, there are some openings for them in the community services, for instance in advising mothers at antenatal and postnatal clinics on the balanced diets required for their babies, and in the nutritional values of meals on wheels.

The first training schools for dietitians were established in the United States in the 1920s, and their students were trained nurses. In 1925 special diet kitchens were opened at one or two hospitals in London, Edinburgh and Glasgow, and they accepted students who had pure science or domestic science qualifications. In 1933, a special training course for dietitians was started at the King's College of Household and Social Science in London, and the therapeutic work of these 'early' dietitians mostly involved weighing and preparing foods. Later, the development of drugs partly overtook the use of dietetics in the treatment of certain conditions. The British Dietetic Association was founded in 1936 and joined the voluntary registration scheme before the institution of requirements for state registration in 1954. Since 1963, the Dietitians Board of the Council for Professions Supplementary to Medicine has been the responsible regulating body. Since the 1990 reforms dietitians are employed by trusts.

12.4.3 Occupational therapists

In 1989, a report from the College of Occupational Therapists[7] defined occupational therapy as the assessment and systematic treatment of people of any age who have physical or mental health problems, in order to restore independence. Occupational therapists (OTs) usually specialize soon after qualifying, treating patients with either physical or mental disorders. In the NHS there are occupational therapy departments in general and mental illness hospitals, day hospitals, and units for mentally and physically handicapped children; other OTs are employed by local authority social services departments. Until the 1930s there were only untrained craft workers in mental hospitals. The Association of Occupational Therapists was formed in 1936, and from then on it registered OTs who had passed examinations after a 3-year course. There are now 31 university courses leading to qualification and registration. The Occupational Therapists Board of the Council for Professions Supplementary to Medicine was set up in 1963, requiring OTs to be state registered in order to practise.

The number of OTs continues to increase to meet expanding

demand: episodes of care went from 770,000 in 1988 to 1.13 million in 1996[8]. Further expansion seems likely, with the current emphasis on care in the community. OTs employed by the NHS have different salary scales and terms of service from those working for social services departments. This, and the division between those who specialize in mental as opposed to physical disorders, has impeded the emergence of a strong professional identity. Although the training syllabus for OTs overlaps in part with physiotherapy, there appears to be insufficient common ground for a joint course to be universally acceptable to both professions.

12.4.4 Physiotherapists

Physiotherapists use physical means to treat patients with injury or disease, and employ a wide range of methods including therapeutic movement, hydrotherapy, manipulation, electrotherapy, ultrasound and ice treatments. They treat most of their patients as hospital out-patients, and see people with bone injuries, chest disease or arthritis, pregnant women and handicapped children, and others referred to them by hospital doctors or directly by GPs. They are the largest group in the paramedical professions. They assess the individual's needs and devise and implement treatment, reporting back to the referring doctor on completion or if problems arise. Long gone are the days when the doctor prescribed what treatment was to be administered. Private practice offers physiotherapists significant opportunities; here patients can refer themselves directly.

Physiotherapists' professional organization evolved from the Society of Trained Masseuses, founded in 1895. It was open only to women until 1920, when it became the Chartered Society of Massage and Medical Gymnastics and began to admit men. It changed its name to the Chartered Society of Physiotherapy in 1943, by which time it was the registering authority for practitioners, conducting examinations and approving training schools. There are now 32 university-based courses. Remedial gymnasts used to be a separate professional group, using active exercise schemes to treat physical conditions. They merged with physiotherapy in 1986 and thus no longer have a separate board within the CPSM.

12.4.5 Speech and language therapists

Speech and language therapists treat defects and disorders of the voice and speech which may arise from a wide range of clinical or congenital disorders. Originally, the work concentrated on stammering, but, after about 1912, hospital departments and local authority clinics began to be set up to offer treatment for a range of disorders. The 1944 Education Act obliged local education authorities to provide treatment for children with speech disorders, so the profession became split between those working in the education and health services. There was a great demand for speech therapists as a result, and the College of Speech Therapists was formed in 1945 to press for independent status of the practitioners.

In 1972, the Quirk report on speech therapy services[9] made proposals for reorganizing and developing the profession so that it could cope with its expanding role in the NHS and the education service. It recommended that AHAs should be responsible for organizing the practitioners in a suitable career structure, and that training courses should be jointly arranged with universities so that the quality of the training might be enhanced. It also proposed a new central council to handle course assessment and registration of qualified practitioners, and that the College of Speech Therapists should remain as a professional body only, its present examining role being taken on by the central council. The government approved the recommendations and, in April 1974, issued guidance to AHAs on how they might begin to integrate their speech services along these lines through the appointment of Area Speech Therapists[10]. It was acknowledged that the transformation of the profession would take some time. In 1982, speech therapists were reorganized on a district basis, but since the 1990 Act they have been based in trusts, dispersing their already small numbers.

The profession has faced serious problems for some time: the small numbers of fully trained members, a small number of training places, and a very wide choice of potential specialization. Statutory demands made on them by the Education Act, 1981 to provide services have put further pressures on them. Speech therapy is not supervised by the CPSM.

12.4.6 Clinical psychologists

The role of the clinical psychologist has become increasingly important. They are crucial in the treatment of mental illnesses, in assessment and in devising appropriate treatment regimens. They formulate training plans for those people with learning disabilities who are being prepared to live in the community. They have a potential contribution to more clinical specialities and particularly family support, child health and rehabilitation. The Trethowan report (1977)[11] emphasized the professional autonomy of clinical psychologists, although they are used to working as part of a therapeutic team. Clinical psychologists have to possess a first degree in psychology, followed by a further 2 years of specialist training. This extended training may be responsible for the relatively small numbers working in the NHS. Clinical psychology is not supervised by the CPSM.

12.4.7 Osteopaths and chiropractors

Osteopaths and chiropractors are skilled at physical manipulation to treat musculo-skeletal disorders and related conditions. They are increasingly seeing patients within the NHS. Both groups are seeking formal recognition. The Osteopaths Act, 1993, set up a General Osteopaths Council and the Chiropractors Act, 1994, set up a General Chiropractic Council. Both bodies are working towards state registration procedures which will confirm their status as a health profession, limiting practice to accredited practitioners and safeguarding patients as a result.

12.4.8 Complementary (alternative) therapists

Complementary (also called alternative) therapies fall into several broad categories: some like shiatsu, Alexander technique and herbalism are physical; others such as hypnotherapy and some types of psychotherapy are concerned with the mind and the emotions. Although there is as yet no overall system of regulation many of the practitioners undergo extensive training and work under supervision. Increasingly, traditional members of the clinical and therapeutic team are prepared to acknowledge that alternative therapies have a place. These treatments are only occasionally available as part of the NHS.

12.4.9 Social work

Medical social work has its roots in the almoner's department of pre-NHS hospitals, which was principally concerned with the financial status of patients, a relevant matter to voluntary hospitals which relied on contributions from patients as well as donations from the general public. This evolved into a general concern for the patients' circumstances, so that social workers in hospital now have a particular responsibility for satisfactory discharge arrangements. In 1974, medical social workers ceased to be employed by health authorities and were transferred to local authority social services departments. This move was brought about by the Seebohm report (1968) which recommended a single social work service with full professional status. Medical social workers, often more highly qualified than social workers coming from the fields of residential care or mental welfare, were reluctant to make the change. In the event, most social services departments have maintained social workers in hospitals and honoured their specialism while enlarging their areas of concern. Social workers are also attached to primary health teams. The Labour government has reiterated the importance of social workers being part of the team looking after patients.

12.5 Scientific and technical staff

The Zuckerman report (1968)[12] proposed a reorganization of the scientific and technical services provided by medical laboratory technicians, some of the professions supplementary to medicine and others in the hospital service. The report included a wide range of technical staff (Box 12.1), some of whom have since changed their name or enlarged their activity.

Many of their recommendations did not survive, and throughout the next 20 years piecemeal alterations to the organization of the services were made. Medical physics, a relatively new profession, developed with the encouragement of doctors, but medical laboratory sciences were not given similar recognition and, where some degree of autonomy was claimed, serious conflict developed. The list includes some staff who have extended training (e.g. physicists) with others who may have

Box 12.1

Hospital scientific and technical staff

Biochemists	Medical physics technicians
Physicists	Radiographers
Other scientific officers	Animal technicians
Audiology technicians	Artifical kidney technicians
Audiology scientists	Contact lens technicians
Cardiology technicians	Electronics technicians
Darkroom technicians	Glaucoma technicians
Electroencephalography	Heart and lung technicians
technicians	Respiratory function technicians
Medical laboratory technicians	Surgical instrument curators

practically no formal training (e.g. darkroom technicians). Three groups need special note: medical laboratory scientists, medical physicists and radiographers.

12.5.1 Medical laboratory scientists

Medical laboratory scientists provide assistance to the diagnosis and treatment of illness through examination of pathological specimens from out-patients and in-patients, and those sent in via GPs. They work under the supervision of consultant pathologists in the hospitals. The Pathological and Bacteriological Assistants' Association was founded in 1912 and in 1921 an examining council of the Pathological Society was set up to develop a system of certification. The Institute of Medical Laboratory Technology (now Sciences) was incorporated in 1942 as the single professional organization. It registered qualified technicians who had worked in approved laboratories and attended part-time courses. The 1954 regulations for medical auxiliaries laid down the requisites for state registration, and, in 1963, the Medical Laboratory Technicians Board of the Council for Professions Supplementary to Medicine became the regulating body.

Entrants to the profession need 'A' levels before proceeding to the Higher National Diploma (HND), and 25% of entrants now have degrees, which entitles them to two years' exemption from state registration as a Medical Laboratory Scientific Officer. Subsequent training, leading to Fellowship, is in one or more sub-specialities, such as biochemistry and haematology.

12.5.2 Medical physicists

The origins of medical physics were in radiotherapy. With the increasing need to give expert support to doctors using technical equipment, an independent profession developed, becoming recognized in the founding of the Hospital Physicists Association (HPA) in 1943. Hospital physicists need a minimum qualification of a degree in physics, engineering or associated subject. The HPA organized a 2-year in-service training scheme, but advancement to the higher grades is unlikely without an MSc or PhD degree.

Registration became a major issue in 1987 when a mistake in calibrating a radiotherapy machine in Exeter resulted in overdoses to patients and extensive litigation. As with other areas of risk, chief executives of NHS trusts now have to assure themselves that the professional accountability of physicists is unambiguous.

12.5.3 Radiographers

X-rays were discovered in 1895 and they are used to help diagnose illness and injury, and to provide treatment for certain malignant and other conditions. Until 1920, non-medical assistants were employed, but, in that year, the Society of Radiographers was formed to organize training courses and examinations and to register qualified practitioners. Both diagnostic and therapeutic radiographers work under the direction of doctors, and there are standard protective and monitoring devices to ensure that they are not excessively exposed to radiation. Radiography is a hospital-based service.

In 1983, the training scheme was increased to 3 years, of which the first part is common to both diagnostic and therapeutic radiography students. After qualification, radiographers are required to register with the Radiographers Board at the CPSM. The majority of radiographers work in diagnostic rather than radiotherapy departments. Computed tomography (CT) scanning, nuclear magnetic resonance and ultrasound have enhanced diagnostic capability, and use techniques that are less invasive and less risky for patients. This has extended the complexity of the radiographer's work so that there is a need for degree-standard training and more postgraduate courses.

12.6 ANCILLARY STAFF

There are well over 300,000 patients in hospital on any one day in the year who have the sheets on their beds provided by the laundry staff, who eat three meals cooked and served by the catering staff in wards cleaned by the domestic staff. Equipment and sterile dressings are provided by the supplies staff, while porters fetch and carry specimens and equipment and conduct patients around the hospital. In addition, certain staff live in the hospital, so some of the 'hotel' services are required for them. Most of the ancillary functions are not exclusive to the NHS, and arise wherever meals and residential accommodation need to be provided. The community health services clearly require these services on a smaller scale since they are mostly concerned with non-residential care. Hostels and homes in the community are the responsibility of social services departments unless they provide medically supervised care, in which case the ancillary staff would be employees of a NHS trust.

In 1970, the DHSS issued advice aimed at improving the management of these support services[13]. New posts of considerable seniority were set up in 1974 for district catering, domestic and linen service managers. By 1982, however, functional management (as it was called) had been discredited largely because of the tension between local unit or hospital administrators and the district functional managers endeavouring to supervise services from a distance. A further change came in 1983 with the government's privatization moves. Districts were directed to check the efficiency of their support services in the open market. When an outside contractor for domestic, catering or laundry work could provide a cheaper service than in-service staff, the employment of such staff was terminated and the outside contractors employed. Money thus saved could be used to benefit patients in other ways. The number of NHS-employed ancillary staff has fallen by 60% since 1980 – mainly as a result of contracting out ancillary services.

Scant training and poor pay has led to high turnover in these occupations, often as much as 50% in one year. In an effort to overcome this problem and to meet the needs of health care assistants (including nursing auxiliaries, physiotherapy aides, occupational therapy helpers and junior clerical staff), it was proposed in 1987 that a more structured national approach should provide a system whereby previously untrained staff could acquire basic competencies under the aegis of the National Council for Vocational Qualifications.

12.7 ESTATES STAFF

This group of staff includes architects, quantity surveyors, engineers, building supervisors, electricians, painters, carpenters, ground maintenance staff and labourers. They deal with the planning, construction and maintenance of the buildings, plant and grounds of the health service and, as with the ancillary staff, they predominantly serve the hospitals. The senior works staff, who used to be based with the regional health authorities, hold professional qualifications such as those of the Royal Institute of British Architects, the Royal Institution of Quantity Surveyors and the various engineering institutions. Senior works staff based in districts prior to the 1990 Act had technical qualifications, but skilled and other works staff tend to belong to a trade union rather than a professional organization.

The stock of hospitals taken over by the NHS in 1948 included many that were obsolete, poorly maintained or in unsuitable locations. In the late 1950s, money began to be specially earmarked for the development of hospital building, and *A Hospital Plan* (1962) acknowledged the shortage of architects and engineers skilled in hospital planning. The Woodbine Parish report[14] published in 1970 made further recommendations for the improvement of building maintenance and the training of supervisory staff. The Ceri Davies report (1983)[15] observed that works departments were too concerned with capital building schemes and with engineering plant at the expense of the wider issue of estate management. The report suggested a change of title from works officer to estates officer.

Pressures to contract out works and estates functions in the same way as the ancillary services, and the introduction of trusts, has effectively privatized the works function, although some trusts retain a small works and maintenance staff.

12.8 AMBULANCE STAFF

Ambulance staff in the UK have traditionally seen themselves as one of the three emergency services (with fire services and the police). Governments have disliked this link, as most of the work is for non-emergencies (in 1997/8, 2.67 million ambulance journeys were doctors' emergencies and 999 calls and 14.9 million were non-emergencies). The matter came to a head in 1989, when extended industrial action failed to promote the ambulance staff's position and, indeed, probably deepened the split between emergency and routine work. Despite this, coterminosity of boundaries between ambulance trusts and the other emergency services has been responsible for stimulating trusts mergers to make bigger trusts.

See further discussion in Section 12.10.3 and Section 5.2.1

Ambulance requests are categorized into three groups: emergency, urgent and planned (see Table 5.1). An emergency ambulance is staffed by an ambulance paramedic, who has special resuscitation skills, and an ambulance technician. The extension of the ambulance person's skills allows patients to be stabilized before or on the way to hospital and helps to ensure that medical staff are not brought to accidents and other emergencies unnecessarily. This avoids depriving their other hospital or surgery patients of appropriate professional attention.

12.9 MANAGERIAL, ADMINISTRATIVE AND CLERICAL STAFF

The early hospital administrators, called 'house governors' in voluntary hospitals and 'stewards' in local authority hospitals, were responsible to the board of governors or to the doctor in charge. With the introduction of the NHS in 1948, the new hospital management committees and regional hospital boards created a new pattern of administrative staffing, separating the senior staff (e.g. hospital secretary, group secretary, finance and supplies officers) from the junior grades (general administrators, clerical officers).

Two important reviews of administrative and clerical staff were conducted in the NHS's first 15 years, resulting in the Noel Hall (1957)[16] and Lycett Green (1963)[17] reports. The latter proposed the setting up of a national staff committee to oversee the development of administrative staff. The Thwaites report (1977)[18] encouraged further systematic training and the Institute of Health Services Management was the first to offer a good foundation in professional hospital management through its diploma course. This course has been superseded by such university-based qualifications as the Diploma in Management Studies (DMS) and a Master in Business Administration degree (MBA). With the advent of general management, there is much more emphasis on training. It is also now accepted that anyone in a managerial position, whatever their professional discipline, needs management training (further details in Section 12.10.3). The Labour government issued a green paper in 1998, *The Learning Age*[19], committed to encouraging creativity, skill and imagination throughout life to equip people to adapt to the changes in their work and in their home life.

Because the NHS is geared to patient care, it is perhaps inevitable that the supporting staff tend to be seen as less important than doctors and other clinical workers. Yet without them the direct care staff cannot function properly. This is all the more so now sophisticated analysis and planning of the use of NHS resources is crucial to success at improving the efficiency and effectiveness of health care. The administrative, clerical and managerial staff, always politically unpopular, have been the main agents for introducing the increasingly frequent organizational changes required by successive governments since 1974. The 1990 reforms, in particular, could not have been implemented without the positive support of administrative and general management staff, who were often left to resolve issues poorly formulated by the Secretary of State and his civil servants.

Managers' pay remained within the Whitley Council until the introduction of general management in 1984, since when conditions of service for this new group are much less protective than had been the case in the NHS and other public services. Tenure is no longer assured and renewal of contracts depends explicitly on satisfactory performance. In return, salaries have risen quite rapidly for senior managers, paying rates for the first time comparable with well-paid jobs in the private sector. Total spending on general management staff remains relatively low, despite a substantial increase in the numbers of managers as a result of the 1990 reforms. In 1998 The NHS Executive announced a new grading structure for managers in health authorities which set out five broad salary bands and signalled the end of mandatory performance-related pay and short-term contracts. NHS trusts will follow similar principles.

The broad banding system had been suggested by the Megaw report in 1982

12.10 PERSONNEL MANAGEMENT

The NHS is a labour-intensive service and its pay bill accounts for at least 75% of its total annual cost. The 1983 Griffiths report criticized, among other things, the paucity of good personnel management in the NHS. In a service so reliant on its staff, the status and number of specialist personnel officers were low; many of them were unqualified. The reason for this was rooted in the management arrangements of the past. It had been customary for each departmental head to be responsible for the employment of staff. Not until the serious pay disputes of the early 1970s did the system begin to change, as specialist personnel officers were brought in.

Personnel (or human resource) managers have several functions. The personnel officer must be up to date with all employment legislation and help managers implement new requirements. He or she must acquire expertise in job evaluation and grading. Deciding how many staff of which disciplines and with what levels of skill are required in order to run a particular ward or department at optimum efficiency demands specialist knowledge and expertise. Human resource planning helps managers to look ahead and estimate future changes in the demand for and supply of labour. Shortages in the labour market mean that NHS employers have to adopt new strategies for recruiting and retaining the staff they need. They have to keep an eye on sickness and absenteeism. The recent report *Improving the Health of the NHS Workforce*[20] presented a worrying picture of staff sickness and psychological distress.

Some aspects of employees' rights have been protected by legislation since the nineteenth century, when laws were first passed in relation to industrial hazards. The Health and Safety at Work Act 1974 consolidated progress and has been supplemented by further regulations and guidance regarding such matters as control of hazardous substances, disposal of clinical waste, and lifting[21]. Most NHS trusts have occupational health departments, some staffed by a full-time doctor, which provide care for people at the workplace, assess for management whether an applicant is fit to take on a particular task and make arrangements for employees whose ill-health is interfering with their capacity to fulfil their duties satisfactorily.

12.10.1 Pay

Pay relativities need to be understood and addressed carefully if large-scale dissatisfaction is to be avoided. Cash limits always restrict NHS employers' discretion to award pay rises, all the more so in periods of significant inflation. The risk of allowing unrestrained local deals is that labour supply can become even more unpredictable as workers move to where they can do the same job for better rates. This exacerbates turnover, which already averages about 23% annually, higher among ancillary staff. A national system of pay was one way of attempting to control the volatility of the employment market. But centralized arrangements were inflexible and localized bargaining was encouraged with the 1990 Act. In the event this proved unsuccessful and a return to centralized control of pay seems likely.

Until recently, in common with the rest of the public sector, the pay of NHS staff was mainly fixed through formal pay bargaining conducted at national level. In the NHS, this was originally through the Whitley Councils. From 1959 onwards, certain professional staff had their pay determined by special national review bodies. By 1990, however, the shortcomings of centralized pay bargaining had become too great to ignore. It is important to examine how this elaborate system operated, to demonstrate that complex and time-consuming though central negotiating is, any successful substitute has to be able to overcome the problems it encountered.

Before the Second World War there had been little attempt to centralize pay bargaining for health workers. The Whitley system had originated in attempts to improve overall industrial relations during and after the First World War. During the Second World War, hospital labour was in short supply. The government intervened by fixing minimum wages for student nurses prepared to work in hospitals where the shortages were particularly acute.

The 1946 NHS Act laid down that all employees of non-teaching hospitals would work under the instruction of their hospital management committee, although their employer at law was the regional hospital board. Schedule 66 of the Act empowered the Minister of Health to make regulations about the qualifications, remuneration and conditions of service of any employee of the NHS. The result was one General Whitley Council and nine functional Whitley Councils (Box 12.2).

Box 12.2

NHS Whitley Councils

- General Whitley Council
- Administrative and Clerical Staffs Council
- Ancillary Staffs Council
- Dental Whitley Council (Local Authorities)
- Medical and (Hospital) Dental Whitley Council
- Nurses and Midwives Council
- Optical Council
- Pharmaceutical Council
- Professional and Technical Staffs Council 'A'
- Professional and Technical Staffs Council 'B'

The functional councils determined pay and all those conditions of service requiring a national decision, affecting directly only those staff within its scope. The General Council's activities were, in practice, limited to matters of general application, e.g. determining travelling and subsistence allowances and the procedure for certain types of leave. The councils each had a staff side and a management side.

On most functional councils, staff organizations with relatively small membership claimed places alongside the major ones, and some trades unions with members in several branches of the health services gained places on more than one council. The composition of the management side reflected the curious position that the hospital authorities were in as a party to collective bargaining. Regional hospital boards and boards of governors were dependent on the government for all the money they spent. Clearly, they could not agree or grant concessions to their staff unless the government was prepared to make money available, but, at the same time, the Ministry wanted to be involved in any discussions that might commit them to increased expenditure on wages. The management sides of the functional councils, therefore, consisted of officials from the Ministry of Health and Scottish Office, representatives from the regional hospital boards, hospital management committees and boards of governors, the executive councils (on Administrative and Clerical) and the local authorities (except on Administrative and Clerical). Health authority membership increased after the McCarthy report, *Making Whitley Work*[22], but decreased again in January 1984 in an attempt to develop a more streamlined and better informed management side.

The way the Whitley Councils worked was for each side to meet separately to determine their attitudes and then, as a joint body, to discuss the issues together. Each side had a chairman and a secretary, the chair of the council alternating between the two sides from year to year while the secretaries were joint secretaries of the full council. The staff side secretary was elected from staff representatives, and the management side secretary was an official of the Department of Health. Regional and national appeals committees existed to hear the cases of employees who were aggrieved in any matter of their employment excluding disciplinary action or dismissal.

Increasingly, however, staff and employers alike became critical of the Whitley system. Why was this? First, it was very cumbersome. The large membership of each council was not an efficient way of conducting business. Secondly, and more seriously, the Whitley system failed to produce coherence or consistency in pay bargaining even within councils and certainly not between councils. There was no national Whitley strategy for NHS staff other than that contained within the government of the day's pay policy. Effective negotiation was often not possible because the management side was given little discretion by the government.

The limitations of the Whitley system led some groups of staff to seek a better arrangement, and as far back as 1963 the permanent Review Body on Doctors' and Dentists' Remuneration had been set up. Electricians and other craftsmen also achieved special direct negotiation arrangements with the setting up of the DHSS Craftsmen's Committee. Finally, the Review Body for Nurses and Midwives and some professional and technical staff was set up in 1983 and the corresponding Whitley Councils were left to deal with conditions of service only.

Despite the recommendations of *Making Whitley Work* aimed at streamlining the system, the reform of the Whitley system made little progress. Only after the creation of NHS trusts in 1991, which in line with the Conservative government's overall market principles largely abandoned the old negotiating system, was there a real change of climate. But problems remain. First, although NHS trusts are empowered to deal with their own personnel issues, they are still part of the NHS and hence their spending appears in the national accounts. For governments concerned with the size of the public sector borrowing requirement (the shortfall between spending and tax revenues), NHS trusts' autonomy must be subordinated to macro-economic policy. Second, NHS trusts need information if they are to negotiate effectively. So a specialist agency, Pay and Workforce Research, endeavours to fill this need. Third, many human resource specialists have had little experience in local negotiations compared with their trades union counterparts. On the other hand, finding a substitute for the Whitley system seems too difficult. Certainly review bodies have not been an acceptable alternative, creating just as many other problems.

12.10.2 Industrial relations

For many years after the introduction of the NHS, staff tolerated comparatively low pay because they felt rewarded by being part of a valued, caring service whose objectives were quite different from those of commercial industry. The NHS was characterized as one large happy family where everyone was content to know their place and work as a team. In the late 1960s, this idealized view was no longer tenable (if it ever had been) as the momentum of dissatisfaction grew. During the 1970s GPs, hospital doctors, nurses, ambulance staff and ancillary staff all took industrial action culminating in the 'winter of discontent' which was very damaging to patients and to the failing Labour government in 1979.

Despite legislation introduced by Conservative governments in the 1980s curbing the rights of trades unions and their members, the potential for unrest in the NHS is a constant factor. The reasons for militancy are complex, but three broad causes are:

* government policy, for instance the inclusion or exclusion of private beds in NHS hospitals, or contracting out support services;
* the problem of pay relativities;
* employment legislation; at times this has caused the pursuit of disputes to the highest level, as was sometimes the case following the introduction of the Advisory Conciliation and Arbitration Service in 1974.

Although the state of industrial relations remains unsettled, and there is continuing dissatisfaction with pay and other conditions of employment, as well as a constant assertion that low morale prevails, most people who work in the NHS have done so all their working lives, including those who have transferable skills and could easily have left. Furthermore, a willingness to work beyond the obligations of their individual contracts is apparent everywhere. This customary loyalty is the paradox of the NHS: the service is generally alleged to be 'collapsing' and yet it goes on being sustained by highly motivated and hard working staff.

12.10.3 Training and development

The importance of appropriate training is officially acknowledged, to ensure patients can rely on competent treatment in all aspects of their care. The formal training for professionals has been referred to earlier in the chapter. But there remains the need for management training at several levels and a myriad of skills and competencies that health staff need to acquire.

To co-ordinate these activities a National Health Service Training Authority (NHSTA, later the NHS Training Directorate, NHSTD) was set up in 1983. It replaced five national staff committees. The NHSTA, based in Bristol, began work in 1985. It had four divisions: the first responsible for developing strategic programmes for responding to the

Appropriated from the opening line of Shakespeare's Richard III, by NUPE's chief, Rodney Bickerstaffe

implications of change. For instance, it determined and organized advance training for the staff likely to be involved with introducing the 1990 reforms. The second division provided training resources. These could be national guidelines, for example on equal opportunities, or actual training materials for use on training courses throughout the NHS. The NHS has rarely evaluated with much rigour the training it does, so there is still little objective assessment of its effectiveness. The third NHSTA division was therefore concerned with setting standards to help trainers measure results. It also had a business division to run the NHSTA as an enterprise. The NHSTA's co-ordinating role brought more coherence into education and training in the NHS. Despite this, it was disbanded as a Special Health Authority in April 1991 and its functions restored to the Department of Health, under the NHS Executive's director of personnel at the NHS Training Directorate. This was superseded in 1996 by the Institute of Health and Care Development operating as an agency.

Management training

In 1986 the DoH published *Better Management, Better Health*[23], which set out the importance of developing managerial skills. Until then, further education for managers had been patchy and had been concentrated on a small élite. Since the mid-1950s, a national General Management Training Scheme has been run for administrators (now managers). It recruits about 60 people a year, some of them graduates, some already working in the NHS, and provides a supervised programme lasting 2 years. An introduction to the service at all levels is followed by working experience in selected posts. The training is supported by an academic department. The trainees are expected to obtain a diploma or master's degree in public sector management and may also acquire NVQ recognition of managerial competence. Following a review of the scheme, individuals are now encouraged to pursue further education throughout their managerial career.

Continuing education is not confined to general managers: HAs and NHS trusts are beginning to see its importance for all staff who have managerial responsibilities within their own disciplines and professions. Working Paper 10[24], emanating from the 1990 reforms, attempted to make sense of the many approaches to training of all kinds and regions set up consortia of employers to develop continuing education arrangements. In 1998 the Labour government set up the Health Care National Training Organization to work with the Training Organization for Personal Social Services to develop a strategic approach to training and to develop national occupational standards.

In recent years there has been greater interest in acquiring NVQs and undertaking postgraduate courses such as DMS and MBA/MSc

CONCLUSION

Notwithstanding considerable technological advance over the last 50 years, the NHS remains fundamentally a personal service reliant on its staff. Although the numbers of staff directly employed by the NHS is declining, the human resource will always remain central to the service and its biggest investment. Some of the professions have a very long history, others are relatively new. Some staff are well paid, others are some of the least well paid in society. The numbers of patients being treated increases and the range of required skills widens. All of these factors make the NHS a unique working environment which needs the highest level of competent management to hold together and deliver effective organization of the service. This chapter has examined just how complex a task that is.

REFERENCES

1. DoH (1997) *Investing in Dentistry* Circular HSG(97)38. DoH, London.
2. Royal Commission on Doctors' and Dentists' Remuneration (1960) *Report of the Royal Commission* (Pilkington Report).
3. Ministry of Health and Department of Health for Scotland(1948) *Report of the Interdepartmental Committee on the Remuneration of General Dental Practitioners* (Spens report). HMSO, London (Cmnd 7402).
4. Ministry of Health and Department of Health for Scotland (1953) *Statutory Registration of Opticians: Interdepartmental report* (Crook report). HMSO, London (Cmnd 8531).
5. Ministry of Health and Department of Health for Scotland (1950) *Medical Auxiliaries, Reports of Committees* (Cope report). HMSO, London (Cmnd 8188).
6. DHSS Circular (1977) *Organisation and Development of Chiropody Services* HC(77)9. DHSS, London.
7. College of Occupational Therapists (1989) *Occupational Therapy: An emerging profession* (Blom-Cooper report). Duckworth, London.
8. DoH (1998) *The Government's Expenditure Plans* op. cit.
9. Department of Education and Science (1972) *Speech Therapy Services, Report of the Committee appointed by the Secretaries of State* (Quirk report). HMSO, London.
10. DHSS (1974) *Speech Therapy Services: Interim Guidance* Health Circular HCS(IS)22. DHSS, London.
11. DHSS (1977) *The Role of Psychologists in Health Services* (Trethowan report). HMSO, London.
12. DHSS and Scottish Home and Health Department(1968) *Hospital Scientific and Technical Services* (Zuckerman report). HMSO, London.
13. DHSS (1970) *Administrative and Clerical Staffs Whitley Council* Advance Letter A/L4/70.
14. DHSS, Scottish Home and Health Department, Welsh Office (1970) *Hospital Building Maintenance* (Woodbine Parish report). HMSO, London, Edinburgh and Cardiff.
15. DHSS (1983) *Underused and Surplus Property in the National Health Service. Report of the Enquiry* (Ceri Davies report). HMSO, London.
16. Ministry of Health (157) *Report of the Grading Structure of Administrative and Clerical Staff* (Noel Hall report). HMSO, London.
17. Ministry of Health (1963) *Report of the Committee of Inquiry into the Recruitment, Training and Promotion of Adminsitrative and Clerical Staff in the National Health Service* (Lycett Green report). HMSO, London.
18. King's Fund (1977) *The Education and Training of Senior Managers in the National Health Service* (Thwaites report). King's Fund, London.

19. Department of Education and Employment (1998) *The Learning Age*, Green Paper. The Stationery Office, London (Cm 3790).
20. Williams, S. *et al.* (1998) *Improving the Health of the NHS Workforce*. Nuffield Trust, London.
21. Health and Safety Executive (1988) *Control of Substances Hazardous to Health regulations 1988 S.I. 1657*. HSE, London.
22. DHSS (1976) *Making Whitley Work* (McCarthy report). HMSO, London.
23. DoH NHS Training Authority (1986) *Better Management, Better Health* (Donne report). NHSTA, Bristol.
24. DoH (1989) *Working for Patients. Working Paper 10: Education and training*. HMSO, London.

13

THE PUBLIC AND THE NATIONAL HEALTH SERVICE

This chapter is concerned with a range of issues that illustrate the relationship between ordinary people and the health services that are provided for them by the State. It starts with statutory and other aspects of the NHS's relationship with the public, and is followed by a discussion of patients' rights.

13.1 COMMUNITY HEALTH COUNCILS

Community health councils (CHCs), an innovation of the 1974 NHS reorganization, have the broad task of representing the views of local users of the health services to the health authorities. There is usually one CHC for each health authority. They provide for about 6000 people nationally to play an active part within the health service as members of statutory bodies for expressing consumer opinion, quite separate from the health authorities and trusts responsible for managing the NHS. The idea of setting them up arose principally because it was felt that health service users had exerted too little influence on the provision and planning of services in an organization that had become dominated by professionals. In the past, the tasks of managing the provision of services and monitoring their quality had been combined. Some members of the old hospital authorities and the former local authority health committees were specifically meant to represent the lay view, but their influence was felt to have been limited. On the AHAs, the lay members were appointed to shoulder managerial responsibilities, and the emphasis was to separate this from the responsibility for representing consumers' views.

> **Key reference:** Levitt, R. (1980) *The People's Voice in the NHS*. King's Fund, London.

CHC membership was worked out principally on the basis of the resident district population, and ranges from 18 in the smallest to 24 in the largest. Half the members are nominated by the local authorities, one-third by voluntary organizations and the remaining one-sixth by the regional offices, who have the job of officially appointing all the nominees, normally for a period of four years, and half the members retire every two years (although they are eligible for reappointment). A limited number of people can also be co-opted. Generally, each CHC has two full-time staff – the chief officer and his or her assistant – who work from offices chosen by the CHC. In some cases CHCs have obtained shop front accommodation, while others work from offices which may be rented from the health or local authorities. Administrative costs have been kept low. The money to pay staff salaries, office costs and all other expenses is made available by the regional offices. The staff of CHCs are employees of a designated health authority in each region. Other support is provided by the appropriate regional office.

Questions of management in an organization as extensive as the NHS are not interesting to the majority of the population. Individuals tend to have views about 'illness' rather than 'health', and find it difficult to consider questions which extend beyond their own personal experience. This is not a criticism but a reflection of the very low priority which governments and authorities have given to explaining issues of policy and management in a clear and honest way. Newspapers, television and radio are the principal sources of information about all aspects of national life for most people, but these are quite inadequate on the whole to enable people to develop a considered view of complex problems.

So, in order to be able to represent the views of their public to the NHS, CHCs were first faced with the task of providing a certain amount of information to interest people and activate awareness. Public meetings, advertisements, exhibitions as well as contact with many local groups and press briefings are some of the ways to do this. Through CHC members' own contacts with voluntary organizations and the local authorities, the work of the CHC can be further explained and developed, but this all requires time and effort, which may be in short supply. CHC members give their time voluntarily in addition to their other commitments, so the degree to which CHCs can become known and hence reflect the needs of local people is very dependent on the determination of the members and the staff.

The meetings of CHCs are open for members of the public to attend (as are those of the health authorities and trusts) and they are given the opportunity to speak. People can also call at the CHC office for help and advice. If they have complaints about the NHS, the CHC can explain how to make best use of the official channels and procedures. Although it is not the responsibility of CHCs to judge or investigate individual complaints, by playing an active part they can support people through what may be complex and bewildering encounters with NHS management, and they can comment constructively on areas of complaint to the health authorities (see Section 13.4).

In terms of their overall influence in the NHS, it may appear that CHCs are relatively powerless; they certainly have no managerial responsibility for the provision of any services. But they do have the right to ask for and receive information, to attend the meetings of the HAs, to visit NHS premises, to be consulted about development plans. Consultation with them on hospital closures and substantial changes of use is required, they can give evidence to official committees, they can enlist the support of MPs and, above all, they can use the media to articulate their views forcibly.

Most CHCs have divided into working groups, each concentrating on a defined sector of health care by meeting regularly to consider information, conduct investigations, make visits and reports. CHCs also have to prepare an annual report to their local region, and there is a statutory annual public meeting with their local health authority. In relation to the family practitioner services, CHCs have more limited official powers. They do not have automatic access to GPs' surgeries. As a result, many councils have found it advantageous to make their own informal contacts with doctors and the local medical committee in order to establish an atmosphere of mutual respect and to improve the exchange of information.

In May 1974, the Secretary of State issued a consultative paper called *Democracy in the NHS*[1], which put forward ways in which the government was prepared to strengthen the principle of delegated authority in the NHS. With reference to CHCs, the two main suggestions were that two members should be appointed to the area health authority, and that a representative body should be created to advise and assist CHCs, with a budget drawn from central funds. The paper announced firm decisions to allow the posts of CHC secretaries to be filled by open competition (instead of being restricted to within the NHS); to oblige district management teams to send a spokesman to CHC meetings when invited, to answer questions in open session; to include CHCs among the bodies consulted by regions before making appointments to the AHAs; to make NHS employees and family practitioners eligible for CHC membership and to give CHCs a key role concerning hospital closures. CHCs, health authorities and other interested bodies were asked to submit their views on the paper's tentative proposals to the DHSS.

In July 1975, the Secretary of State announced that, in the light of these representations, each CHC would be allowed to send one member to attend AHA meetings with the right to speak but not to vote. In 1976, the DHSS amended its advice about appointing CHC members. It indicated that regions should include a trades council representative and a disabled person among its own nominees, and pointed out that all members of CHCs should be 'prepared to devote a considerable amount of time and energy to their Council's work. It is important that appointing bodies should take account of this, and confirm with prospective members that they can undertake the necessary duties before putting forward nominations.'

By the end of the 1970s there was a feeling that CHCs were not worth their annual level of expenditure, small though that was. This attitude resulted from both too much CHC activity and too little. In a few cases, notably inner city areas, some CHCs had spearheaded an attack on government policy and had disrupted AHA meetings. But in many other areas the CHCs were relatively ineffectual, duplicating some work done by health authority members themselves.

In many places CHCs were not very successful in making their presence felt, partly because, being made up of many separate representative interests, it has been difficult to formulate a clear point of view, particularly one which may be critical of government policy. Even hospital closures have been difficult for CHCs to fight, conscious as they have to be that they will be expected to suggest alternatives if their opinion is to be considered seriously. CHCs are reliant on HAs and their staff for information, and this tends to reduce their power to do much more than give a second opinion on plans.

The Royal Commission unequivocally supported the continuation of CHCs, but *Patients First*[2] was less sure and committed the government only to a further review. In the event, Circular HC(80)8[3] announced that CHCs would continue for the time being, and this was followed by a more detailed circular, HC(81)15[4], revising membership numbers to make most CHCs smaller, and clarifying other matters concerning the role of the CHC and the method of appointing members. In 1990, following the reconstitution of districts, the role of CHCs in the NHS was confirmed, but more narrowly defined. They no longer had to be consulted whenever the health authority intends to introduce a substantial change to local services, but only if the HA considers 'it would be expedient and in the interests of the health service to do so'[5]. CHCs do have access to trusts, but they are still excluded from examining GPs' services as of right.

The idea of a national body for CHCs was discussed for some time, until a meeting of CHC representatives decided, in November 1976, to proceed with its establishment. The first annual general meeting of the Association of Community Health Councils for England and Wales (ACHEW) was held in June 1977, attended by representatives of more than 70% of CHCs who had decided to join. At the request of the DHSS, in 1975, a national information service for CHCs, including a regular publication called *CHC News*, was set up and sponsored by the King's Fund. This proved to be successful, and in 1976, the DHSS assumed responsibility for its costs. The withdrawal of financial support caused the end of its publication in June 1984.

The reorganization of the NHS in 1974 and the creation of CHCs occurred at a turning point in the history of health service provision. Continued growth and expansion was for the first time seriously in doubt, and the public expenditure cuts of successive governments in the 1970s had a significant effect on the NHS. CHCs were not, therefore, in a position to expect demands for increased overall spending to be met, but they could pioneer attempts to encourage shifts in spending, particularly away from the hospital services towards the community services. Despite the reservations outlined above, they are, through their knowledge of the way the NHS works and through their involvement in the planning cycle, potentially able to promote the more effective use of limited resources, particularly in relation to the needs of the local community. However, health authorities and trusts do not always use this knowledge, and even when they do, they see the CHC's voice as only one among many. Other expressions of public opinion are equally important to them.

13.2 Public opinion

Public satisfaction with the NHS has tended to decline since the beginning of the 1980s. This may be both because the quality of the service is falling and because expectations are rising. Certainly there is discussion in the media about the NHS and its performance almost every day. Indeed the ethos of consumerism underpinning the National Health Service and Community Care Act 1990 has encouraged patients and the public generally to make their views known. The 1997 Labour government continued to stress the need for the NHS to be responsive to patient opinion.

The media can be helpful in explaining issues, but can also foster negative attitudes by sensationalizing shortcomings. NHS managers can no longer afford to disregard the importance of public relations. The methods used in industry and commerce to promote a positive image are disliked in the public services, yet the NHS allows images to persist that too often reduce the confidence of patients and the morale of the staff. Management therefore has to make sure that the services provided have public and patient support and will be promoted appropriately by the NHS's own ambassadors, the staff.

Since the 1990 reforms of the NHS there has been an increase in the number of locally conducted opinion polls, focus groups and citizen's juries and a surge of interest in trying to make the whole consultation process more reliable. Three factors are responsible. First, the setting up of the new corporate boards has abandoned the more traditional public accountability which the nominees on district health authorities had shouldered. The new non-executive directors are not intended to be formal representatives of their communities.

Second, and more importantly, the new commissioning role given to health authorities has exposed the hitherto implicit priority setting and rationing process which has always existed in the NHS, and this has perhaps prompted authorities to ease the path of difficult decisions through public consultation and opinion surveys. But increasingly it seems that priority-setting (or rationing) creates as many problems as it solves. Early in the 1990s managers followed with interest the experiment in the US State of Oregon, where public meetings and surveys were used extensively as part of a process to try and elicit a priority ranking for services to be provided within a limited Medicaid budget. The experiment has had limited success because it has been felt that rationing contravenes citizen's constitutional rights.

In the UK, the case of 'Child B' exposed some of the dilemmas of rationing. In 1995 the health authority concerned refused continuing treatment for a child with a rare cancer on the grounds that the likelihood of success was minimal. But the father and much of the press felt that the child's rights were being infringed by this decision and sought to have it reversed. In the end a private donor was secured but the child died within the year[6].

> **Key reference:** Hunter, D.J. (1997) *Desperately Seeking Solutions – rationing health care*. Longman, London.

Third, health authorities have carried out surveys of the attitudes of patients and the public about local health services, to obtain additional information to help purchasers respond to the wishes of their local populations[7]. Citizen's juries originated from the work of Birmingham University's Institute for Local Government Studies to improve local democracy. Pilot schemes showed these could be a useful way of gathering local opinion which was not unduly biased by self interest[8]. Trusts have also undertaken patient satisfaction surveys to check their own performance and also to acquire evidence to influence the health authorities with whom they make service agreements.

> **Key references:** McIver, S. (1999) *Healthy Debate? An independent evaluation of citizen's juries in health settings*. King's Fund, London; Davies, S. *et al.* (1999) *Ordinary Wisdom – reflections on an experiment in citizenship and health*. King's Fund, London.

In August 1998 the Secretary of State announced a national survey of 150,000 patients covering all English HAs. This ongoing programme will concentrate on primary care each year and on other selected areas such as heart disease and cancer services.

13.3 *Patient's Charter*

The implementation of the *Patient's Charter* and the political importance attached to it have probably given further impetus to the process of finding out what the public think, what they want and what patients feel about their services. In July 1991 the government published the *Citizen's Charter*[9]. The intention was to improve quality and standards in all public services through such mechanisms as privatization, contracting out services, greater competition, performance-related pay for public servants, published performance targets, more effective complaints procedures and so on. This emphasis on privatization and contracting out summed up the Conservative government's attitude to public services as inherently inefficient and unresponsive to users' needs and demands. The *Citizen's Charter* set out the overall framework for other specific charters, with examples of targets and policies for different public services, such as the railways (then in public ownership), the police and the inland revenue. Each service had to produce its own charter.

The NHS published the *Patient's Charter*[10] in 1991. It set out seven existing rights for patients:

- To receive health care on the basis of clinical need.

- To be registered with a GP.
- To receive emergency medical care at any time.
- To be referred to a consultant if thought necessary by a GP.
- To be given a clear explanation of any treatment proposed.
- To have access to one's own medical records.
- To choose whether or not to take part in medical research.

Three further rights were implemented by 1 April 1992:

- To have detailed information about available local services, quality standards and maximum waiting times.
- To be guaranteed admission to hospital no later than 2 years from the day a patient joined a waiting list (subsequently reduced to 18 months and then a target of a year).
- To have any complaint investigated and to receive a full and prompt written reply from the chief executive of a trust or health authority.

The general standards of service outlined in the *Citizen's Charter* also apply to the NHS. From April 1992, local charter standards also required trusts and health authorities to minimize out-patient waiting times and all front-line staff to wear name badges.

Having a charter is one thing, keeping to it is another. The *Patient's Charter* has not been particularly successful in improving standards. The government published a consultation document *A First Class Service*[11] in June 1998, aimed at bringing together the various initiatives for improving performance and responsiveness (see also Chapter 10).

13.4 COMPLAINTS

One aspect of consumer relations that has received considerable attention is the complaints procedure. The first official advice from the Ministry of Health on how to handle complaints about hospital care was set out in Circular HM(66)15[12]. It differentiated between minor complaints that could be dealt with on the spot and more substantial cases of dissatisfaction. However, health service staff were generally unsympathetic to complaints and were inclined to dismiss them. The Davies Committee was set up to examine hospital complaints procedures. Its report (1973)[13] suggested a detailed code of practice and the establishment of investigating panels. Although the government welcomed the report, only in 1976 did it announce that a uniform code of practice would be implemented for hospital and community services. This did not cover complaints about GP services.

13.4.1 Clinical complaints

In 1981 further guidance was issued, and it included an important new procedure for handling complaints about hospital clinical matters. This had always been difficult for patients and their relatives because they had only two choices: either accept the management's explanation or sue. The new procedure was set up in September 1981 and after 16 months a report was presented to the Secretary of State[14], who concluded that the new arrangements were working well. Overall the procedure was welcomed, as it dealt more satisfactorily with complaints arising from diagnosis and treatment. The total number of complaints remained very small, given the millions of patient contacts each year. However, the new arrangements did not ensure that all health authorities dealt with complaints adequately. The Hospital Complaints Procedure Act, 1985, required health authorities to establish a designated complaints officer who prepares regular reports for the health authority.

By 1993, the Secretary of State had responded to mounting criticism by setting up a new inquiry into complaints procedures. Hospital patients still felt that they were not always receiving a fair hearing. GPs' patients were often thwarted by the rigid procedure and timescales. They found GPs very reluctant to be open with them. The result of this was the 1994 Wilson report *Being Heard*[15], commissioned by the Secretary of State. The report was accepted by government in their guidance *Acting on complaints*[16]. Essentially every effort should be made to resolve the complaint locally and promptly, certainly within 6 months. If that fails, an independent chairman can convene a panel of independent people to consider the complaint and call expert witnesses to advise. The chief executive is responsible for informing the complainant of the result and of informing him or her of her of their right to take the matter to the Health Service Commissioner (ombudsman) if they remain dissatisfied.

13.4.2 Health Service Commissioner

Originally the Commissioner was unable to deal with clinical complaints but this was changed by the Health Service Commissioners (Amendment) Act 1996. This Act also allowed staff who felt they had encountered injustice to appeal to him. The Commissioner serves three separate offices for England, Scotland and Wales and issues an annual report to Parliament. He has his own staff and also has recourse to expert advisors. The process of investigation is lengthy – only 15% of cases are resolved in under 36 weeks; 43% exceed a year. The Commissioner has the power in law to require NHS staff and documents to be available. In his annual report for 1996/97[17] his office dealt with 2210 complaints, which showed a 24% increase on the previous year. Despite this many of the cases are not accepted and referred back for local resolution. The main topics of complaint included poor communications, poor record keeping, poor handling of relatives of dying patients and poor management of the initial complaint. Of complaints of poor treatment 43 were upheld and 63 rejected.

Given the millions of patient contacts with the NHS each year the complaint level still remains very low. Nevertheless, it is clear that there are many who could complain who do not consider it worthwhile, and of those who do, many find the way their complaint is handled unsatisfactory. The staff, for their part, feel beleaguered by the workload, intimidated by the aggressive attitudes of some patients and fearful that a complaint may lead to legal action against them, or their trust. It is a difficult matter to balance all these factors.

13.5 THE WORK OF VOLUNTARY ORGANIZATIONS

As the historical summaries in earlier chapters have shown, many of the existing health services have their origins in the work of volunteers and voluntary organizations. Outstanding examples are the voluntary hospitals themselves, district nursing and health visiting, the blood transfusion service, occupational therapy and family planning services, and there are many others.

The term 'voluntary organization' covers those non-profit-making associations of individuals (or organizations) which are not created by statute. Depending on their constitution or statement of objective, they may be registered charities, registered companies, chartered bodies or have some other legal status. The contribution of voluntary organizations alongside the statutory provision of health and social services is considerable. Governments continue to recognize that this co-operation is mutually beneficial, since in some cases the work of the voluntary organizations supplements that provided by the state, while in other cases the voluntary organizations fill in the gaps of state provision.

There is, however, an important distinction between voluntary and statutory services. Voluntary organizations often identify particular areas of need and specialize in educating public opinion on the deficiencies and potential improvements in statutory services, and they can often do this more flexibly and experimentally than a statutorily prescribed organization.

Those organizations registered under the Charities Act, 1960 (probably the majority in the health and welfare area), enjoy a number of financial benefits. Much of their income is derived from donations, legacies, government grants and fund-raising activities. They are entitled to direct relief of tax payable on this, as well as being able to reclaim the tax paid by individuals on donations given as a covenant and considerable relief on the local tax payable on their premises. Some of the larger charities also derive a part of their income from their capital assets. Money is required to cover staff wages and administrative costs, advertising campaigns, research support and direct grants. The increasing inflation of recent years has put considerable financial pressure on many charities, particularly those whose income from year to year is less predictable. *Care in Action*[18] encouraged the use of voluntary organizations as agents of the health authorities, because they could be more sensitive to new demands. Many existing voluntary bodies could not exist, however, without money from health and local authorities. The voluntary and statutory services are mutually dependent – many hospitals employ a co-ordinator of voluntary work.

The role of the voluntary sector has been debated a good deal, especially since the Conservatives came to power in 1979. Circular

HC(80)11[19] encouraged health authorities to involve themselves in fund-raising if this seemed beneficial: previously, direct fund-raising had not been allowed. In the discussions leading up to the 1982 reorganization, the Secretary of State, Patrick Jenkin, suggested that much more could be provided by the voluntary sector, leaving the statutory bodies as a 'safety net' to ensure no one was left without support[20]. Such a view was anathema to the Labour Party. Even less acceptable was the idea that voluntary work was a suitable alternative for paid work at times of unemployment. Indeed, despite periods of high unemployment, volunteers have not always been easy to recruit. Health services have long been supported by leagues of hospital friends and numerous other bodies, but they cannot rely on raising large sums of money on a recurring basis to become a sufficient, realistic alternative to central funding.

As well as voluntary bodies and CHCs, pressure groups enable the public to influence the NHS. They are set up with a specific purpose, such as saving a hospital from closure or campaigning for services for a particular group of patients or for a new facility. The newspapers, television and radio have become increasingly interested in health matters, notably aspects of high-technology medicine and hospital life. Informed television and radio programmes involve and educate the public about medical research and new treatments. Popular television series such as *Casualty* cover many areas of concern, from how best to care for the elderly to epilepsy and solvent abuse.

Since the 1974 reorganization, health authorities and their staff have become more responsive to their role as agents of the public they serve, and a more open attitude to the media has resulted. The media, in their turn, can do much to protect the rights of the public. This is particularly important in matters of research and to ensure patients' rights are not abused in other ways.

13.6 MEDICAL RESEARCH AND INTERVENTION

Research into new and more effective forms of treatment is a necessary and expected activity, and the benefits of its results are well known. However, a strong body of opinion is opposed to the conduct of certain techniques and experiments on animal and human subjects. The state finances research directly through the Medical Research Council and through grants to individuals, and indirectly through its funding of academic institutions which carry out research. Most of this work is carefully done, but concern has arisen over cases where the rights of the subjects may appear to have been disregarded. To overcome this, ethical committees were set up to vet all new proposals for clinical research. This acknowledged that the responsibility for deciding on the ethics of an experiment should not rest with the investigator alone. Yet a review of ethical committees sponsored by the King's Fund and undertaken by Julia Neuberger in 1992[21] demonstrated that not all such committees worked satisfactorily.

The drug thalidomide was first synthesized in Germany in 1956 and marketed as a sedative and hypnotic. In 1958 it was manufactured and marketed in Britain, under licence to Distillers Company Biochemicals Ltd, under several brand names including 'Distavel'. It was found to be a particularly effective sedative which did not have some of the disadvantages of the barbiturates, and was prescribed for pregnant women to reduce feelings of tension. In November 1961, a German paediatrician reported the suspected connection between congenital deformities in babies and the use of thalidomide in early pregnancy. On 2 December 1961, Distillers announced withdrawal of the drug. About 8000 deformed children were born as a result of the use of thalidomide, over 400 of them in Britain[22]. Legal actions against Distillers were pursued by a number of the children and settlements were made in other cases, some following an investigation by Sir Alan Marre, largely completed in 1978

The Medicines Control Agency's purpose is to safeguard the public by ensuring that new medicines are safe and appropriate. They rely on the expert advice of the Medicines Commission and the Committee on the Safety of Medicines. It still remains true that animal and human subjects have to be used at an early stage, before a medicine can be known to be safe and effective or not. The case of thalidomide, although 40 years ago, has acted as a cautionary tale about what can happen if not enough research is done. The affair was one of the factors contributing to revised legislation on testing new drugs and advertising their properties.

Even so, there have been other cases where significant numbers of patients have been adversely affected by a drug. Furthermore, even after drugs have been declared suitable for use, doubts about their longer term safety can persist, as for example with certain steroid preparations and the contraceptive pill. In addition there is increasing concern with the safety of foods. For some time people had urged the UK, like the USA, to have a national agency concerned with the safety of food. The Food Standards Agency was finally set up in 1999 as a semi-autonomous body by the Minister of Agriculture.

Within the NHS the increasing pressure to achieve accountability for clinical decisions (see Chapter 10) is helping to create the climate in which only those medical interventions which have been proved effective and beneficial are undertaken. But the question about how to handle innovation remains. When heart transplants were first performed in the 1960s they captured the interest of the press, but the success rate remained relatively disappointing. The high cost of the procedure and the problems of finding suitable donors at the right time limited what could be achieved in this area. Kidney transplantation has proved more successful. Before transplantation, people with chronic renal failure are kept alive by being attached to a kidney machine for intermittent dialysis. Demand for this treatment far exceeds the availability of kidneys. The transplant operation itself is technically less difficult than for the heart, and, if a suitable donor can be found and the considerable problems of tissue rejection managed, a patient with a transplant can recover to lead a fully active and normal life. The untreated disease is fatal, and life with a kidney machine is far from easy, so transplantation can offer the best solution for many sufferers. In 1972 the DHSS launched a public donor campaign to encourage people to decide to allow their kidneys to be used for transplantation if they died. Response to further campaigns remained disappointing and, although many hospitals were fully equipped to perform the operation (except for shortages of technical staff in some places), people with the disease are still dying prematurely because there are insufficient donors.

13.7 ETHICS

Handling innovation and research are two of the ethical dilemmas facing clinical staff and managers in the NHS. The decision whether to prolong a patient's life or not can be extremely difficult to make, especially when facilities for continuing care are in short supply. The increasing incidence of degenerative and terminal illnesses in old people bears witness to considerable mastery over the infectious and damaging diseases and the poor social conditions that limited life expectancy for earlier generations, but this brings its own problems. One observer has written:

> It is clearly pointless to keep a patient with an inoperable brain tumour breathing when a fatal outcome is certain, and in the case of recurrent chest infections in the elderly respiratory cripple there may come a time when it is unkind to rescue the patient yet again from an acute episode only to restore him to distressing permanent disablement. The decision to submit a patient to resuscitation or intensive therapy must be informed, deliberate and responsible[23].

A report from the Royal College of Physicians in May 1994 accused health authorities and providers of discriminating against elderly patients, on the assumption that the elderly should be at the end of the queue because they had less time to live[24]. The Royal College of Physicians recommended that:

> The guiding principle upon which the provision of acute medical care to elderly people is based must be that there is no distinction or negative discrimination on grounds of age.

Whether this means that it is justifiable to discriminate on the grounds of life expectancy – which would tend to mean preference given to younger rather than older people – is unclear. Or should every patient receive maximum treatment even if this prolongs their life by only a few days and deprives someone else of resources which would prolong their life by years? These ethical choices are extremely difficult and the rigid application of any one set of principles may be costly in terms of human lives.

Cases of serious and possibly irreversible brain damage following road accidents, or the birth of babies with congenital abnormalities exercise the judgement of doctors and families to the extreme, and the definition of meaningful survival and the cost of intervention, both financial and emotional, have to be made somehow. The Helsinki Agreement on Guidelines for Research in 1964 stimulated concern about the ethical aspects of health care.

As well as the limitation of resources, and the rationing that may result, other ethical issues more in the domain of health services management include:

- proper employment practice;
- honouring the rights of patients;
- carrying out the government's will even when the consequences may be uncertain;

- accountability to patients, public, the media, politicians and to conscience.

All these are matters of concern[25]; doing what is right is not only a matter for clinical staff. Managers and the population at large need to contribute to the ethical debate

CONCLUSION

Matters raised in this chapter lead to the question 'Is the NHS sensitive enough to the public it serves?' Health authorities and trusts, the CHCs, voluntary bodies, pressure groups and the media all help to inform and protect the public interest. Unlike some countries, in the UK litigation is a relatively insignificant factor in bringing about changes. In the early 1980s, the government took the view that subjecting the NHS to more competition might improve standards, so private hospitals were enabled to develop more rapidly. But the private sector still provides only a small part of total patient care. Such provision did draw to health authorities' attention the scant concern most hospitals and community units had shown for fostering better staff attitudes towards patients, and the widespread complacency about waiting times in out-patient departments and waiting-lists for admissions.

Policy statements by government ministers have emphasized the pressing need for the NHS to show it really is concerned about the consumer. In 1992 *Local Voices*[26] and more recently *Patient partnership: building a collaborative strategy*[27] and the setting up of *NHS Direct*, a 24-hour help line staffed by nurses to give advice to patients, have stressed the importance of listening to the public's concerns and demonstrating commitment to satisfying their needs. The very titles of white papers – *Patients First, Working for Patients, Caring for People* and the NHS version of the *Citizen's Charter*, the *Patient's Charter* – underline this desire to portray the NHS more in the image of a commercial service committed to pleasing its customers, and less like a welfare institution where the recipients of care are expected to be grateful for whatever they are fortunate enough to receive. Health authorities and their providers of health care have been set a challenge by the 1990 Act; it remains to be seen whether the confidence of the public in the NHS can be maintained.

REFERENCES

1. DHSS (1974) *Democracy in the National Health Service*. HMSO, London.
2. DHSS and Welsh Office (1979) *Patients First*. HMSO, London.
3. DHSS (1980) *Health Service Development: Structure and Management* Circular HC(81)8. DHSS, London.
4. DHSS (1981) *Health Service Development: Community Health Councils* Circular HC(81)15. DHSS, London.
5. DoH, NHSME (1990) *Consultation and Involving the Customer*. DoH, London.

6. Ham, C. and Pickard, S. (1998) *Tragic Choices in Health Care*. Kings Fund, London.

7. For a useful collation of a number of opinion surveys and a useful discussion of their interpretation see Judge, K. and Soloman, M. (1993) Public Opinion and the National Health Service: Patterns and Perspectives in Consumer Satisfaction. *Journal of Social Policy* **22**(3): 229–327.

8. McIver, S. (1998) *Citizen's Juries in Health Authority Settings: an evaluation of six pilot studies*. Health Services Management Centre, Birmingham/King's Fund, London.

9. Cabinet Office (1991) *The Citizen's Charter*. HMSO, London (Cmnd 1599).

10. DoH (1991) *The Patient's Charter*. HMSO, London.

11. DoH (1998) *A First Class Service – Quality in the new NHS*. The Stationery Office, London.

12. Ministry of Health (1966) *Methods of Dealing with Complaints by Patients* Circular HM(66)15.

13. DHSS and Welsh Office (1973) *Report of the Committee on Hospital Complaints Procedure* (Davies report). HMSO, London and Cardiff.

14. DHSS, Scottish Home and Health Department and Welsh Office (1983) *Report on the Operation of Procedures for Independent Review of Complaints involving the Clinical Judgement of Hospital Doctors and Dentists*. HMSO, London, Edinburgh and Cardiff.

15. DoH (1994) *Being Heard* (Wilson report). HMSO, London.

16. DoH (1995) *Acting on Complaints* Executive Letter EL(95)37. NHS Executive, Leeds.

17. Health Service Commissioner (1997) *Health Service Commissioner: Annual Report for 1996–97*. HMSO, London.

18. DHSS (1981) *Care in Action – A Handbook of Policies and Priorities for the Health and Personal Social Services for England*. HMSO, London.

19. DHSS (1980) *Health Services Management. Health Services Act 1980: Fund Raising by HS Authorities* Health Circular HC(80)11. DoH, London.

20. Jenkin, P. (1981) Article in *The Guardian*, 26 January.

21. Neuberger, J. (1992) *Ethics and health care – the role of research ethics committees in the UK*. King's Fund, London.

22. Ministry of Health (1964) Deformities Caused by Thalidomide. *Reports on Public Health and Medical Subjects, No 112*. HMSO, London.

23. Miller, H. (1973) *Medicine and Society* p. 2. Oxford University Press, Oxford.

24. Royal College of Physicians (1994) *Ensuring Quality of Care for Elderly People*. RCP, London.

25. Wall, A. (1989) *Ethics and the Health Services Manager*. King's Fund, London.

26. DoH (1992) *Local Voices*. HMSO, London.

27. DoH (1996) *Patient Partnership: building a collaborative strategy*. NHS Executive, Leeds.

14

THE NHS IN AN INTERNATIONAL CONTEXT

Health care is needed to combat diseases, accidents and disasters. Air and water-borne infections, poor nutrition and housing, pollution, and genetic deficiencies are some of the principal causes of disease. Equally significant are the disasters – natural (such as earthquakes, floods) and man-made (such as war). Health services are characteristic of their countries in many ways. They evolve from particular histories and circumstances and have to deal with particular health needs. Nevertheless, while every health service encounters this distinctiveness, all countries' health services face a number of similar organizational problems and basic issues. Setting priorities within a limited budget means the same in Mozambique as in Germany or the UK. The order of magnitude and the choices involved, and their implications, may differ – malaria control versus a TB vaccination programme, compared with the latest portable bone scanner versus a community psychiatric nurse. But the need to make the choice is there. Different countries also share considerable overlap of aims and objectives of their respective health care systems and institutions: equity of access, efficiency and effectiveness are commonly cited in a number of countries.

Recognizing such similarities is not to ignore the existence of obvious differences, but all health care services have much to learn from each other's good and bad practices. The World Health Organization was set up in 1948 as an agency of the United Nations. It enables professionals from its 170 member countries to share their expertise and to devise means of helping each other. The WHO's current priorities cover a wide agenda (Box 14.1).

Box 14.1

WHO priorities

- Health of mothers and children.
- Combating malnutrition.
- Controlling malaria, TB and leprosy.
- Combating AIDS.
- Mass immunization.
- Improving mental health.
- Providing safe water supplies.
- Training health personnel.

Managers, clinicians and academics from more and more countries look abroad to see how others do it, whether it works and how it would work back home. The health care systems in many countries are currently tackling similar reforms. This chapter looks abroad to examine the way other countries organize and fund their health care services, and assesses their relative success in achieving equitable, high quality and efficient services for their populations.

14.1 EQUITY OF PROVISION

There are many ways to define equity of provision of health care. At one extreme equity could refer to equality of outcome of medical intervention. However, some notion of fairness concerning access to health care services is a commonly accepted definition. The fundamental belief underlying this is that people in equal need of care should have equal access to care, and this means minimizing barriers to care and treatment. This belief is common to all health care systems[1].

In the UK, except for medicines, dental treatment and spectacles and some aspects of nursing home care for the elderly and severely disabled, health care is free to all at the time of use. In the USA, although health care is paid for more directly like a conventional economic commodity, the government spends billions of dollars every year to underwrite a degree of equity of access for those on low incomes and the elderly. Other countries, such as Canada, New Zealand, Sweden, Denmark, Spain and Germany, have few, if any, payment requirements at the time of use, but fully equitable access to health care has still never been achieved. Differences between countries in access to health care appear to be unrelated to the existence of universal public health care coverage. A pan-European study[2] suggested that in the Netherlands and Switzerland, where comprehensive public cover is limited, there is little income-related inequity. Inequitable access (defined in terms of the shares of health care spending devoted to different income groups) is common. In the UK, inequity favours the well off. Empirical work to test the existence and degree of inequity of health care delivery can be very sensitive to the variables chosen to represent health (i.e. need).

14.1.1 What is 'need'?

Health economists define 'need' in the context of equity as the ability or capacity to benefit from medical intervention. From this perspective, equality of access for those in equal need can discriminate between people experiencing exactly the same health problem, whose capacity to benefit differs. The health economists' argument is that while two people may have the same poor health status, if choices have to be made between allocating scarce resources, then using those resources efficiently should not be completely dominated by the goal of equality of access. Given the obligation to make a choice, a person with poor prospects of survival from an operation to remove a malignant tumour should receive less of the scarce care resource (or perhaps none at all) than someone with the same problem whose prospects of survival are better.

Opponents of the economists' view of need argue that every human life is equally valuable, and that it is therefore immoral to discriminate using the criterion of the capacity to benefit from medical treatment (just as it is wrong to discriminate on the grounds of income). Economists

One or two examples of patient selection on the grounds of their capacity to benefit hit the headlines every year. In 1993, for example, surgeons at a hospital in the north of England refused a heart operation to a patient who smoked. The clinicians involved justified their refusal on the grounds that the patient would not benefit from treatment as he refused to give up smoking, and that the resources involved could be better spent on someone else

argue that, if followed rigidly, such a position would entail an enormous waste of resources and hence unnecessary loss of life and additional suffering. Most economists recognize that both stands, if taken to their extremes, are undesirable and would produce irreconcilable ethical disputes. Despite some vehement critiques of the health economists' position[3], their view hardly differs from actual medical practice. In formalizing what actually happens, the economists thereby expose some of the extremely difficult (and, to many, unpalatable) ethical decisions being taken by clinicians every day.

One answer is to leave matters as they are, with doctors and others muddling through, and simply accept the inconsistencies and potential loss of equity/efficiency that inevitably arises[4]. This position distinguishes between access to the system as a whole and access to a particular amount or level of care once inside the system. Discrimination with regard to the former is highly discouraged. The latter is accepted as unfortunate but necessary (and should be left largely to doctors to sort out). Whether this is a tenable resolution of the issue, in the light of the greater transparency of decision-making and the need to make choices following the 1990 reforms in the UK, remains to be seen. These ethical dilemmas inherent in the application of concepts of need and equity are universal; all countries continuously grapple with competing judgements and views in these matters.

14.1.2 Social class, income and equity

In practice, inequitable access to the health care system as a whole generally arises for three reasons: social or ethnic group, financial status and geography. The Black report[5] and numerous previous and subsequent research studies established that people in the UK belonging to lower occupational classes suffer more ill-health. The Black report suggested that if the mortality rates of class I (professional people and their families) were applied to classes IV and V (manual workers and their families) during 1970–72, as many as 74,000 lives would not have been prematurely lost. The association of poor health with low social status persists, and this is largely outside the scope of the health services because it includes low income, poor housing, less education and, consequently, a comparatively deprived lifestyle.

How far are these findings applicable in other countries? The Black report wrestled with the difficulties inherent in making international comparisons[6] where statistics do not have a common base. It concluded, in its study of infant mortality, that socio-economic factors were usually influential, although the different rates between countries stimulate more questions than answers. It is still not clear why the results are so much better in Sweden and Norway than in England. How has France improved its position so markedly in a relatively short period?

In the UK, the NHS is available to all irrespective of their social class. In practice, different classes have different patterns of use and consumption of health care from the NHS which cannot be explained completely by differences in their health status. Some other countries demonstrate more entrenched or formalized class-related services. In the USA, middle-class people widely use private sources of care based on a fee for services system. But the poor, estimated at over 30 million people, including ethnic minorities and those living in inadequate conditions in inner cities, have to rely on a public system, mostly based on the local county or city hospital. Unlike the middle-class, middle-income patients who have potentially limitless choice, the disadvantaged have little or no choice. Germany has a tiered hospital system in which paying more money buys a better level of service and access to more experienced and senior doctors. This is reminiscent of pre-1948 Britain, where access to the voluntary hospital often required a member of the management board to sponsor the individual, while patients could be admitted to municipal hospitals directly (see Chapter 2).

A fundamental principle embodied in the creation of the NHS was that patients should be treated equally, entirely irrespective of their financial means. Despite the increase in private medicine, which allows people to buy prompt treatment instead of having to queue on the waiting list, this principle has remained largely intact. But a hidden discriminator remains. Studies have shown that middle-class people use the NHS more, and more effectively, than working-class people[7]. This is true in the preventive field too, where voluntary screening programmes fail to reach those most at risk. High socio-economic status is associated with more knowledgeable individuals who are better able to make beneficial use of the available services. The same effect is observed in other countries. In America, those with money can afford as much health care as they like, those without have limited choice, but are also restricted to more stringently controlled services where even the number of consultations or referrals to hospitals are regulated.

14.1.3 Geography and equity

Does distance from a hospital lead to poorer levels of health care? Apparently not. Sweden achieves some of the best results in the world with, for instance, an infant mortality rate of under 5 per 1000 births compared with the UK's figure of 6.0 per 1000 births (1996). Furthermore, the most remote county in Sweden has the lowest rate in Sweden itself.

The Royal Commission on the NHS undertook a study, in 1978, to examine whether location within the UK was a significant influence on people's view of their access to health care[8]. This study looked at a rural community in Cumbria and a London borough, and found that patients in both places were satisfied with their access to care, at least at the primary level. The public support for retaining local hospitals in the UK suggests that physical proximity is an important consideration. But how do other countries manage where distances are much greater?

The actual distribution of hospitals tends to be determined by the population distribution characteristic of that country. It has been estimated that despite the continuous increase in urbanization, half the world's population is still rural. In the United Kingdom, 10 miles may be regarded as too far from the nearest hospital, while in rural Sweden 100 miles might be considered reasonable. But in rural Africa 100 miles would be far too far given that the most likely means of transport is on foot. Sweden's population is only 8.2 million, of which 3 million live in three cities, and the remainder are spread thinly over an area bigger than Italy, Austria and Switzerland combined. As in Canada, health facilities in Sweden have to be widely spaced. In France, legislation between 1958 and 1968 developed a three-tiered system of university hospitals, general hospitals and local hospitals. Other countries such as Germany, the Netherlands and the USA have a less structured system, but through planning regulations they are attempting to rationalize hospital provision and reduce maldistribution.

14.1.4 Availability of health care services

In the developing world the WHO has defined a district hospital as one which serves a recognizable population defined by both geography and culture[9]. It may be the first stop for care or may supplement primary care either through outreach or by general co-ordination of health care workers. The WHO has done much to encourage developing countries to provide a sustainable infrastructure of care and not to go for high technology where the basics such as a safe water supply or a reliable power source are not yet in place.

The variations in access to health care associated with class, financial and geographical factors are important, but equally significant is the actual availability of health services. The policies controlling distribution of doctors and other health care workers, hospitals and clinics are crucial. In the developed world, access to treatment is principally determined by doctors. There are marked differences between Western countries. One of the successes of the NHS is the much more even distribution of family doctors than before. GPs have an average of around 1800 patients on their lists and, because of the system of regulation (see Chapter 11), the number of doctors working in each area is controlled. In Germany, a system of incentives was introduced in 1976 to encourage doctors to practise in unpopular areas, but these doctors were not general practitioners in the English sense. Indeed, only Denmark and the Netherlands have a system of general practice remotely comparable to the English system. In other countries, there is no difference between general practitioners and hospital doctors. A doctor will first see a patient in the surgery and then, if hospital care is needed, will treat the patient in hospital or refer the patient to a colleague.

Outpatient departments are not found in some countries. In Germany, out-patient departments have only recently been established, and then only in university hospitals. In Sweden, community health centres, covering a population of between 20,000 and 50,000, provide both primary care and out-patient consultation. Norway has smaller health centres, so the out-patient element is less significant, but the Municipal Health Act of 1984 has promoted locally controlled primary care services.

The most common system, found for example in Germany, the USA and France, allows patients to attend surgeries of their chosen specialist doctor or, in some cases, as referred by their employer. The doctor then decides how best to treat the patient. This system is often criticized in these countries because it has several disadvantages. First, patients may make the wrong choice and consequently be at risk from inappropriate treatment from a doctor not in an appropriate speciality. Second, their care consists of unco-ordinated treatments for single episodes of illness. Third, this encourages waste, as the more affluent patients may go to more than one doctor for the same symptoms. In Germany and Sweden, where the number of hospital beds per population is generous, patients may be admitted to hospital unnecessarily, but they will not wait. Nowhere else has the UK's problem with waiting lists.

Waiting lists are discussed in Section 9.7.3

14.1.5 Doctor numbers

The total number of doctors affects the situation too, and there are wide variations (Table 14.1).

Germany	332
France	350
Sweden	360
USA	420
UK	560
Australia	560
New Zealand	645

Table 14.1

People per doctor (1990)

In those countries, the number of doctors has increased and often doubled in the last 30 years, to the point where some countries believe they have too many doctors. In the UK, numbers entering medical schools have been regulated, although in the 1960s the government expanded the number of medical schools, thinking there might otherwise be too few doctors. Recent regulation of medical student intake in France has been unpopular. In the USA, regulation of medical schools started in 1910, and current estimates suggest that the country as a whole is becoming over-doctored, although distribution continues to be uneven. In France the government has been trying to tackle maldistri-bution problem because 35,000 of the 46,000 doctors are private practi-tioners and the regulation of these has brought about major conflicts.

14.1.6 Doctors' pay

Doctors are paid differently from country to country. In the Netherlands there is increasing pressure to employ doctors directly on salaries. In Sweden, where 85% of doctors are publicly employed, this is popular, even among doctors, because it has eradicated major differences in doctors' earnings. In this respect, Sweden is the most radical of all Western countries. It abolished fees for hospital care in 1959 and for ambulatory (out-patient or community) care in 1970. Recent proposals

As Chapter 11 indicates, the original NHS Act and the 1966 GP Charter were a political trade-off for improving general practice primary care. Following the 1990 contract, GPs continued to be paid by basic capitation fees, together with certain incentive payments. The 1997 Primary Care Act allowed for salaried GPs

to reform payment methods and employment terms for doctors encountered widespread opposition.

In the USA, various attempts are being made to curb the increasing level of doctors' fees. Health Maintenance Organizations (HMOs), introduced in 1973, enable doctors to set up pre-payment group practice. In this way, they can provide more comprehensive care with less reliance on hospitals and at correspondingly lower cost. The reforms in the USA proposed by the Clinton administration in the early 1990s were designed to address many of the criticisms of inequity, inefficiency and expense levelled at the US health care system. The libertarian tradition in the USA which encourages personal freedom of choice caused the failure to support these reforms, at least for the time being. Other attempts have been made to curb costs. 'Managed health care', building on the apparent success of the HMO movement, attempts to limit the cost of care through planning the patients' clinical progress through the health care system (see also Section 14.3.1).

14.1.7 Hospital beds and throughput

The work of doctors is determined not only by the needs and demands of the public but also by the availability of hospital beds and other facilities and the medical profession's attitudes to treatments. In the UK, a shortage of beds is often cited as the reason for long waiting lists, whereas it is the throughput of cases for these beds that compares unfavourably with some other countries. The USA and other countries which rely on a payment system for occupied beds per day have a vested interest in maximizing the use of beds, and management of the beds tends to be affected by these considerations. Whether the patient needs to be in the bed is a separate issue. Operation rates vary widely between England and the USA because some surgical procedures are much more readily undertaken in the USA.

Continental European countries also have a higher level of bed provision than the UK. The Netherlands has about 5.5 beds per 1000 population for short-term care (comparable to what the UK calls acute), Germany has 7.7 beds, whereas Department of Health guidance allows only 2.8. The allocation of beds for the elderly in England is 8.5–10 per 1000 population over 65, eight times lower than in Sweden. Since the mid-1970s, admissions overall have increased in all countries at the same time as the length of stay has shortened dramatically. Yet there are still wide discrepancies in throughput which are difficult to explain; no one knows how to define the 'correct' number of beds. Influential factors are the supply of community and primary care, the availability of out-patient facilities, the extent of market competition between hospitals, the historical distribution of beds and variations in medical practice.

The number of beds has a major effect on the cost of the service. The UK's relatively low annual cost as reflected in its proportion of the GNP (see Figure 14.1) is the consequence of its relatively low number of beds. Most countries are worried about the high cost of hospital services and

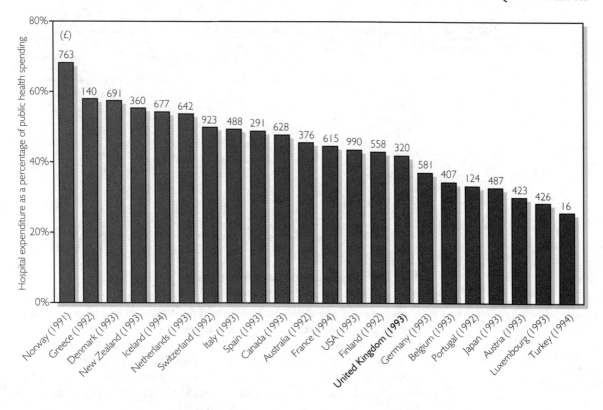

Source: compiled using material from the *Organisation for Economic Co-operation and Development Health Database 1997*. OECD, Paris

acknowledge that they have too many beds or that these tend to be wastefully used. To a certain extent this is due to the way doctors exercise control over hospital resources.

Figure 14.1

Hospital expenditure per person as a percentage of public health spending in OECD countries, circa 1993.

14.2 QUALITY OF SERVICE

What do we actually mean by a 'quality' health service? Ultimately, of course, the quality of a service is reflected in the outcome of treatment. In this sense, quality really means (medical) effectiveness and appropriateness so that a patient receives a treatment that works and benefits from it. Methods for improving quality and hence the outcomes of services range from hospital and doctor accreditation to organizational and managerial 'quality' marks, guaranteeing that a particular process, shown to deliver good outcomes, is always used.

Is the public confident that the expenditure and the organization of health care does provide appropriate benefits? Table 14.2 shows the considerable differences in public attitudes between ten developed countries. By monitoring the quality of the services provided and, in particular, the work of doctors themselves, it is possible to see where there is specific scope for reform.

Chapter 10 examines the problems associated with achieving and assessing quality in health care

Table 14.2

Public attitudes to health care
services

	Minor changes needed (%)	Fundamental changes needed (%)	Completely re-build system (%)
Canada	56	38	5
Netherlands	47	46	5
West Germany	41	35	13
France	41	42	10
Australia	34	43	17
Sweden	32	58	6
Japan	29	47	6
United Kingdom	27	52	17
Italy	12	46	40
United States	10	60	29

Source: adapted from Harvard-Harrris-ITF, 1990 Ten-Nation Survey. In, Blendon, R. *et al.*,
DataWatch: Satisfaction with health systems in ten countries. *Health Affairs*, **10**(2), 185–92.

14.2.1 The quality of doctors' work

Countries vary in their attempts to control the quality of doctors' work.
Until recently the NHS lagged behind in this respect. How do other
countries regulate their doctors? Although health services in the USA are
apparently allowed to flourish in the open market of free enterprise,
hospitals and doctors are in fact closely regulated. All doctors have to be
licensed practitioners, and beyond this there is a system for further
professional accreditation after postgraduate training. Hospitals
themselves are also subject to accreditation procedures.

The Joint Commission on the Accreditation of Hospitals (JCAH)
assesses hospitals every 2 years on their organizational structure, physical
environment and the staffing levels. More recently JCAH has started to
examine medical audits undertaken within hospitals by their own staff.
Hospitals appoint specialist staff to carry out the accreditation, and those
failing to meet the standards face withdrawal of federal or state funds
and a consequent loss of financial viability. In 1972, the US Department
of Health Education and Welfare introduced Professional Standards
Review Organizations (PSROs) to undertake reviews of the use of facilities. These are conducted by physicians and examine individual medical
practice in detail. PSROs have been unpopular, and some critics doubt
whether they have materially controlled the inflation in hospital costs[10].

France has a well articulated system of inspection. About 4000 physicians, employed by the social security administration, have to authorize
costly procedures and scrutinize lengthy stays in hospital. The system is
bureaucratic and resented, but the inspectors are well paid and there is
no difficulty in recruitment. Hospitals themselves are inspected by a
smaller body of civil servants at département level. Nationally a further
body, usually staffed by administrators, undertakes special studies and
issues an annual report. Auditors have the right to examine any aspect of
the country's administration, and recent reports from them have drawn
attention to poor standards in some French hospitals, particularly for
longer-stay patients.

The European Union provides for the free movement of health care professionals across the EU but this has been limited partly by problems of recognition of qualifications and partly because of natural language barriers. Movement will increase particularly if one country is short or provides better working conditions than another.

There are many opportunities for health professionals from the developed world to work on short or long-term contracts in developing countries. For instance, in the UK, Voluntary Service Overseas (VSO) sends health care workers with varying levels of experience to Africa, Asia, the Pacific and the Caribbean. The DoH also supports health care development elsewhere in the world.

14.3   FINANCING HEALTH CARE

Financing health care is a problem in all countries. All governments find themselves spending more than they wish, all complain of waste and poor control, all are worried for the future. Significantly, since the 1980s most have introduced major legislation to control health care costs and financial allocations. It seems that whatever the ideological stance of the government, more state involvement and more state control is inevitable in financing health care. In the UK, the 1990 reforms showed an increased interest in cost-sharing through privatization and the introduction of a limited form of provider competition to promote the more efficient use of resources, together with the determination to hold management more accountable. These issues are echoed in many other countries and by their governments. Despite the problems facing the NHS, the services produced for the resources provided still make it relatively cost effective.

Methods of financing health care vary considerably, but in all developed countries there is a mix of state funding, insurance and direct payments. Table 14.3 shows the variations in funding sources in nine European countries. A major concern of all governments is to control costs whatever their methods of financing health care. In the UK, the NHS review leading to *Working for Patients*[11] studied the various options for financing health care. After some interest in switching to an insurance-based scheme, it was concluded that the present method, largely dependent on taxation (see Chapter 8), was probably better than any other. Certainly the British system is simpler, and this is reflected in the lower administrative costs of the service. It is said that administrative costs in the USA are over 20%, in France 10%, but in the UK less than 5%.

14.3.1   Equity in financing

All countries profess to be committed to equity in both the provision and financing of health care. In fact these commitments vary considerably. Given that health care consumes resources, what is the fairest way of paying for health care? Because the NHS is funded largely from general taxation, and because the (direct) tax system is mildly progressive

Table 14.3

Sources of health care funding: selected countries

Country	Taxation	Social insurance	Private insurance	Out-of pocket payments
Denmark	1981	General central and local government tax revenues used to fund public health care.	None.	Usually provides cover only for public sector copayments.	Copayments for prescription drugs, dental care, physiotherapy.
France	1985	Some revenues from tax on car insurance used to cover social insurance fund deficit.	Three separate occupational health insurance funds covering 98% of population. Contributions related to earnings but vary across schemes. Compulsory in case of employees and split between employee and employer. Ceiling on contributions recently removed for *Régime Général*.	Supplementary insurance paid to *mutuelles* and private insurance companies. Premiums to *mutuelles* related to earnings and provide cover for *ticket modérateur*. Premiums to private insurees related to risk.	*Ticket modérateur* covers 25% of cost of GP visits and 30% of cost of medicines. Private and *mutuelle* policy-holders can obtain at least partial reimbursement except for some medicines. Some groups and some medicines exempt from ticket *modérateur*. Some small copayments for inpatient care.
Ireland	1987	General central government tax revenues used to fund public health care. Tax deductability of private insurance.	Small health-specific social insurance contribution goes towards funding of public health care.	Mainly taken out by persons in middle and upper income groups whose public cover is limited. Private insurance tax deductible.	Middle income group liable for copayments for inpatient and outpatient treatment, and payment in full for GP visits and prescription medicines. Top income group liable for copayment for inpatient hotel facilities, and payment in full for consultant services, outpatient and primary care, and prescription medicines.

Table 14.3 continued

Country	Year	Taxation	Social insurance	Private insurance	Out-of pocket payments
Italy	1987	General central government tax revenues paid into national health service fund in respect of fiscalization and under other headings. Taxes also used ex-post to cover health services fund deficit.	Compulsory earnings-related contributions to social health insurance fund. Some general social insurance contributions also used to fund public health care. In both cases, contributions schedules vary across professional groups.	Taken out as supplementary cover to health service cover. Includes compulsory scheme for managers.	Ticket modérateur payable for prescription drugs, with disabled, etc., exempt. Direct payments to private sector by persons with and without private insurance.
Netherlands	1987	General central government tax revenues used to subsidize sick funds and to finance preventive care.	Compulsory contributions payable by all to AWBZ scheme for catastrophic expenses. Additional insurance contributions payable to sickness funds by persons with income less than Dfl49 150 for non-catastrophic expenses. In both cases contributions proportional to earnings but subject to ceiling.	Taken out by persons with income in excess of Dfl49 150 to cover non-catastrophic expenses.	Copayments deductibles paid by persons with private insurance. Direct payments by persons without insurance cover for non-catastrophic expenses. Copayments by sickness fund-insured.
Portugal	1981	General central government tax revenues used to fund public health care and subsidize occupational health insurance schemes operating in public sector.	Some compulsory occupational schemes providing double cover to public sector employees. Contributions related to earnings.	Taken out as supplementary cover to public sector cover.	Copayments to public sector for consultations, diagnostic tests, and medicines. Direct payments to private sector by those with and without private/occupational insurance.

Table 14.3 continued

Country	Year	Taxation	Social insurance	Private insurance	Out-of pocket payments
Spain	1980	General central government tax revenues used to cover social insurance deficit and to fund some public care.	Compulsory contributions to social health insurance fund. Contributions proportional to earnings but subject to ceiling which varies across professional groups.	Taken out by persons without public cover and as supplementary cover by persons with public cover.	40% ticket modérateur for prescription medicines, but pensioners exempt. Payments to private soctor for some services available in public sector and for other services.
Switzerland	1981	General federal, cantonal, and communal government tax revenues used to subsidize basic cover provided by sickness funds and to fund public hospitals.	Compulsory contributions to the national accident and disability insurance.	Non-compulsory health insurance premiums paid to sickness funds. Premiums not related to earnings, but vary according to age at time of entry into sickness fund, gender, and (mainly) comfort of inpatient care. Sickness funds are private but subsidized and regulated by the federal government.	
UK	1985	General central government tax revenues used to fund NHS.	Some general social insurance contributions used to fund NHS.	Taken out as supplementary cover to NHS cover.	Charges for prescribed medicines, dental care, and opthalmic care.
USA	1981	Federal and state general revenues used to fund Medicaid and some Medicare, and general assistance. Some state and local revenues used to support public hospitals.	Some social insurance contributions go towards funding of Medicare.	Provided mostly as fringe benefit to employees. Participants in Medicare also purchase supplementary cover.	Copayments for inpatient and primary care payable by the privately insured and Medicare enrollees.

Source: adapted from van Doorslaer, E., Wagstaff, A. and Rutten, R. (eds) (1993) *Equity in the Finance and Delivery of Health Care: an International Perspective.* Oxford Medical Publications, OUP, Oxford

(that is, the rich pay proportionately slightly more in tax than their total share of pre-tax income), NHS funding is also mildly progressive. The Dutch and US systems, in contrast, tend to be regressive – lower income groups contribute proportionally more to health care funding than their share of pre-tax income[12].

Sweden

Although Sweden and the UK have state-financed systems, the Swedish health service allows for 23 county councils (average population 350,000) and three county boroughs to raise 75% of the total finance through local taxation. The Federation of County Councils negotiates with the National Board of Health and Welfare. Around the 1960s, the high standard of living and relative social equality in Sweden led to an explosion in health care facilities and expenditure, but subsequent slower economic growth rates have required costs to be controlled more rigorously, particularly central vetting of new capital building and manpower developments. There is some interest in fixing costs through the use of Diagnostic Related Groups (DRGs; see Section 8.6.2) and introducing some competition into the system. In common with other countries, the number of elderly in Sweden has increased, as have demands for high-technology medicine.

Netherlands

The system in the Netherlands before the 1990 Dekker reforms had marked differences from the NHS. A large proportion of health care was provided by the private sector, but controlled through a series of acts of parliament, such as the Hospital Facilities Acts of 1972 and 1979 and the Health Charges Act, 1984. Private fees account for 25% of the total budget of health care, and the rest comes from the Sickness Fund Insurance Scheme set up in 1964 (43%), the Special Sickness Expenses provisions (27%) and a small proportion of direct state funding.

Germany

The German system is acknowledged to be complicated. Insurance covers over 90% of the population, of whom 57% are compulsorily insured, 13% voluntarily insured and 30% retired but insured. State employees claim 50–70% refunds for services received, but many take out private insurance to cover costs not reimbursed by the State.

France

Under the French system, patients first pay in full and then claim back about 75% of the cost. Within that, 80% of in-patient costs are charged direct to the patient's insurance fund, leaving the remainder to be met by the patient. The costs themselves vary geographically and are related to doctors' fees. Insurance cover is by no means universal, and in the early 1970s it was estimated that 80% of the population under the age of 35 was covered, but of the over 80s only 51% of men and 29% of women were covered. A social aid programme therefore exists to support those not covered, and those suffering from such chronic illnesses as tuberculosis or mental disorder.

USA

In the USA, health care is predominantly an insurance-based system, financed in four different ways. First, from private practice on a fee-for-service basis; second, by local government, particularly for the poor inner-city and minority groups; third, through the Veterans Administration system and fourth by the military authorities. Only the last of these could be said to be well organized and integrated, because it deals with a finite population and the organization is subject to clear procedures. The Veterans Administration is mainly a hospital service and looks after retired and disabled people who previously served in the forces; it is therefore largely for men, and receives considerable consumer and political attention.

The local government programme in the USA is heavily supported by federal funds in the form of Medicaid, set up in 1965 to provide a safety net for those too poor to be eligible for private health care insurance schemes. Medicare is also funded by federal government and provides cover for all people over 65. County and city hospitals, private hospitals and many nursing homes recover the daily cost of treating patients under these two schemes. The system allows quality of service standards in these institutions to be scrutinized and, if they are found unsatisfactory, funds may be withdrawn. For instance, a South Carolina hospital, slow to integrate black and white patients, was threatened with the withdrawal of federal funds. If implemented, this would have closed the hospital: integration therefore took place[13].

Private care in the USA is available for anyone capable of paying or who has private insurance. The heavy reliance on this system and inadequate financial control of health care charges has inflated costs, so that by 1994 over 15% of GNP was being spent on health care in the USA, and yet the services remained ill co-ordinated and under-planned. This is despite the National Health Planning and Resources Development Act which, in 1974, had provided a major impetus to efforts to cut some of the waste inherent in the multiplicity of health care systems. Up to the mid-1960s, government funds contributed only about 25% of the total health care budget, but by the mid-1980s this had increased to 40%. The Reagan administration, in the early 1980s, became increasingly unhappy with this commitment and endeavoured to shift expenditure from federal government to the states, and to encourage more cost sharing with the consumer while preserving a basic minimum level of service. For the poor inner-city dweller, the minimum standard may be very low indeed, even in this highly developed country. In 1993/4 the Clinton administration attempted, unsuccessfully, to tackle some of the inefficiencies, high costs and inequalities in the US health care system.

14.4 DEVELOPING COUNTRIES AND EASTERN EUROPE

Momentous recent political and economic upheavals in the former Soviet Union and many of the countries of Eastern Europe have deeply affected health care services in these societies. Converting command economies into ones driven primarily by market forces has created enormous economic and social problems which remain largely unresolved. This has provided an unstable environment for the implementation of health services reforms. Many former Soviet bloc countries exhibit an uneasy mix of the sophistication of industrialized countries alongside basic problems still common in the developing countries. As all countries strive to improve their economies and raise the standard of living of their citizens, they face difficult dilemmas about the amount of health services to provide and the way to pay for these.

14.4.1 World Bank

The influence of the World Bank and the International Monetary Fund (IMF) in the economies of many developing and Eastern European countries expanded in the 1980s and 1990s, to the point where the Bank's loan strategy embraces social and political as well as economic goals. Because the effects of structural adjustment policies have, controversially, spilled over into other areas such as health and education, the World Bank has increasingly taken an interest in how countries accepting loans organize and fund their public services. In its *World Development Report* for 1993[15], devoted to health and health care, the World Bank set out detailed policies for the organization of health care services in developing countries.

> The term 'structural adjustment' has been used to describe a clutch of economic policies promoted by the World Bank and the IMF in return for loans. These policies include relaxation of exchange rates and reductions in public spending and are designed to liberalize the economies of 'borrower' countries. Although associated mainly with African countries, the UK was subject to IMF adjustment policies when the British government took out a loan in the late 1970s. For a clear exposition of structural adjustment see Ref. 14

Many of these policy ideas, such as the promotion of a diversity of competing health care providers and greater use and development of information on cost-effectiveness and provider performance, are familiar to those working in the NHS. But the Bank's ideas also raise issues which the NHS has only more recently begun to consider. One of these is that governments should specify in detail, and fund, a basic package of health care which is available to all. The question of what particular services the NHS should provide and what it should not has never been overtly or systematically addressed. The greater explicitness in purchasing arising from the UK National Health Service and Community Care Act 1990 will increasingly force commissioners of health to consider this.

CONCLUSION

This chapter has been, of necessity, a selection of 'snapshots' of health care systems. No two systems are the same (although all have elements in common), and nearly all are experiencing change. Getting the best health care out of a finite budget is a universal concern, as are notions of justice and fairness in terms of access to, and financing of, health care. A policy theme common to many countries is the idea of a mixed economy of health care, and limited or controlled forms of market or managed competition.

REFERENCES

1. See, for example, van Doorslaer, E. and Wagstaff, A. (1992) Equity in the delivery of health care: some international comparisons. *Journal of Health Economics* **11**(4): 389–411.

2. Ibid.

3. Harris, J. (1987) QALYfying the value of life. *Journal of Medical Ethics* **13**: 117–23.

4. Hunter, D. (1993) *Rationing Dilemmas in Health Care*, Research Paper No. 8. NAHAT, Birmingham.

5. DHSS (1980) *Report of the Working Group on Inequalities in Health* (Black report). HMSO, London.

6. This chapter faces the same difficulties, but the literature of international comparisons is expanding. Useful books are McLachlan, G. and Maynard, A. (1982) *The Public/Private Mix for Health*, Nuffield Provincial Hospitals Trust, London; Maxwell, R. (1976) *Health Care: the Growing Dilemma*, 2nd edn, McKinsey & Co.; Maxwell, R. (1981) *Health and Wealth: an international study of healthcare spending*, Lexington Books, New York; Mizrahi, Mizrahi, and Sandier, S. (1983) *Medical Care, Mobility and Costs*, Pergamon, Oxford; Ham C. Robinson, Benzeval (1990) *Health Check*. King's Fund, London.

7. See, for example, Le Grand, J. (1982) *The Strategy of Equality: Redistribution and the Social Services*, Allen and Unwin, London.

8. Simpson, R. (1978) *Access to Primary Care*, Research Paper No. 6, Royal Commission on the National Health Service. HMSO, London.

9. WHO Technical Report no 819 (1992) *The Hospital in Rural and Urban Districts*. WHO, Geneva.

10. For an account of PSROs see Williams and Towers (1980) *Introduction to Health Services*, pp. 345–6. John Wiley & Sons New York.

11. DoH (January 1989) *Working for Patients*, HMSO, London (Cm 555).

12. Wagstaff, A. and van Doorslaer, E. (1992) Equity in the finance of health care: Some international comparisons. *Journal of Health Economics* **11**(4): 361–87.

13. For a full account of this, see Hepner, J. O. (ed.) (1980) *Hospital Administrator–Physician Relationships*. C.V. Mosby, St Louis.

14. Melamed, C. (1994) *Adjusting Africa*. Worldview, Oxford.

15. World Bank (1993) *World Development Report 1993: Investing in Health*. Oxford University Press, Oxford.

THE NHS AND THE FUTURE

15

The NHS, now past its first half century, has been the proud epitome of the welfare state. But the principles upon which it was founded are increasingly being challenged. Some people think it is no longer appropriate for the state to act in this way because, they say, it robs people of their personal autonomy and provides no incentive for them to take charge of their own lives. Furthermore, they believe that monolithic state organizations are intrinsically bureaucratic and, therefore, inefficient and insensitive to the people they are set up to serve. In addition to these political criticisms, the NHS also faces changes arising from advances in medical technology, changes in expectations, patterns of disease and illness and external economic forces. This chapter discusses key issues now facing the NHS, and explores the likely effects of the changes brought about by the legislation of the last decade. First, the issue of priority-setting is examined, then there is a discussion on resources, and, finally, an examination of the organizational and political responses to views on how the NHS should be run in the light of all the forces which together shape the nation's health services.

15.1 PRIORITY SETTING

In looking at other countries' health care systems, Chapter 14 noted that while there are obvious differences between systems there are also universally shared themes, issues and problems. One is the inevitable need to make choices in health care, to set priorities. At the national level, the competing demands come from health care and education, or defence, or roads, or any other service or good (public or private) that consumes resources (land, labour, etc.) which we would like to enjoy. The need to choose arises from the impossibility of completely satisfying all demands, wants or needs. In the pure ideal free market, demand would equal supply, there would be no unemployment and no need for government intervention. In the rather dismal language of economics, sacrifices have to be made and opportunities forgone. Some demands and needs may be infinite and insatiable. There is an observable tendency to set demands just beyond the total resources available at the given time, whatever these are. Why people behave like this is not simple to explain. It might seem easier to organize things if everyone were more readily satisfied. For the foreseeable future the need to make choices appears inescapable, not only nationally but within health care systems too.

Behaviour and expectations play an important part in priority-setting. It is important to see that these are neither totally malleable nor carved in stone. For the NHS, the issues of needs, demands (what we want our health services to do) and the role of expectations are intrinsic factors which exert an enormous influence over the services and treatments provided by the NHS and over the way it is organized, the way services are delivered, to whom and in what way. It is essential to consider these fundamental issues in looking at the future of the NHS and the way it may set priorities.

15.1.1 Need, demand and expectations

Need and demand are interrelated, not the same. Need is based on an objective assessment against known criteria. So, for example, the needs of very elderly people can be gauged by assessing their level of physical disability and social isolation. From this, appropriate ways of reducing the effects of disability and loneliness can be designed. Demand, on the other hand, is more volatile and is based on expectations, realistic or not. The increasingly sophisticated knowledge of the population in matters of health and illness, fuelled in part by coverage in the media, excites expectations that may be unreasonable because of uncertain outcome or excessive cost.

Heart transplants for babies attract great popular interest, even though this expensive procedure is rare and has, as yet, a relatively poor success rate. On the other hand, greater understanding of the causes of heart disease ought not to lull people into thinking that the risk of avoidable illness or premature death has thereby been eliminated. Many screening programmes have proved to be surprisingly costly and sometimes ethically dubious. These schemes, which may identify only one positive in many thousands of negatives, prompt the question, how much money can justifiably be spent on finding those at risk? The mass screening of women for cervical cancer finds proportionately few positive cases. The cost, estimated at over £300,000 per positive result, may be thought unreasonably high if that money could be more effectively used on other services with unequivocally beneficial outcomes. Also, if screening reveals disease that is then untreatable for medical or financial reasons, is it right to have put the individual under that degree of distress? The incidence of AIDS pinpoints this dilemma: what benefit does a test that establishes a patient as HIV positive provide to that person if nothing can yet be done to cure him or her, and if it exposes them to discrimination?

The arguments are emotive and the public expects more and more, while at the same time tolerating less risk or failure. Childbirth provides a clear illustration. Twenty years ago it was not possible to save a very low weight baby or one who failed to recover quickly from trauma at birth. Naturally all parents want a healthy baby and they now consider that almost their right. When this does not happen it is readily assumed that the pregnancy and the delivery were mishandled. The increase in litigation is most marked in maternity cases. Yet doctors and midwives can take much of the credit for the greatly improved care of pregnant women and their newborn infants, in contrast to those mothers whose smoking or diet gives their baby a poor start in life.

Another example of the shifting tolerance of risk was demonstrated in recurrent scares about unsafe food, from salmonella in eggs to CJD and beef. Of course, this is not to say that matters are satisfactory or that experts should become complacent. Some food producers have been shown to be lax and too ready to put profit above public safety. Equally many food producers and retailers have led the way in improving food hygiene standards.

It is important for the public to be able to understand risk and assess what can be tolerated realistically. Regarding all risk as unacceptable is unrealistic and puts professionals, who are often working at the limits of knowledge and expertise, in a difficult position. Should they do the best they can, taking a few risks in the process, or should they play safe, knowing that the price of this is to slow down innovation and limit the expansion of their own clinical skills? Moreover, if patients get more and more into the habit of going to law when things go wrong, defence costs will claim more of the money that could be available to treat other patients. In the end society may be the worse off. The increase in patients' medical knowledge, and the pride of place given to consumerism both put the NHS itself at some risk. There needs to be the maturity to expect the NHS to do its best, which means that there will always be some imperfections. The USA provides clear evidence that higher expenditure does not necessarily assure better health.

15.1.2 Health service objectives

The public has not yet grappled with the full implications of these difficult issues and, until it does, demand, as enshrined in the now fashionable concept of consumerism, will try to dominate the debate about health care. As it would be extremely unwise to allow demand to overrule need, how should the NHS decide what to do? Should it target disadvantaged groups? Should it ignore accusations that it interferes in the rights of individuals? Can it justify spending large sums to screen the population in order to identify only small amounts of disease? In 1979, the Royal Commission on the NHS[1] listed seven main objectives of the service, and they are still appropriate:

1. Encourage and assist individuals to remain healthy.
2. Provide equality of entitlement to health services.
3. Provide a broad range of services of high standard.
4. Provide equality of access to these services.
5. Provide a service free at time of use.
6. Satisfy the reasonable expectations of its users.
7. Remain a national service responsive to local needs.

The policies and actions of successive governments clearly have not always honoured these. Health promotion (see Chapter 9) has often elicited half-hearted responses, compromised by conflicting interests. Certainly the NHS generally provides a wide range of care and treatment for all, but it has allowed long waiting lists to become an endemic problem. In 1998 there were well over one million people waiting for admission to hospital, many of them obliged to wait well over 12 months for treatment. This is a severe embarrassment for any government, by so obviously displaying the NHS's persistent failure to reach this very widely known target, particularly when other countries have avoided the problem.

Equality of access to care is a more complicated objective: who should have priority? The Black report[2] (and many others since) produced a detailed description of social inequality and related this to ill health (see Chapter 14). The report's finding, that there is a much higher incidence of disease among the poorest and most deprived, may now seem unsurprising, but it still poses challenges for any government wishing to correct the inequality. At times when the welfare state is criticized for supposedly weakening individuals' self-reliance, governments may find it politically incorrect to direct the NHS to single out disadvantaged groups for special favour. Yet failure to do so increases the prevalence of avoidable ill health. Similarly, immunization is a successful and simple way of eliminating certain diseases and is now, on the whole, accepted as a voluntary duty, while other preventive measures are resisted. Official exhortations to combat poor diet, reduce alcohol intake and cigarette smoking and regulate certain aspects of food production are regarded by some as improper trespasses upon the liberty of the individual.

Very few copies of the Black report were printed when it was published in 1980 and discussion was effectively suppressed by the Conservative government, even though the report had been officially commissioned in 1977 and was conducted by an eminent senior figure in the medical profession. He presented his findings in careful, sober terms. The 1997 Labour government took up the need for a coherent approach by setting up health action zones. In these, all aspects of the public services work together to eliminate particular social problems. This experiment has to demonstrate whether such government initiatives can produce results; it needs to define the limits of effective government intervention in the everyday lives of individuals.

Demands for health services come not only from patients; doctors have been the most powerful claimants for NHS resources. Technological advances now permit them to make highly complicated interventions. These include such sophisticated diagnostic techniques as computed tomography (CT) scanning and nuclear magnetic resonance, both of which are real improvements on the older, more invasive forms of radiological investigation. Joint replacement surgery and microsurgical techniques have greatly increased the range of possible treatments. New drugs, too, though often extremely expensive, have unquestionably alleviated hitherto medically untreatable conditions. Doctors have not been slow to share their successes with the public and this, in turn, has boosted expectations. At the same time, the rising number of infirm elderly in the population is currently accompanied by a shortage of those most likely to look after them. Elderly people's use of health services in general is relatively high, although only about 10% of them actually need residential or hospital care at any one time. The types of community-based services they need compete weakly for resources with glamorous, headline-making high-technology hospital medicine.

15.1.3 Future choices

If one thing is certain in the future, it is the necessity to make choices between competing demands for scarce resources. This remains true with or without the NHS. If the NHS did not exist, then choices would transfer to individuals, who would then have to engage in trade-offs between different health-giving activities and commodities, subject to limits on their personal resources, such as time and money. Traditionally, the NHS has tackled the question of priority-setting through a combination of political and administrative processes. At the level of choice for individual patients, it has relied on doctors to shoulder the ethical and moral burden of selecting who should receive treatment (and how much) and who should not. Generally, this arrangement (particularly the doctors' role) has been covert. This is changing, now that questions about priority-setting and its related activity of rationing become much more public. The separation of purchasers (commissioners) – whose main role is to maximize health gain or, put another way, choose whom not to buy care for – and providers has highlighted the essential priority-setting task and more clearly identified purchasers as responsible for undertaking it.

How are commissioners of health services best to tackle this? One possibility is to adopt the health economists' technical answer to the problem, that is to redefine the objectives of health care in terms that allow them to make rational (and justifiable) purchasing decisions. Although appealing in its logical simplicity, this priority-setting method not only requires the resolution of complex value judgements and trade-offs with other objectives but also implies a huge data collection and research exercise to establish the evidence and evaluate the outcomes of medical interventions.

An alternative course would be to pursue the traditional method of 'muddling through elegantly', to use Hunter's phrase[3], in a way that maximizes society's agreement rather than maximizing the health care outcomes, however measured. In return, this will produce (as it has done in the past) numerous examples of inconsistency and variation between clinicians, geographical areas and over time. The dilemma for the NHS is that there is no agreed rule for opting between different ways of choosing. In these circumstances, an important role for the NHS is to educate the public about the issues involved and to be open about the costs as well as the benefits of whatever methods are used to make the choices.

15.2 THE RESOURCE QUESTION

The NHS is mainly financed from general taxation, with National Insurance contributions and charges contributing under 20% of the total budget. It is, therefore, inextricably linked with the state of the economy. Chapter 8 showed that the proportion of the gross national product (GNP) spent on health services was lower than in most other comparable countries, but that, despite this, value for money was relatively high. One reason for the 'low' level of expenditure is the fact that doctors and other professional workers are paid comparatively less than their counterparts in other countries. Yet it is still broadly true that most patients who are acutely ill will be able to receive the treatment they require.

Why then should so many UK governments have investigated other ways of paying for the resources the NHS consumes? Their first concern is control: the pressure from unrestrained demand would soon become intolerable. Experience in other countries demonstrates that, however much money is invested in health care, the trend is always for it to require more. In the UK the principal method of financing (general taxation) and the system for determining the level of financing (imposition of an overall budget determined by the government) have remained largely unchanged over the years. Though alternatives have been canvassed and explored, the costs of change and the new disadvantages they bring have never been deemed worth the benefits of solving other problems. For example, insurance-based schemes inflate costs and exclude those who are likely to be bad financial risks. Millions of people in the USA are uninsured and, according to the criteria adopted by the insurance companies, uninsurable. Voucher schemes are an imperfect method because, while they equalize the potential for access, they do nothing to ensure actual needs are met. A patient requiring extended care may run out of entitlement, while a healthy person could choose to spend his or her vouchers on inessential treatment.

However, within the NHS itself, various initiatives have been explored to address the resourcing issue. One is to control wasteful use within the system. In the case of hospital ancillary services, this was attempted first with the bonus schemes for ancillary staff in the early 1970s and then by the government's enforced introduction of competitive tendering in the 1980s. Both these events caused a fall in the number of staff required and in the costs of the service. They were also effective in curbing union power. But these were only marginal gains in efficiency and did not address the core activity, clinical patient care. The introduction of local professional clinical and management audit and studies by such government agencies as the Audit Commission and the National Audit Office have put specific health services and activities in the spotlight. No longer can wide variations in the costs of clinical procedures be explained away as permissible manifestations of doctors' clinical autonomy. Why should the same operation in one hospital cost double in another? The Audit Commission has now extended its remit to look at nurses working in the community, where there are also marked variations in costs and results[4].

The introduction of the internal market following the 1990 reforms of the NHS was meant to promote efficiency and make available resources go further. In theory, high-cost hospitals should suffer financial penalties because patients are referred to competing units, where the same treatment can be obtained for a lower price. In practice, the extent to which this basic market principle actually operates in the NHS is unknown and depends on whether prices ever properly reflect or transmit all the characteristics of a provider's services. Another skewing factor is that purchasers are likely to use other criteria in choosing providers, such as how close they are situated to the populations they will serve.

Although some changes seem to have been brought about by the market, for instance the distribution of health services in London, the market has not proved to be a satisfactory way of getting the best use of health resources. Indeed, competition in some places may have led to over-provision of some services or the development of services which are relatively unimportant. Ironically, given that the genesis of the reforms lay in calls to tackle underfunding, the answer – a competitive market – may have done more to expose the extent of this underfunding than any other approach.

15.3 ORGANIZATIONAL STRUCTURE

The NHS is one of the largest employers in the world, with 940,600[5] staff directly employed and many thousands more working as contractors. An organization as big as this is likely to concern governments, not only because of the huge resources it requires but also because its day-to-day business is ultimately beyond a government's grasp. If health authorities were to challenge government policy en masse, the political consequences could be dramatic. Recent reorganizations and reforms have been designed partly to reduce the risk of organizational anarchy by strengthening lines of accountability and imposing stringent checks and balances. The new duality of purchasers and providers has established countervailing forces, intended to render the previous monolithic structure obsolete. The theory of the new market in the NHS was that neither purchasers nor providers could dominate, because they were locked into mutual dependency and were obliged to negotiate with one another.

However, experience shows that while there have been gains there have also been losses, which a proper study of the original economic model would have foreseen. Only under the most idealized of conditions do markets reach a state of competitive equilibrium, in which demand equals supply and no one can be made better off without making someone else worse off. Even a small deviation from the ideal, perfect market means that not only will equilibrium not be reached, it can be missed completely. In other words, the market fails to allocate resources efficiently. This has been known by economists for years[6].

The recent reorganization of the NHS Executive and the regional offices was meant to set up a regulatory framework to manage the market so that it would not fail, and the publication of *Local Freedoms, National Responsibilities* in 1994 attempted to address problems of market regulation[7]. It is still unclear exactly how regulation can achieve that goal. The DoH does not have adequate measures readily to identify even the most blatant of (potential) market failures. With monopoly providers in many cases there are no real alternatives.

The introduction of trusts and the extent of their freedoms added an uncertain element. If several of them all concluded, for sound financial reasons, that they would not offer all the basic services the conveniently situated health authorities wished to buy from them, would that signal the end of comprehensive local care under the NHS? Or would the market regulators, in the form of the regional offices, have the power to force providers to comply with the wishes of purchasers? There has been some evidence that trusts will stimulate the markets in the easier areas, avoiding the high-cost and difficult-to-provide services if they can. If forced to provide them they may make sure that the commissioning health authority pays a price which safeguards the trust's risk. This may inflate costs for the same service.

On the commissioning side, the 100 health authorities have progressed beyond purchasing to a wider strategic view of need. But working with other agencies to assess that need has been made more difficult by the reform of local government. In many parts of the country this has increased the number of local government bodies, where unitary authorities have replaced the previous counties with whom HAs dealt. This has led some to revive the proposal that the only effective way of arranging the commissioning of health care is to put the management of the health service under local rather than central government. However, the potential loss of control of national initiatives, and the lack of credibility of local government, scarcely improved by several notorious examples of corruption in both Labour and Conservative councils, make this an unsatisfactory solution for the time being. Another possibility would be to create a joint health and social services organization as in Northern Ireland. The most likely development in England meriting constructive discussion is the potential for regional government. The NHS could be run for regions of England of similar population sizes to that of Scotland, that is around 5 million.

The incoming Labour government of 1997 introduced changes only where it thought these were immediately necessary. This led to some compromises and some organizational confusion, particularly in the proposals to set up primary care groups. If these succeed in time they will make community trusts redundant and may also reduce the scope of HAs. Ironically, they could become more and more like the district health authorities that the 1990 Act swept away, although their design seems to give more power to clinicians than general managers.

Nevertheless, the influence and authority of managers will have to continue. From their role as subordinate, facilitating administrators at the start of the NHS, managers have gained significant responsibility for controlling and planning health services. This has been greatly resented by some clinical staff and by politicians and the public. But someone has to manage the complexity of the NHS's organizational development and growth competently and fairly. It makes little sense for clinicians to try to take on the general managerial role. Managers who are professionally trained and experienced will continue to carry the major organizational responsibility, in order to find ways to accommodate the demands of clinicians, politicians, patients and the public.

CONCLUSION

Whatever the organizational changes still to come, the NHS seems likely to remain, in most respects, a public, state-financed service. The 1990 Act provided opportunities for greater innovation and enterprise, but also for more local regulation through accreditation and monitoring. The increased emphasis on standards, on quality, on evaluating outcomes and ensuring greater efficiency and effectiveness present important challenges to the managers and professionals on whom the service depends. After 50 years of the NHS and 30 years of virtually continuous reorganization, the NHS is still able to make a remarkably good attempt at honouring its prime objective of providing a comprehensive service aimed at improving the overall health of the nation.

REFERENCES

1. Royal Commission on the National Health Service (1979) *Report of the Royal Commission*, HMSO, London (Cmnd 7615) para.2.6, p. 9.
2. DHSS (1980) *Report of the Working Party on Inequalities in Health* (Black report). HMSO, London (also published in amended form by Penguin Books in 1982).
3. Hunter, D. J. (1997) *Desperately Seeking Solutions*. Longman, London.
4. Audit Commission (1997) *Survey of Trusts employing District Nurses*. Audit Commission, London.
5. DoH (1997) *The Government's Expenditure Plans 1998–1999*. HMSO, London (Cm 3912).
6. There are many somewhat technical papers by economists dealing with the inherent weaknesses of the competitive equilibrium theory: see Radner, R. (1968) Competitive Equilibrium under Uncertainty, *Econometrica* **36**; 1:31–58.
7. DoH (1995) *NHS Responsibilities for Meeting Continuing Health Care Needs* Health Circular HSG (95)8/LAC (95)5. NHS Executive, Leeds.